Sex and Gender in Acute Care Medicine

Until the past decade, clinicians and researchers assumed that both the medical evaluation and treatment of women and men were the same. This archaic and dangerous notion persisted in spite of the clear anatomic and physiologic differences between the sexes. Today, we fully understand that this paradigm is false. In all specialties of medicine, practitioners and researchers are beginning to consider the influence of sex and gender and how this should inform the care of their patients. This book focuses on the issue of sex and gender in the evaluation and treatment of patients specifically in the delivery of acute medical care. It serves as a guide both to clinicians interested in the impact of sex and gender on their practice and to researchers interested in the current state of the art in the field and critical future research directions.

Alyson J. McGregor, MD MA FACEP is Associate Professor of Emergency Medicine at The Warren Alpert Medical School of Brown University. Dr. McGregor is Co-Founder and Director for the Division of Sex and Gender in Emergency Medicine (SGEM) at Brown University's Department of Emergency Medicine. She also serves as the Co-Director for the SGEM Fellowship and currently serves as Topic Editor for the journal *Clinical Therapeutics in Women's Health and Gender Medicine*. Dr. McGregor is Co-Founder and member of the Board of Directors for the national organization Sex and Gender Women's Health Collaborative. Her research focus is on the effects of sex and gender on emergent conditions, and she has been an advocate for this model nationally through talks such as "Why Medicine Often Has Dangerous Side Effects for Women" on TED.com.

Esther K. Choo, MD MPH is Associate Professor in the Department of Emergency Medicine in The Warren Alpert Medical School of Brown University and the Department of Health Services, Policy and Practice at the Brown University School of Public Health. She serves as faculty in the Rhode Island Hospital Injury Prevention Center and as Associate Director of the Division of Sex and Gender in Emergency Medicine, and is Co-Director of the division's Sex and Gender in Emergency Care Fellowship. Her research focuses on women's health, intimate partner violence, substance use disorders, and technology-based health interventions. She lectures nationally and has authored more than 50 peer-reviewed publications and 5 book chapters focusing on these topics.

Bruce M. Becker, MD, MPH, FACEP is Professor of Emergency Medicine and Behavioral and Social Science at The Warren Alpert School of Medicine of Brown University. He has practiced and taught Emergency Medicine for more than 30 years in the United States and around the world. He has extensive research experience with more than 80 peer-reviewed publications, book chapters, and texts. He has participated in many nationally funded research projects including more than 20 NIH grants. His areas of research focus include preventive health, addiction and behavioral change, alternative and complementary medicine, and geriatrics.

Sex and Gender in Acute Care Medicine

Alyson J. McGregor
Warren Alpert School of Medicine, Brown University

Esther K. Choo
Warren Alpert School of Medicine, Brown University

Bruce M. Becker
Warren Alpert School of Medicine, Brown University

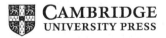

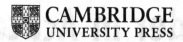

CAMBRIDGE
UNIVERSITY PRESS

Shaftesbury Road, Cambridge CB2 8EA, United Kingdom

One Liberty Plaza, 20th Floor, New York, NY 10006, USA

477 Williamstown Road, Port Melbourne, VIC 3207, Australia

314–321, 3rd Floor, Plot 3, Splendor Forum, Jasola District Centre, New Delhi – 110025, India

103 Penang Road, #05–06/07, Visioncrest Commercial, Singapore 238467

Cambridge University Press is part of Cambridge University Press & Assessment, a department of the University of Cambridge.

We share the University's mission to contribute to society through the pursuit of education, learning and research at the highest international levels of excellence.

www.cambridge.org
Information on this title: www.cambridge.org/9781107668164

First published 2016

A catalogue record for this publication is available from the British Library

Library of Congress Cataloging-in-Publication data
McGregor, Alyson J., editor. | Choo, Esther K., editor. | Becker,
Bruce M., editor.
Sex and gender in acute care medicine / [edited by] Alyson J.
McGregor, Esther K. Choo, Bruce M. Becker.
New York, NY : Cambridge University Press, 2015. | Includes
bibliographical references.
LCCN 2015036045 | ISBN 9781107668164 (paperback)
| MESH: Emergency Treatment. | Sex Factors. | Acute Disease – therapy. | Diagnosis,
Differential. | Symptom Assessment.
LCC RT48 | NLM QZ 53 | DDC 616.07/5–dc23
LC record available at http://lccn.loc.gov/2015036045

ISBN   978-1-107-66816-4   Paperback

Contents

List of contributors   vii

Foreword   ix
Judith E. Tintinalli

Preface   xi
Alyson J. McGregor

Acknowledgments   xiii

1. **Know the Difference: Sex and Gender in Acute Care Medicine**   1
   Alyson J. McGregor and Esther K. Choo

2. **It's not all Chest Pain: Sex and Gender in Acute Care Cardiology**   6
   Morgan Soffler, Alyson J. McGregor and Basmah Safdar

3. **You've Come a Long Way, Baby: The Effects of Sex and Gender on Asthma, COPD, Smoking, and Smoking Cessation**   24
   Stacey Poznanski and Rita Cydulka

4. **Sex and Gender-Specific Differences in Alcohol and Drug use Among Patients Seeking Treatment in the Acute Care Setting**   49
   Esther K. Choo, Marna Greenberg and Grace Chang

5. **Sex and Gender; Pharmacology, Efficacy, Toxicity, and Toxicology**   63
   Annette Lopez and Robert G. Hendrickson

6. **A Sex and Gender Based Perspective on Traumatic Injury**   77
   Jason Cohen, Stefan Merrill and Federico E. Vaca

7. **Sex and Gender Differences in the Presentation and Treatment of Cerebrovascular Emergencies**   87
   Tracy Madsen and Karen Furie

8. **From Title IX to the Q angle: Sex and Gender in Acute Care Orthopedics and Sports Medicine**   101
   Neha Raukar and Kimberly Templeton

9. **Are Women More Sensitive? Sex and Gender Differences in Pain Perception, Clinical Evaluation and Treatment**   122
   James Miner

10. **Digesting Sex and Gender: Gastroenterology**   136
    David J. Desilets

11. **Overcoming Resistance: Importance of Sex and Gender in Acute Infectious Illnesses**   147
    Erica Hardy, Mitchell Kosanovich and Arvind Venkat

12. **Diagnostic Imaging: Focusing a Lens on Sex and Gender**   163
    Christopher L. Moore

13. **Special Populations:**
    a. **Old, not Neutered: A Sex and Gender-Based Approach to the Acute Care of Elders**   179
       Elena Kapilevich and Bruce Becker

b. **Girls and Boys: Sex and Gender in Pediatrics** 193
Therese L. Canares, Marleny Franco and George M. Lazarus

c. **Acute Medical Care for the Transgender Patient** 216
Elizabeth Samuels and Michelle Forcier

14. **Sex and Gender in Medical Education: The Next Chapter** 230
Marjorie R. Jenkins

Index 237

Contributors

Morgan Soffler, MD, Clinical and Research Fellow, Massachusetts General Hospital/Beth Israel Deaconess Medical Center

Basmah Safdar MD, Associate Professor, Department of Emergency Medicine, Director, ED Chest Pain Center, Yale University School of Medicine

Stacey Poznanski, DO, M.Ed., Associate Professor, Wright State University Boonshoft School of Medicine, Director of EM Undergraduate Medical Education

Rita K. Cydulka, MD MS, Professor, Case Western Reserve University School of Medicine

Marna Rayl Greenberg, DO, MPH, Associate Professor, University South Florida, Morsani College of Medicine, Lehigh Valley Health Network, Director of Emergency Medicine Research

Grace Chang, MD, MPH, Professor, Department of Psychiatry, Harvard Medical School

Annette M. Lopez, MD, Adjunct Assistant Professor, Department of Emergency Medicine, Medical Toxicologist, Oregon Poison Center, Staff Physician, Portland VA Medical Center

Robert G. Hendrickson, MD, Professor, Department of Emergency Medicine, Oregon Health and Science University, Program Director, Fellowship in Medical Toxicology

Jason Cohen, DO, Assistant Professor, Department of Emergency Medicine, Albany Medical Center, Medical Director, LifeNet of New York

Stefan Merrill, MD, Department of Emergency Medicine, Albany Medical Center

Federico E. Vaca, MD, MPH, Professor and Vice Chair, Department of Emergency Medicine, Yale University School of Medicine

Tracy Madsen, MD, ScM, Assistant Professor, Department of Emergency Medicine, Alpert Medical School of Brown University

Karen L. Furie, MD, Chair, Department of Neurology, Alpert Medical School of Brown University

Neha P. Raukar, MD, MS, CAQ Primary Care Sports Medicine, Assistant Professor, Director, Division of Sports Medicine, Department of Emergency Medicine, Alpert Medical School of Brown University

Kimberly Templeton, MD, Professor, Department of Orthopaedic Surgery, University of Kansas Medical Center, Past-President, US Bone and Joint Initiative, President-Elect, American Medical Women's Association

James R. Miner MD, Professor of Emergency Medicine, University of Minnesota, Chief of Emergency Medicine, Hennepin County Medical Center

David J. Desilets, MD, PhD, Assistant Professor of Clinical Medicine, Tufts University School of Medicine, Chief, Gastroenterology, Baystate Health

Erica J Hardy, MD, MA, MMSc, Clinical Assistant Professor of Medicine, Alpert Medical School of Brown University, Women & Infants Hospital, Associate Director, Women's Infectious Disease Consultation Service

Mitchell Kosanovich, MD, Department of Emergency Medicine, Allegheny General Hospital

Arvind Venkat, MD, Vice Chair for Research and Faculty Academic Affairs, Department of Emergency Medicine, Allegheny Health Network, Clinical Professor of Emergency Medicine, Temple University School of Medicine (adjunct), Associate Professor of Emergency Medicine, Drexel University College of Medicine

Christopher L. Moore, MD, Associate Professor, Chief, Section of Emergency Ultrasound, Department of Emergency Medicine, Yale University School of Medicine

Elena Kapilevich, MD, University of Rochester Medical Center, School of Medicine and Dentistry

Therese Canares, MD, Assistant Professor, Division of Pediatric Emergency Medicine, Department of Pediatrics, Johns Hopkins University School of Medicine

Marleny Franco, MD, Assistant Professor, Department of Pediatrics, Perelman School of Medicine at the University of Pennsylvania, Attending Physician, Division of Emergency Medicine, Children's Hospital of Philadelphia

George M. Lazarus, MD, Associate Clinical Professor, Department of Pediatrics, Columbia University College of Physicians and Surgeons

Elizabeth Samuels, MD, Department of Emergency Medicine, Alpert Medical School of Brown University

Michelle Forcier MD MPH, Clinical Associate Professor, Department of Pediatrics, Alpert Medical School of Brown University

Marjorie Jenkins, MD, Professor of Medicine, Founding Director and Chief Scientific Officer for the Laura W. Bush Institute for Women's' Health, Associate Dean for Women in Science, J. Avery Rush Endowed Chair for Excellence in Women's Health Research, Texas Tech University Health Sciences Center

Foreword

Women such as Ellen Johnson Sirleaf, Christine Lagarde, Angela Merkel, and Janet Yellen are steadily, confidently, and appropriately occupying positions of national and international power in government, business, and academia. But most of the 3.5 billion women in the world do not have the opportunity, resources, or social supports to reach such commanding heights.

Worldwide, women have been consigned to narrow roles and behaviors; subject to oppressive cultural values; and forced to accept economic, educational, social, and health care disparities that have limited their potential. The US Agency for Healthcare Research and Quality,[1] the World Health Organization,[2] and the United Nations[3] have launched major initiatives to improve gender-related health inequities. This text, *Sex and Gender in Acute Care Medicine*, is the first to organize women's health care issues as they pertain to emergency practice. The scope of the book is broad and will, I believe, help us understand the differences between women and men as we diagnose and treat their acute illnesses and injuries.

I hope this text will inspire and challenge us as emergency physicians and researchers to think twice: once about our individual patient and once about health care systems and public health initiatives. This book will stimulate us to identify gaps in our knowledge, to ask questions, and to find answers. This book can become the foundation for global thinking about the emergency care of both women and men: How can we use our understanding of sex and gender to improve access to care, increase the availability and quality of mental health services, initiate effective preventive health interventions, and use our powerful and expensive diagnostic and therapeutic armamentarium to provide the most benefit to our patients?

> Someday there will be girls and women whose name will no longer mean the mere opposite of the male, but something in itself, something that makes one think not of any complement and limit, but only life and reality: the female human being.
> Rainer Maria Rilke, letter, May 14, 1904, *Letters to a Young Poet*

Respectfully submitted,

Judith E. Tintinalli, MD, MS
Professor and Chair Emeritus
Department of Emergency Medicine
University of North Carolina at Chapel Hill

---

[1] Healthcare Quality and Disparities in Women: Selected Findings from the 2010 National Healthcare Quality and Disparities Report. Agency for Healthcare Research and Quality. 2011. Available at: http://www.ahrq.gov/research/findings/nhqrdr/nhqrdr10/women.html.

[2] World Health Organization: Gender, Women and Health. Available at: http://www.who.int/gender/en/.

[3] Women and Health. WomenWatch: Information and Resources on Gender Equality and Empowerment of Women. United Nations. Available at: 1) www.un.org/womenwatch/directory/women_and_health_3003.htm.

Preface

We come to work each day. The sliding doors to the department open and we face fluorescent lights, beeping monitors, piercing sirens approaching the hospital, and a waiting room filled with patients complaining of headaches, chest pains, weakness, and fever. These are common scenes in any acute care treatment facility. As you, the practitioner, begin your busy clinical shift and enter into the first of many patients' rooms, have you ever taken a moment to consider how your patients' sex and gender affect their presentation, the symptoms and signs of their illness or injury? Or whether sex and gender considerations should influence your workup and management plan? Consider your patients with traumatic injuries, such as the all-too-common fall from standing in elder women and men, head injuries and concussions in girls and boys playing sports, motor vehicle crashes involving intoxicated teenagers or middle-aged baby boomers. How can understanding the medical implications of your patient's sex and gender assist you in creating more effective, personalized health care plans? Additionally, what about your own sex and gender? We health care providers often think of ourselves as neutral entities making decisions for our patients without any subconscious and unrecognized personal bias, bias that is as unavoidable as our chromosome count or our ethnic and sociocultural background, instilled by our families, the media, and our own unique histories. Do our unrecognized and unacknowledged perspectives and prejudices about sex and gender determine our rapid clinical decision-making strategies as strongly as our medical training?

The study of sex- and gender-specific "evidence-based" medicine was initiated to rectify the long-standing neglect in the medical world of the clinical differences between women and men. While sex- and gender-specific medicine was initially a reaction to the historical, patriarchal, and sexist perspective that women's health was uniquely about reproduction, pregnancy, and women's genital organs, this new field has begun to delineate and magnify the unique clinical needs of both men and women. Uncovering biologic similarities and pathophysiologic differences will lead inevitably to quantum improvements in the health of women and men, disrupting and changing outmoded patterns of diagnosis, treatment, and prognosis and creating individualized paths to care that will improve patients' outcomes.

Despite the promulgation of the importance of preventive health maintenance, modern medicine is often delivered in an acute care setting. Emergency department (ED) visits are steadily rising in the United States with more than 136 million patients treated in EDs in 2015, according to the Centers for Disease Control and Prevention. The important role of acute care medicine in the health care delivery system and the role that acute care services play in the real-world treatment of patients who are ill or injured underscore the importance of recognizing and embracing this new field of investigation, education, and clinical practice, which promises to have a major impact on the health of so many women and men.

Information about sex- and gender-specific medicine for the acute care practitioner is, at best, scattered piecemeal throughout most standard medical textbooks and educational resources. We chose to write this textbook to synthesize the current knowledge base, highlighting the impact of sex and gender on common subspecialty areas within acute care medicine. By bringing all of this current information together, this text serves as a primary teaching resource for medical students, residents, and specialists alike. Each chapter addresses specific answers to questions proposed by authors as well as relevant research questions designed to stimulate readers to develop their own lines of investigation.

While reading this text, please be aware of two assumptions that may challenge your understanding of this work:

1) This field of study was born out of discovering differences that exist between men and women. Of course, there are indubitably aspects of biology and medicine where no differences exist, such as no difference between men and women for a particular presentation, drug effect, or case fatality rate for a particular disease. Nevertheless, we must never assume. Conversely, we should assume that there is a difference and, then, carry out investigations to determine if that difference exists and if so its basis in physiology, pharmacology, and cell biology.

2) Sex differences are not the same as gender differences. Sex differences are biologically based and represent variance across the cell lines of individuals. Gender differences are molded by sociocultural forces and, therefore, are malleable and reflect the culture and the society in which the patient has been raised and/or now lives. An understanding of the role of both sex and gender on illness and injury will lead clinicians to optimize strategies that promote health and prevent disease in their patients.

Practitioners of acute care medicine are well positioned to embrace the concept of sex- and gender-specific medicine in their practice. Acute care medicine has expanded over the past 40 years, crossing and melding all subspecialties. For practitioners who apply the knowledge and information in this book, their evaluation and treatment in the acute care setting will have the unprecedented opportunity to transform these advances into life-saving outcomes for their patients.

Alyson J. McGregor MD MA FACEP
Director, Division of Sex and Gender in
Emergency Medicine
Associate Professor of Emergency Medicine
Warren Alpert Medical School of Brown
University

Acknowledgments

The editors would like to thank the editorial staff at Cambridge University Press for recognizing the potential that the impact of sex and gender confers on medical practice in the acute care setting; the contributors, who brought a vision and enthusiasm to this new field and will be its leaders; Zachary Becker (freelance medical illustrator) for creating the cover art; and Dr. Jeanette Wolfe and Dr. Gus Garmel for helping us initially navigate the academic book world.

Know the Difference: Sex and Gender in Acute Care Medicine

Alyson J. McGregor and Esther K. Choo

Defining Sex and Gender

The Institute of Medicine (IOM) has stated that "Sex, that is being male or female, is an important basic human variable that should be considered when designing and analyzing studies in all areas and at all levels of biomedical and health related research" (IOM 2001, p. 3). "Sex" refers to biological differences between men and women, such as chromosomes (XX or XY), internal and external sex organs, and hormonal profiles. "Gender" refers to the socially constructed roles, values, and personality traits that vary from society to society and over time. Every cell has a sex. Whether a cell contains an XX or XY chromosome may have an impact on everything from regulation of gene expression in a cell line to efficacy or toxicity of a pharmaceutical in a living human.[1]

The IOM report also listed several barriers to research progress, including "the inconsistent and often confusing use of the terms 'sex' and 'gender' in the scientific literature and popular press."[2] Often, the terms are used interchangeably in scientific writing with both terms referring to whether individuals are biologically male or female.[3] Sex and gender are associated and interactive but are not the same. Each variable has significant health implications, is worthy of dedicated study, and can lead to insights into mechanisms underlying morbidity, mortality, and health behaviors.

In real life, there is a continuous interaction between the two: Health is determined by the biology of being male or female and the social context of gender. Therefore, the significance of sex, gender, and their interaction should be considered in the daily practice of patient care.

Identifying the Problem: Do Sex and Gender Matter?

In its 2001 report entitled "Exploring the Biological Contributions to Human Health," the IOM called on biomedical researchers to increase their investigation of sex and gender as critical variables affecting health.[2] It described the rapidly growing evidence for significant differences between males and females in every aspect of health and disease and urged the scientific community to increase its understanding of the impact of sex and gender to advance the practice of medicine.

The evidence-based research that served as the basis for the practice model used today was primarily conducted on male cell lines and male rats and translated to middle-aged, average-sized Caucasian males. The lack of inclusion of sex differences in health and disease, largely as a result of the greater accessibility and convenience of male subjects, is considered a failure of science.[4]

Cardiovascular disease (CVD) research provides a good case example of how sex and gender differences may have meaningful implications for clinical care and health outcomes. Research regarding therapy and prevention of heart disease had largely been performed on men. For instance, in 1988, the Physicians' Health Study, aimed at examining the benefits and risks of aspirin and beta-carotene in the prevention of CVD and cancer, consisted of 22,000 male participants.[5] The study's finding that a daily aspirin could prevent myocardial infarction (MI) was widely adopted into clinical practice, despite not being studied in women. Today, the US Preventive Services Task Force (USPSTF) recommendations provide gender-specific recommendations regarding aspirin. Questions still remain about the recognition and treatment of cardiac disease in women, particularly with repeated media reports of undiagnosed chest pain, missed MIs, and negligence on the part of physicians.[6, 7]

Another well-publicized example of the impact of sex and gender is the US Food and Drug Administration's (FDA) process of evaluating new drugs as safe and effective, approving drugs for marketing, and providing post-market surveillance to determine if adverse effects are detected after initial approval.

The US General Accounting Office (GAO) reviewed 10 prescription drugs withdrawn from the market between January 1997 and December 2000 and found that 8 out of the 10 drugs were withdrawn because of adverse events occurring predominantly in women.[8] Women were found to be at a greater risk of Torsades de Points from the antihistamines terfenadine and astemizole; a public health advisory was placed when women were found to make up 70% of reports of Torsades de Pointes thought to be induced by these QTc-prolonging medications.[9] The FDA is also responsible for determining indications and dosing for approved drugs. On May 14, 2013, the FDA issued a safety communication approving label changes to zolpidem for treatment of insomnia and recommended significantly lower doses in women for extended-release products because women are more susceptible than men to the risks posed by "next-day impairment of driving and other activities that require full alertness."[10] Concerns remain as to why these sex-determined adverse events were discovered after the drug was approved and on the market. Because of this lack of participation of women in clinical trials, Congress mandated the formation of the FDA's Office of Women's Health (OWH), which was established in 1994. The OWH supports research that examines biological differences and advocates for inclusion of sex and gender as a critical study variable in research within and outside the National Institutes of Health (NIH).

Evolution of Women's Health

To understand the evolution of sex and gender within the scientific and medical environment, it is important to recognize the historical transition in the conceptualization of women's health (Figure 1.1).[11]

The female reproductive system was the focus of women's health care in the early nineteenth century. Even mental illness was connected to the female menstrual cycle, such that the word "hysteria" came from the Greek word meaning "uterus."[12] Throughout the twentieth century and with the rise of modern medicine and scientific methods, a number of forces conspired to prevent equal inclusion of men and women in clinical research. One important factor was the federal government's paternalistic approach toward women, particularly pregnant women. This attitude was fueled by the disastrous outcomes that resulted from new medications prescribed to pregnant women: diethylstilbestrol, prescribed in the 1950s for pregnant women to prevent miscarriage, led to gynecologic cancer in the daughters of the women who took it; thalidomide, an antiemetic medication given to pregnant women to alleviate morning sickness, caused severe limb abnormalities in developing fetuses.[13, 14] In the face of these events and pressure from the public, the FDA implemented a policy that would eliminate all women of childbearing potential from clinical trials to do away with any risk to the fetus.[12–14] The FDA's 1977 Guidance of General Considerations for the Clinical Evaluation of Drugs essentially had the effect of excluding women of childbearing potential from participation in industry-sponsored clinical trials.[15] It also led to a reluctance of women themselves to serve as study participants.

Another factor influencing the exclusion of women from research was investigators' concerns that women subjects would make the study population less homogeneous, leading to increased sample size requirements, more complex analyses, and correspondingly higher study expenses.[13] A related concern was that biologic factors, such as hormonal fluctuations resulting from menstruation, pregnancy, oral contraceptive pills, menopause, and hormone replacement therapy, created a web of baseline variables that would be difficult to consider when analyzing research.[13, 14, 16]

The most fundamental obstacle to sex- and gender-specific research, however, was the simple lack of recognition of their impact as independent

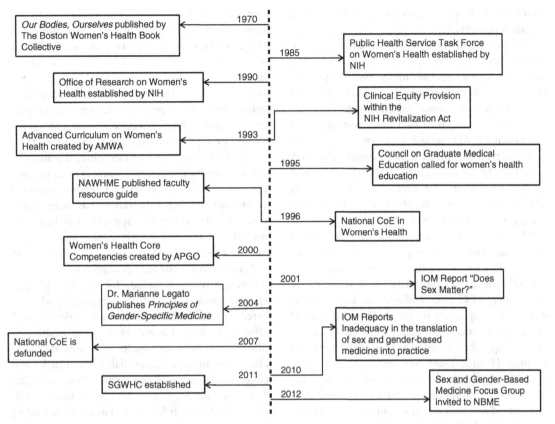

Figure 1.1 Key historical contributions to the evolution of sex and gender in medicine. Reproduced with permission from Biology of Sex Differences

variables in medicine. Ultimately, scientists needed not only to accept the validity of sex-related differences but also to translate this acceptance into how they designed studies and recruited participants into clinical trials.[16, 17]

Compounding considerations of risk, complexity, and cost was the implicit assumption that outcomes in men would be adequate proxies for outcomes in women, despite the fact that physiologic, anatomic, and metabolic differences between men and women argued against this assumption.[11] In the latter half of the twentieth century, with women's individualism brought to the nation's consciousness by the feminist movement, the concept of "sex" in human biology began to shift. In the 1980s, the NIH established a Public Health Service Task Force on Women's Health. Recommendations for increased attention to women's health issues led to the development of specific guidelines and processes regarding the inclusion of women as subjects in NIH-funded extramural research.[18]

Identifying a Difference

In 1986, the NIH set up an advisory committee that recommended but did not mandate that grants include women as subjects in clinical studies.[19] Nevertheless, the Congressional Women's Caucus commissioned the GAO to evaluate the implementation of this policy advising the inclusion of minorities and women in clinical studies.[19] In the 50 NIH grant applications reviewed during this audit, 20% did not mention gender, more than 30% did not provide breakdown percentages, and some all-male studies gave no reason for women's exclusion.[20] This led to the creation of the NIH Office of Research on Women's Health (ORWH) in 1991.[13] In 1992, the GAO reported that more than 60% of trials submitted by the pharmaceutical companies to the FDA lacked female representation.

As the recognition of the research gap for women became more apparent, the FDA policy was reevaluated; modifications issued in 1993 encouraged drug companies to include minorities and women and provide subgroup analyses.[13, 21] In addition to inclusion of women, this Revitalization Act, signed into law by President Clinton, required that the NIH ensure that cost would not be an acceptable reason for exclusion.[22]

Yet, even after 1993, there were more reports of unexpected adverse events in women than men during post-market surveillance.[23] In 1994, the IOM established a Committee on the Ethical and Legal Issues Relating to the Inclusion of Women in Clinical Studies.[22] In November 1999, the IOM formed a Committee on Understanding the Biology of Gender Differences. This was the first major step taken by the IOM in the area of sex-based science and policy. The 2001 report "Exploring the Biological Contributions to Human Health: Does Sex Matter?" presented scientific evidence in support of the biologic basis of sex differences, promoted sex- and gender-related research questions, identified barriers, and clearly solidified sex as an important variable of health.[24]

Calls to action have not been adequate to radically change researchers' behaviors. In 1997, the FDA implemented the Modernization Act, stating that further guidance was necessary in the inclusion of minorities and women in research trials.[17, 25] More than 15 years later, the NIH acknowledged that basic science studies still lack equal consideration of males and females: A recent joint statement by NIH Director Francis Collins and ORWH Director Janine Collins addressed ongoing neglect of sex inclusion in basic science studies.[26] Multifaceted strategies, coupled with funding, need to be in place to address the gaps in women's health and ensure that sex is taken into account when addressing health and disease.

Why Focus on Emergency Care?

The emergency care setting provides access to a vast array of disease conditions at critical periods in their management. The concept of a treatment "window," during which definitive action within minutes to several hours is critical to improve

clinical outcomes, is almost exclusive to the field of emergency medicine. The Emergency Department (ED), therefore, is an ideal place to observe where and how men and women diverge in their presentations and responses to treatment. Furthermore, with its access to a large proportion of the population, any sex- or gender-specific clinical practice within emergency care has the potential to have a large impact.

As with every area of medicine, the study of sex and gender in emergency care is in its infancy; the lack of attention to sex and gender within the emergency medicine literature has been documented.[27] However, the specialty has begun to mobilize its research efforts around sex and gender in a coordinated manner, notably through a 2014 national consensus conference aimed at defining a research agenda for sex- and gender-specific research regarding emergency and acute care.[28] Hand in hand with these early research efforts, we must review the existing multidisciplinary literature and make informed decisions about how to apply the available scientific knowledge around sex and gender to clinical practice. The future holds promise for a better understanding of sex-based differences in acute care, leading to new, personalized approaches to prevention, diagnosis, and therapy.

This book is designed to bridge the gap between our traditional clinical practice of considering the differences between men and women within the confines of reproductive health to our growing certainty about the profound significance of sex and gender in every aspect of disease.

References

1. Klinge IWC. Sex and gender in biomedicine. In *Theories, Methodologies, Results*. Gottingen: Universitatasverlag; 2010.

2. Wizemann TPM. Exploring the biological contributions to human health: does sex matter? *Journal of Women's Health & Gender-Based Medicine* 2001; **10**:1–267, at 2, 174.

3. Haig D. The inexorable rise of gender and the decline of sex: social change in academic titles, 1945–2001. *Archives of Sexual Behavior* 2004; **33**:87–96.

4. Moncher KL, Douglas, PS. Importance of and barriers to including women in clinical trials. In *Principles of Gender-Specific Medicine*. Amsterdam and Boston: Elsevier; 2004:275–82.

5. Final Report on the Aspirin Component of the Ongoing Physicians' Health Study. Steering Committee of the Physicians' Health Study Research Group. *New England Journal of Medicine* 1989; **321**:129–35.

6. Kannel WB, Abbott RD. *Incidence and Prognosis of Myocardial Infarction in Women: The Framingham Study.* New York: Haymarket Doyma; 1987.

7. Malacrida R, Genoni M, Maggioni AP et al. A comparison of the early outcome of acute myocardial infarction in women and men. The Third International Study of Infarct Survival Collaborative Group. *New England Journal of Medicine* 1998; **338**:8–14.

8. Sandberg K, Verbalis JG. Sex and the basic scientist: is it time to embrace Title IX? *Biology of Sex Differences* 2013; 4:13.

9. Makkar RR, Fromm BS, Steinman RT, Meissner MD, Lehmann MH. Female gender as a risk factor for Torsades de pointes associated with cardiovascular drugs. *Journal of the American Medical Association* 1993; **270**:2590–97.

10. United States Food and Drug Administration (FDA). FDA Drug Safety Communication: FDA approves new label changes and dosing for zolpidem products and a recommendation to avoid driving the day after using Amben CR. 2013.

11. McGregor AJ, Templeton K, Kleinman MR, Jenkins MR. Advancing sex and gender competency in medicine: sex & gender women's health collaborative. *Biology of Sex Differences* 2013; 4:11.

12. Laurence L, Weinhouse B. *Outrageous Practices: The Alarming Truth about How Medicine Mistreats Women.* New York: Fawcett Columbine; 1994.

13. Bull J. *Women and Medical Research – What We've Learned and Where We're Going.* Washington, DC: Society for Women's Health Research; 2000: 7–9.

14. Chervenak FA, McCullough LB. Ethical considerations in research involving pregnant women. *Women's Health Issues* 1999; **9**:206–7.

15. US Department of Health and Human Services (USDHHS). *Guidance for Industry.* Rockville, MD: US Government Printing Office; 1977.

16. Charney P, Meyer, B, Frishman, W. et al. Gender, race, and genetic issues in cardiovascular pharmacotherapeutics. In *Cardiovascular Pharmacotherapeutics.* New York: McGraw-Hill; 1997:1347–62.

17. Dietrich EB, Cohan C. *Women and Heart Disease.* New York: Crown; 1992.

18. Health NIo. *NIH Guide for Grants and Contracts.* Bethesda, MD: National Institutes of Health; 1986.

19. Hamilton JA. *Guidelines for Avoiding Methodological and Policymaking Biases in Gender-Related Health Research.* Rockville, MD: US Public Health Service; 1985.

20. Health NIo. *Problems in Implementing Policy on Women in Study Populations.* Washington DC: US General Accounting Office; 1990.

21. Administration USFaD. FDA clinical testing guidelines will represent women. 1992.

22. Mastroianni AC, Faden R, Federman D. *Women and Health Research.* Washington, DC: National Academy Press; 1994.

23. Office USGA. Drug Safety: Most drugs withdrawn in recent years had greater health risks for women. 2001.

24. Institute of Medicine CoUtBoSaGD. *Exploring the Biological Contributions to Human Health: Does Sex Mater?* Washington, DC: National Academy Press; 2001.

25. Mastroianni AC, Faden R, Federman D. *Women and Health Research.* Washington, DC: National Academy Press; 1994.

26. Clayton JA, Collins FS. Policy: NIH to balance sex in cell and animal studies. *Nature* 2014; **509**:282–83.

27. Safdar B, McGregor AJ, McKee SA et al. Inclusion of gender in emergency medicine research. *Academic Emergency Medicine* 2011; **18**:e1–e4.

28. *Gender-Specific Research in Emergency Care: Investigate, Understand, and Translate How Gender Affects Patient Outcomes.* Academic Emergency Medicine Consensus Conference, 2014. http://www.saem.org/meetings/past-annual-meetings/2014-aem-consensus-conference.

It's not all Chest Pain: Sex and Gender in Acute Care Cardiology

Morgan Soffler, Alyson J. McGregor and Basmah Safdar

An Introduction to Gender in Acute Care Cardiology

This chapter focuses on the gender differences in epidemiology, pathophysiology management pearls, and prognosis of cardiovascular disease with a clinical focus on acute coronary syndrome (ACS), non-ischemic cardiac syndromes, structural heart disease, and arrhythmias. We also discuss cardiac diseases with increased prevalence in women, such as Takotsubo's cardiomyopathy and Syndrome X.

Section 1   Acute Coronary Syndromes

Patient A   A Case of Acute Coronary Syndrome

A 54-year-old woman with history of diabetes and high blood pressure presents to the Emergency Department (ED) with a sensation of burning in her chest for the past week each time she walked upstairs. She thought the burning would subside as it had previously; however, on the day of presentation, the burning worsened and was associated with shortness of breath and fatigue. She attributed her symptoms to anxiety resulting from increased financial stress but came in at the urging of her son. She has a history of diabetes for which she takes metformin 1000 mg twice daily but otherwise reports no other significant medical issues and takes no other medications. She smokes about 10 cigarettes per day. She has no significant family history of coronary artery disease (CAD), stroke, or sudden death. On initial exam, she is afebrile with a blood of

pressure 145/85, a heart rate of 98 beats/min, with normal respirations and oxygen saturation of 96% on RA. In general, she is in mild distress without jugular venous distention and has clear lung fields. Her cardiac exam demonstrated a regular rhythm, without murmurs, rubs, or gallops. PMI was non-displaced. Her abdominal exam was benign and extremities were without edema with 2+ pedal pulses. Work-up revealed an EKG with sinus rhythm and T-wave inversions in leads I and AVL. Initial troponin was negative. Chest X-ray was normal.

Clinical Questions

- How would you approach a cardiac work-up in this patient?
- What are the gender-specific elements in diagnosis and management that you should consider?

The following section summarizes the most recent literature on key gender-specific differences in epidemiology, presentation, physiology, diagnostics, treatment, and prognosis for ACS.

Prevalence of Acute Coronary Syndrome in Women

ACS should be the first diagnostic consideration for this patient with chest pain, as CAD is the most common cause of death for women and men in the United States.[1] The onset of CAD in men occurs 10 to 15 years earlier than in women. Nevertheless, heart disease remains a leading cause of death in women. Over the two decades, the mortality rate from CAD has been declining at a slower rate in women than in men and, in fact, has increased for women in mid-life (35–54 yrs).[2]

Gender-Specific Diagnostic Approach to ACS

In accordance with 2012 American College of Cardiology (ACC) and American Heart Association (AHA) guidelines, the initial approach for evaluating this patient should include risk stratification through a gender-specific lens. Early detection relies on three basic pillars for identifying critical CAD based on risk estimation. These are history of presentation (including cardiac risk profile), serial ECG, and biomarkers, which should be determined before conducting an anatomical or functional stress test.[3]

Elements of the History of Presenting Illness

Warning Signs Only about one-third of women with ischemic heart disease experience warning chest pain prior to presentation. Compared with men, women are more likely to complain of shortness of breath, profound fatigue, and weakness in the month preceding their myocardial infarction.[4]

Presentation Earlier reports suggest that women with CAD present more often with atypical symptoms. However, a recent prospective study of 2,475 ED patients showed that chest pain or discomfort was the most common presenting complaint in both men and women and accounted for almost 90% of acute myocardial infarction (AMI) cases regardless of age.[5] The difference in presenting complaints between men and women with CAD can be found in their description of chest discomfort as well as an increase in reporting associated atypical symptoms (excessive fatigue, nausea, jaw/shoulder pain, etc.) by women.[4] Gender-specific variation also appears in symptoms based on whether the primary event is a ST-elevation myocardial infarction (STEMI) or a non-STEMI. In general, women under-recognize their symptoms and delay seeking care (on average by 2–3 hours).[6] Women are also overrepresented in a third of AMI group that presents without chest pain (42% women vs. 21% men),[7] further delaying the initiation of definitive care.

Role of Cardiac Risk Factors

There is gender-specific moderation of traditional and nontraditional cardiac risk factors. Traditional factors such as diabetes and smoking differentially increase the risk of MI in women as compared to men. The Copenhagen City Heart Study demonstrated this by prospectively following 13,000 patients with type-2 diabetes for 20 years and found a twofold higher risk of MI in women as compared to men.[8,9] Similarly, smoking increases the risk of CAD in women by 25% compared to men.[10] Even small amounts of tobacco use, as little as 1.4 cigarettes per day, have been shown to increase cardiovascular risk in women.[10] On the other hand, hypertension and dyslipidemia increase the risk in men to a greater extent than in women.[11]

Nontraditional risk factors, such as depression and autoimmune conditions, present with greater frequency in women as compared to men.[12,13,14] Depression has been associated with a fourfold increase in mortality post AMI.[15] Similarly, metabolic syndrome (impaired glucose tolerance and any two of the following: [1] BP $\geq$ 130/85 mmHg, [2] TRG $\geq$ 150 mg/dL, [3] HDL < 40 for men and < 50 for women, [4] central obesity or BMI > 30 kg/m^2, and [5] microalbuminuria [30–300 mg/24 hours]) may result in a differential higher risk of mortality and CAD in women.[16,17]

Knowledge of the gender-specific risk attribution by these conditions is important in overall risk stratification of symptomatic patients. While some authors debate the role of cardiac risk factors in ED chest pain patients, evidence suggests that these factors have a predictive role, especially in patients <55 years.[18,19]

Investigative Studies

Serial ECGs are recommended for ruling out ACS regardless of gender. The frequency of ST-segment abnormalities in women with ACS is similar to that for men, but women more often have T-wave inversions.[3] The prognosis of these T-wave inversions in the absence of positive stress tests needs further investigation.

Biomarkers While several cardiac and inflammatory biomarkers are elevated in ACS, the 2012 ACC/AHA guidelines recommend serial testing of troponin in suspected cases. New data indicate that the 99th percentile for troponin assays are consistently lower for women as compared to men; changing the diagnostic threshold would increase the precision of diagnosis in women as compared to men if high-sensitivity troponin assays are obtained. The upcoming results of the High STEACS (High-Sensitivity Troponin in Evaluation of Patients with Acute Coronary Syndrome) study would likely change our current practice. Additional prognostic value has been attributed to elevated beta-natriuretic protein and C-reactive protein (CRP), especially in women, but larger trials are needed before these tests become standard of care in acute ACS.

Risk-Stratification Scores

Several risk-stratification tools divide patients with chest pain into low-, intermediate-, and high-risk groups to guide outpatient management. Traditional scores such as the Framingham Score (FRS) or the ATP-III score have been shown to underestimate the 10-year risk of CAD in asymptomatic women as compared to the Reynolds Risk score.[20,21] The latter score is derived from 24,000 women and is unique in considering sex-differential factors such as metabolic syndrome and CRP in its algorithm. Age also affects the accuracy of traditional scoring instruments by gender. Whereas young women have a low pretest probability of developing CAD, a recent study of young women (<55 yrs) reported a high burden of cardiac risk factors in these patients when compared to the general population. Nevertheless, traditional scores underestimate their risk. Choi et al.'s paper called for 30-year risk scores to better accommodate the age- and gender-specific nuances of risk stratification.[19] Also, none of these scores is predictive of acute events.

In patients with acute chest pain, measures such as the Thrombolysis in Myocardial Infarction (TIMI) risk score, the Global Registry of Acute Coronary Events (GRACE) risk score, the HEART (History, ECG, Age, Risk factors, Troponin) score, the Vancouver Chest Pain rule, the Quantitative Pretest Probability (QPTP) ACS instrument, and the Emergency Department Assessment of Chest Pain Score (EDACS) provide a more immediate assessment for risk of AMI or death. Of these contemporary risk scores, however, only the EDACS score includes patient gender as a variable in the final model and has been validated in at least one study thus far.[22] As high-

sensitivity troponins become more widely used over time, it is likely that risk scores for ED chest pain patients will require additional refinement and validation.

Stress Testing and Other Diagnostic Modalities

Symptomatic patients who have not sustained a myocardial infarction should undergo provocative imaging to rule out critical CAD. In 2005, a consensus group reviewed the sensitivity and specificity of commonly available tests and recommended stress testing for intermediate- to high-risk women.[23] The 2013 ACC and AHA guidelines recommend no differences in testing recommendations for men and women. The sensitivity and specificity of diagnostic tests are influenced by the lower prevalence of CAD in premenopausal women and the fact that single-vessel disease is less common in women. This is why the exercise treadmill test has diminished accuracy (61%–70%) in women as compared to men (70%–80%).[23] Nuclear perfusion studies have comparable accuracy in women and men (near 80% specificity) and are comparable to stress echo (85% specificity). In non-obese patients with a low and stable HR, coronary CT angiogram (cCTA) provides excellent image quality.[24] There is, however, a non-negligible lifetime attributable risk of cancer associated with cCTA. This risk appears to be largest in women who are younger and have combined cardiac and aortic scans; rates are as high as 1/715 women and 1/1,911 men age 60.[25] The risk of contrast-induced nephropathy must also be taken into consideration.

In summary, both men and women with ACS present often with chest pain, but their descriptions of pain and associated symptoms may differ. Variable risk of cardiac risk factors, non-specific ECG changes, and lower cutoff levels of troponin should be incorporated in gender-specific risk stratification. Risk scores should be validated in gender-specific clinical models. Decisions for optimal imaging strategy should incorporate risk stratification, weight, functional capacity, sensitivity and specificity, institutional expertise, and the radiation risk associated with each modality.

Gender-Specific Pathophysiology for Ischemic Chest Pain

Varying gender-specific mechanisms of pathophysiology influence the clinical course of ACS in men and women. Observations that support pathophysiologic differences include the following: (1) Women have less obstructive disease than men; (2) among women, chest pain symptoms and disability do not correlate with the severity of coronary artery stenosis; (3) women show higher rates of adverse outcomes after acute MI than men of similar age despite having less severe stenosis, smaller infarcts, and more preserved systolic function; and (4) women have higher rates of other disorders suggestive of vascular dysfunction such as Raynaud's phenomenon and migraine headache.[26] The gender-specific causes of cardiac chest pain are varied; they are summarized in Figure 2.1 and outlined next.

Obstruction of the coronary artery (>50%) is the most common cause of ischemic chest pain regardless of gender. However, clinicians now

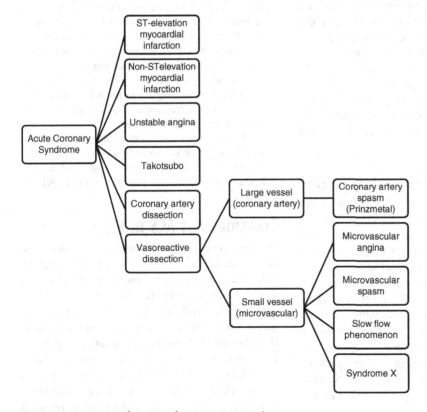

Figure 2.1 Gender-specific causes of acute coronary syndrome

understand that there can be multiple alternate mechanisms of cardiac chest pain, which are more prevalent in women than in men. Syndrome X represents vasoreactive dysfunction and can be categorized as (1) large vessel (coronary) dysfunction commonly seen as coronary artery spasm[27] and (2) small vessel (microvessel) dysfunction. Small vessel dysfunction represents a heterogeneous group of disorders including slow flow phenomenon,[28] microvascular angina,[29] microvascular spasm,[30] and cardiac Syndrome X.[31] Two theoretical explanations of sex-specific differences in coronary pathophysiology may be found in microvascular and endothelial dysfunction as illustrated in Figure 2.1. Microvascular dysfunction can be further differentiated on the basis of exertional/rest angina, timing of pain, presence or absence of typical cardiac risk factors, changes in coronary flow reserve, lactate measurements in the coronary sinus, and microvascular resistance.[32] Higher vasoreactive dysfunction occurs in women for several reasons: Women have a higher proportion of vascular conditions including hypertensive disorders of pregnancy, peri-partum dissection, migraine, vasculitis, and Raynauds. Women also have smaller coronary vessels and more diffuse disease patterns.[33] They have stiffer aortas and more dysfunctional microvessels than men.

In addition to ischemia, two other sex-specific mechanisms of chest pain include coronary artery dissection and Takosubo cardiomyopathy, both of which are discussed in more depth in the section titled "Transient Left Ventricular Apical Ballooning."

Non-obstructive Coronary Artery Disease

The Women's Ischemia Syndrome Evaluation (WISE) Study showed that up to 47% of women undergoing elective angiography have <50% obstruction of one or more coronary arteries as opposed to 17% of men as reported in historical cohorts. Vasoreactive dysfunction often coexists with non-obstructive CAD causing angina despite so-called negative angiography. At least 20% of women with normal or non-obstructive angiography have myocardial ischemia as assessed by perfusion imaging.[34] These patients are often labeled as having Syndrome X, even though the original description of Syndrome X was different.[35]

Testing for Microvascular Angina

Even though endothelial dysfunction of large and small vessels has been described for more than three decades, there is no consensus on uniform definitions for each of these two types of dysfunction.[28] The lack of consensus and definition has made diagnosis a challenge. Classically, administration of intravenous ergonavine, acetylcholine, or adenosine during angiography was considered the gold standard for measurement of endothelial reactivity, but it is no longer performed routinely. More noninvasive forms of testing, such as hemodynamic measurements of coronary flow reserve by cardiac PET scan or MRI have shown some promise. Their widespread use, however, has been limited by cost and availability. At present, the diagnosis of Syndrome X is often made clinically based on classic symptoms, presence of risk factors, and non-obstructive CAD demonstrated by an anatomical study with or without a positive functional test.

> **Clinical Pearls**
>
> Obstructive CAD is the most common cause of ischemic chest pain in both men and women. Other causes of ischemic chest pain such as Syndrome X and microvascular disease are more prevalent in women than men.
>
> Women with chest pain who undergo coronary angiography are more likely than men to have non-obstructive CAD (<50% stenosis of one or more coronary arteries).
>
> Microvascular angina is a clinical diagnosis based on symptoms, risk factors, and often a finding of non-obstructive coronary artery disease. However it can also exist with and without CAD.

Treatment of ACS in Women

For patients with STEMI, immediate reperfusion is recommended for both men and women. Percutaneous coronary intervention (PCI) is shown to be superior to fibrinolysis in women with STEMI, reducing the incidence of subsequent cardiovascular sequelae more effectively than in men.[36] However, the timing of treatment is considered more important than the choice of strategy.[3] For NSTEMI patients, the treatments do not demonstrate gender-specific advantages. However, the recommended dose of anticoagulant medication is less in women because of a higher risk of bleeding that could be related to lower body weight. PCI was associated with a 33% decreased risk of death, MI, or repeat ACS in biomarker-positive women, whereas women who were biomarker negative had a greater risk; this difference in risk of adverse outcome was not evident in men.[20] Thus, invasive therapy is recommended for all men, but only for intermediate-high–risk women; optimal medical management is recommended for low-risk women. No randomized control trials compare percutaneous coronary intervention to CABG in men versus women. Gender-specific analysis of these data will shed more light on this debate.

Standard medical therapies such as beta-blockers and aspirin have been shown to have equal efficacy in women and men in acute MI treatment.[37,38] In contrast, treatment of non-obstructive CAD depends on improvement in symptoms and/or vascular function. No evidence-based guidelines address management for these patients. However, we recommend optimization of their cardiac risk factors. These patients often have persistent chest pain resulting from some form of microvascular angina and often require a trial of one or more options. Exercise has been shown to ameliorate symptoms and improve vascular function. Other options include tricyclic antidepressants such as imipramine for patients with abnormal cardiac pain perception and normal angiograms, beta-blockers, calcium channel blockers, ACE-inhibitors/ARB, statins, and new antianginal drugs such as Ranolazine.[39]

Prognosis of ACS in Women

Women who have had an MI have higher morbidity and mortality rates than their male counterparts – both acutely[40] and long term.[41] The overall mortality rate during hospitalization is about 17% for women and 12% for men. Sex differences in mortality after ACS are emphasized in younger women (<50 yrs) and those presenting with STEMI.[42] This trend applies across the spectrum of coronary disease. Women with stable angina are twice as likely as men to suffer death or nonfatal MI during a one-year follow-up of stable angina symptoms, and younger women (<75 yrs) have higher coronary mortality ratios.[50] Women with ACS have higher rates of cardiogenic shock,

bleeding, and vascular complications.[44] Possible explanations include increased age and number of comorbidities at the time of infarction, delay in presentation, and increased rate of associated complications.[45,46]

Adverse events have also been reported for non-obstructive disease. Studies indicate an annual cardiac event rate of 2.5% in patients with persistent chest pain.[47,48] In a study comparing five-year cardiovascular event rates in women presenting with chest pain with either non-obstructive CAD or normal coronary arteries, women with non-obstructive CAD (stenosis 1%–49%) had a 16% five-year adverse event rate compared to a 7.9% adverse event rate in women with normal coronary arteries.[48] Up to 30% of women with chest pain, a "normal" angiogram, and endothelial dysfunction developed obstructive CAD in a 10-year follow-up.[20] The extent of non-obstructive CAD is a significant estimator of all-cause mortality in women. In one study, the relative hazard for mortality was 1.3 per non-obstructive lesion found in women. For men, the number of non-obstructive lesions was not a significant estimator of mortality.[49]

Some reports indicate that the prevalence of both angina and non-ischemic chest pain is higher in women than men.[50] Symptomatic women are more likely to have persistent chest pain symptoms with a greater likelihood and duration of hospitalization compared to men, thereby increasing the costs of care.[20] The aggregate lifetime cost for patients with persistent chest pain is estimated to be $767,288.[51] Furthermore, patients with non-obstructive disease have a higher 10-year rate of development of obstructive CAD.[20]

Clinical Pearls

Medical and interventional treatments for STEMI and NSTEMI are equally efficacious in men and women.

The treatment of non-obstructive CAD surrounds symptom management and improvement in vascular function.

Women with acute MI have higher morbidity and mortality rates than their male counterparts.

Women with non-obstructive CAD have higher incidence of future CAD than women who are found to have normal coronary arteries on angiography.

Patient A Conclusion and Rationale

In summary, this woman has atypical symptoms of ACS and significant risk factors including diabetes and smoking. While her initial negative troponin is reassuring, her ECG does show evidence of ischemia in the lateral leads. She was treated with aspirin and a beta-blocker and admitted to an observation Chest Pain Unit for monitoring on telemetry and repeated troponin measurements and ECG studies. Exercise treadmill testing was indeterminate. An echocardiogram showed mild diastolic dysfunction with preserved systolic function. She was discharged with cardiology follow-up. On follow-up, she described worsening of her symptoms. Cardiac catheterization was performed and ultimately showed non-obstructive CAD. Further medical optimization and treatment with tricyclic antidepressants and regular exercise ultimately decreased her discomfort and improved her functional capacity over the next several months.

Transient Left Ventricular Apical Ballooning

Introduction

Takotsubo cardiomyopathy (TC) is a reversible cardiomyopathy, often precipitated by emotional stress; Japanese authors first described the condition in the early 1990s.[52] Its name is derived from the Japanese word for "octopus trap," as the heart looks like a Japanese octopus trap when imaged by echocardiogram. Takotsubo's is now referred to as "Apical Ballooning Syndrome" or "Broken Heart Syndrome." Further prospective studies have demonstrated the same clinical phenomenon in the United States.[53,54]

Clinical Presentation

The majority of patients are women, typically postmenopausal and white.[53,54] Studies suggest that Takotsubo's cardiomyopathy accounts for 1.5%–2.2% of patients presenting with symptoms that initially were thought to be ACS.[53–56] In a systematic review, women accounted for 82%–100% of patients with an average age of

62–75 years.[52] In a prospective study of 22 women with Takotsubo's cardiomyopathy, 20 patients had initial clinical findings consistent with ACS, including abrupt onset of substernal chest pain, ST-segment elevation, and hypotension. Patients typically present with signs and symptoms of an ACS with a history of a recent strong emotional stressor. Approximately 27% of patients reported severe emotional stress prior to symptom onset.[52,56]

Abnormalities on ECG are common at the time of presentation. Anterior ST-segment elevation has been reported in greater than 90% of these patients. They may also develop evolutionary deep symmetrical T-wave inversions within 24 to 48 hours and may have prolongation of the QTc interval.[52] Cardiac enzyme elevation is variable but is commonly abnormal.[52,53,55,57]

Cardiac Catheterization and Angiography

When cardiac catheterization is performed, patients with Takotsubo's cardiomyopathy do not have evidence of obstructive CAD causing their depressed cardiac function (Table 2.1). Prospective studies show systolic dysfunction in all of these patients with ejection fractions ranging from 9% to 29%. Wall motion abnormalities typically involve akinesia or hypokinesia of the distal one-half to two-thirds of the LV chamber.

Table 2.1 Diagnostic Criteria of Takotsubo's Cardiomyopathy [52,53,58]

Diagnostic Criteria
There are no strict criteria for the diagnosis of Takotsubo's cardiomyopathy. Proposed criteria include the following: (1) Transient LV wall motion abnormalities involving the apical and/or mid-ventricular myocardial segments with wall motion abnormalities extending beyond single epicardial coronary distribution. (2) Absence of obstructive epicardial CAD or angiographic evidence of acute plaque rupture as explanation for the observed wall motion abnormality. (3) New ECG abnormalities such as transient ST-segment elevation and/or diffuse T-wave inversions, or troponin elevation.

The resulting cardiomyopathy has a distinctive apical ballooning appearance with associated basal hypercontractility at end systole.[54]

LV outflow obstruction can result from the apical and mid-ventricular wall motion abnormalities and mitral valve systolic anterior motion. In one prospective study, the administration of dobutamine was associated with hemodynamic collapse related to LV outflow obstruction but resolved with discontinuation of the drug.[54]

Mechanisms

Several mechanisms are proposed for TC. They include transient multi-vessel epicardial spasm and microvascular ischemia.[52,55,59] The reason for the predisposition to TC among women is unknown but is thought to be related to gender differences in myocardial sensitivity to catecholamines and subsequent intra-myocyte calcium overload.[60,61] Takotsubo's has mechanistically been linked to other forms of non-ischemic myocardial stunning reported in non-cardiac disease such as subarachnoid hemorrhage, which is also linked to a neutrally mediated trigger of acute LV dysfunction.[54]

Management

The acute management of patients with TC is the same as with ACS. If the ECG shows ST elevations, the initial ED management is the same as that for STEMI and includes emergent angiography, beta-blocker therapy, nitrates, aspirin, intravenous heparin, and hemodynamic support (Table 2.2).

Clinical Course

Takotsubo's cardiomyopathy has a favorable prognosis. The in-hospital mortality is low (about 1%–3%).[52,56,62] Complications are uncommon but can include hemodynamic instability, often related to LV outflow tract obstruction, arrhythmias, heart failure, and cardiogenic shock. The most common causes of mortality with TC are cardiogenic shock and systemic embolization.[52]

Recurrence

Data on recurrence rates for Takotsubo's cardiomyopathy are limited. TC recurs within the first few years in 2%–10% of patients according to some studies.[52,54,63]

Table 2.2 Management Considerations in Patients Presenting with Stress-Related Cardiopmyopathy[52]

(1) Monitor patients on telemetry and evaluate for signs and symptoms of heart failure.

(2) Perform echocardiogram or MRI to evaluate LV function, valve dysfunction, LV mural thrombus, and dynamic LV outflow obstruction.

(3) Evaluate for dynamic obstruction in the LV outflow tract in those with new systolic murmur, hypotension, and/or new mitral regurgitation.

(4) Consider anticoagulation with heparin to prevent LV mural thrombus formation in those with apical involvement and no contraindications for anticoagulation.

(5) Initiate standard medical therapy for LV systolic dysfunction including beta-blocker therapy and ACE-inhibitor therapy +/− diuretic therapy.

(6) Repeat echocardiography prior to discharge to reassess LV function and repeat echocardiogram at one and three months if LV dysfunction persists.

Clinical Pearls

Takotsubo's cardiomyopathy is a reversible cardiomyopathy with clinical presentation similar to acute ischemic heart disease but with normal coronary arteries on angiography. It is often precipitated by stress.

Initial management of TC is similar to acute management of STEMI.

The prognosis of TC is almost uniformly favorable.

Spontaneous Coronary Artery Dissection

Spontaneous coronary artery dissection (SCAD) is a rare cause of AMI.[64] Approximately 82% of cases occur in women and the mean age of presentation is 43.[65] SCAD is thought to be caused by an intimal tear in or bleeding from the vasa vasorum in the endocardium.[66] Traditional cardiovascular risk factors are not associated with increased risk for this cause of myocardial infarction. Researchers at the Mayo Clinic collected the largest cohort of patients with SCAD studied to date (87 individuals). Chest pain was the presenting complaint in 91% of these patients; 49% of the cohort presented with STEMI and 44% with NSTEMI. Life-threatening arrhythmias were present in about 14% of the patients. Many of the patients in this cohort reported exertion prior to their event; another large contingent was postpartum (average 38 days).[65] The left anterior descending was the most common vessel affected. In-hospital mortality was small.

SCAD is treated like ACS; patients should receive emergent coronary angiography followed by PCI or CABG. Some evidence shows that PCI may be associated with increased rates of complication as compared to CABG.[65] In the subgroup of patients with SCAD presenting with STEMI, fibrinolytic therapy has demonstrated some benefits;[64] however, reports indicate an extension of the coronary dissection in a few patients treated with thrombolytics.[67] While the in-hospital mortality rates are favorable, the 10-year recurrence rate was found to be around 30%, and these patients have an estimated 10-year rate of cardiovascular morbidity or mortality of approximately 47%.[65,67]

> **Clinical Pearl**
>
> Spontaneous coronary artery dissection is a rare cause of AMI most commonly seen in young women.

Section 2   Heart Failure and Structural Heart Disease

Introduction: Importance of Heart Failure

Heart failure (HF), a major cause of cardiac death, is a complex clinical syndrome that can result from a number of structural or functional cardiac disorders. ED visits for heart failure saw a 20% increase from the 1990s to 2005.[68] Heart failure is the most common ED discharge diagnosis particularly in elderly women, and this disease creates a significant economic burden.[69]

Definition and Types of HF

Heart failure is characterized by a defined set of symptoms and physical findings. Echocardiography is routinely performed in patients with HF to measure the ejection fraction (EF) and to classify patients with HF into two groups: those who have reduced systolic function (HFREF; HF with reduced EF) and those with preserved systolic function (called HFPEF; HF with preserved EF). Patients with normal EFs can have marked diastolic impairment.[70] The leading cause of HFREF in the United States is CAD most studies show that more men than women have HFREF. In contrast, previous myocardial infarction is seen less frequently in patients with HFPEF, which is more common in women.[71] Clinically, some patients with diastolic dysfunction do not have the typical symptoms that are associated with HF; nevertheless, HFPEF is associated with marked increases in all-cause mortality.[70]

Lack of Evidence in Women

Although equal numbers of men and women live with HF, women are underrepresented in clinical studies of HF.[72] Not surprisingly, then, evidence elucidating pathophysiology, etiology, clinical presentation, treatment, and outcome of HF is predominantly based on data collected from men.[73] The underrepresentation of women in this dataset has made it difficult to delineate the differences in clinical characteristics of men and women with HF. Furthermore, researchers have not had the opportunity to analyze sufficient clinical and laboratory data to be able to identify markers and potential determinants of survival of women with HF.[74]

Sex Differences in HF: Physiology

Women are twice as likely as men to develop HFPEF.[75] Many potential factors contribute to the discrepancy in HFPEF pathophysiology between men and women, including sex effects on the natural course of aging of the cardiovascular system. Beginning at puberty, left ventricular chamber size and mass are 15% to 40% smaller in women than in men, and these size and mass differences persist even after adjustment for average body size in women, which generally is smaller than that in men.[76] Interestingly, men experience loss of myocardium at the rate of 1 g per year across the lifespan, whereas left ventricular mass is preserved in women.[77]

Recent studies shed light on some of the contributors to this difference. Women display significant differences in central hemodynamics when compared to men, although peripheral hemodynamics are similar. Left ventricular diastolic dysfunction significantly correlates with arterial stiffness in women, but not in men.[78] Arterial stiffness and early wave reflections lead to augmentation of the central aortic pressure wave amplitude and increased LV afterload, resulting in impaired relaxation.[79] There are also fundamental differences in the left ventricular response to chronic load alteration. Women are more likely to develop *concentric* remodeling with stress, whereas men are more likely to develop *eccentric* left ventricular remodeling.[80] The extent of concentric ventricular remodeling in women may be associated with greater loss in systolic and diastolic function in older women, as each of these sex dimorphisms becomes more pronounced after menopause.[71] These data suggest that sex-specific differences in the way that older women's hearts adapt to hypertension may explain the greater risk of HFPEF.

Gender Differences in Acute HF Presentation

Two constellations of presenting characteristics appear in patients with acute heart failure. Women present with hypertension, valvular diseases, supraventricular arrhythmias, and preserved LV function more often than men. Male patients are younger and more often smokers and have CAD and dilated cardiomyopathy. Women more frequently have concomitant diabetes, anemia, and thyroid disease; men more often have renal failure, peripheral arterial disease, and chronic obstructive pulmonary disease.[81] These variances in findings emphasize the importance of personalized management of acute HF. A better understanding of sex-specific risk factors will improve clinicians' abilities to formulate effective strategies to improve outcomes for these patients.

HF as Risk Factor for Atrial Fibrillation

Atrial fibrillation (AF) and HF have been recognized as the two major clinical epidemics of modern cardiovascular medicine.[82] These conditions frequently coexist: HF is a major risk factor for AF

in patients with abnormal diastolic dysfunction as opposed to those patients with normal diastolic function. AF is the most common arrhythmia in contemporary clinical practice.[69] The prevalence of AF increases with age; the elderly are the fastest-growing demographic in the United States today to be diagnosed with AF. Structural heart disease influences the clinician's approach to management, for example, rate versus rhythm control, and the variety of treatment options available. It has become increasingly evident in the past decade that gender differences in cardiac structure and function affect the presentation and clinical course of many arrhythmias and are reflected in cardiac electrophysiology.

Clinical Pearls

Women are more likely than men to develop HFPEF.

Women tend to present with hypertension, valvular disease, supraventricular arrhythmias, and preserved LV function more often than men.

Diabetes, anemia, and thyroid disease are common comorbidities in women, whereas men more often have renal failure, peripheral arterial disease, and chronic obstructive pulmonary disease.

Heart failure is a major risk factor for AF. Patients with abnormal diastolic function have an increased risk of AF when compared to patients with normal diastolic function.

Section 3 Atrial Fibrillation and Other SVTs

This section focuses on the gender differences in the epidemiology, etiology, treatment, and prognosis of arrhythmia, with an emphasis on atrial fibrillation.

Patient B A Case of Atrial Fibrillation and Heart Failure

A 74-year-old women presented to the Emergency Department complaining of increasing shortness of breath, dizziness, and the sensation of a "racing heart." She has a history of long-standing hypertension. Her heart rate was 160bpm, her blood pressure was 100/50mm Hg, her respirations were 26 breaths per minute, and her oxygen saturation was 88% on room air.

Electrocardiogram showed atrial fibrillation with a rapid ventricular response. Crackles were present in the bases of both lungs. Peripheral pulses were diminished and irregular.

Basic lab work, including thyroid studies, was normal. A chest X-ray revealed bilateral pleural effusions. After determining that she had no known allergies to medications, diltiazem 20 mg IV and lasix 20 mg IV were given.

Clinical Questions

- How do the clinical characteristics of men and women presenting with heart failure and supraventricular tachycardia differ?
- When choosing medications to control the heart rate or restore sinus rhythm in these patients, are there special considerations depending on the sex of the patient?

Almost 2.3 million people in the United States have atrial fibrillation, with more than 5.6 million cases expected to be diagnosed by the year 2050.[83] The absolute number of men and women with AF is about equal.[84] After adjustment, men have a 1.5 times greater risk than women of developing atrial fibrillation.[85] Women who present with atrial fibrillation are generally older than their male counterparts and have additional comorbidities.[86]

Triggers

Both men and women presenting with new onset atrial fibrillation are responding to the same triggers regardless of gender. These triggers may include hypertension, myocardial infarction, structural heart/valve disease, hyperthyroidism, and underlying infection. Women with AF are significantly more likely than men to have valvular disease as a major risk factor, whereas myocardial infarction and hypertension are more significantly associated with the development of atrial fibrillation in men.[85]

Treatment

The treatment of atrial fibrillation is similar for men and women. Studies have examined the impact of sex on the advantages of choosing rate or rhythm control. Mixed-sex studies have shown no difference in stroke risk for patients receiving rate versus rhythm control.[87] However, one study revealed that women with persistent atrial fibrillation whose treatment focused on rhythm control (i.e., chemical or electrical cardioversion) had more cardiovascular morbidity and mortality than women whose treatment focused on rate control.[88]

Current therapeutic options for patients with concomitant heart failure and atrial fibrillation include control of their heart rate and anticoagulation or medical therapy aimed at restoring and maintaining sinus rhythm. Women generally have higher heart rates at rest and longer corrected QT intervals than men. Women are at greater risk for developing QT prolongation and Torsades de Pointes than men in response to certain classes of anti-arrhythmic drugs. This propensity must be considered when choosing anti-arrhythmic drugs and may affect the selection of drugs available for rhythm control and the success of that control in women with AF.

An equal proportion of men and women with atrial fibrillation are anticoagulated.[86] Some studies, however, have demonstrated that anticoagulants are prescribed less frequently for older women with atrial fibrillation when compared to older men despite comparable risk profiles.[89] Researchers have not uncovered a difference in the quality or sufficiency of anticoagulation between the genders.[90]

Prognosis

Findings about the role of sex as a predictor of stroke in AF are somewhat inconsistent in the literature; however, studies have shown an increased risk of stroke in women with atrial fibrillation.[86] Women stopping their Warfarin appear to be at higher risk than men for AF-related thromboembolism.[90,91] According to one study, strokes occurring in women with atrial fibrillation appear to be more disabling, with a relative risk for fatal stroke in women versus men of 3:1.[90] Women with atrial fibrillation–associated HF more often have preserved left ventricular systolic function, when compared to men with AF-associated HF.[86]

Complications of Therapy

Rates of bleeding complications from anticoagulation therapy for atrial fibrillation also demonstrate a sex specificity. Studies have indicated a significantly higher risk of major bleeding in women on Coumadin when compared to men, suggesting the need for more intensive monitoring of anticoagulant efficacy in women.

Patient B Conclusion and Rationale

In response to the IV diltiazem, the patient's heart rate initially slowed to a rate of 110 to 120 bpm but rapidly returned to a higher rate. After 15 minutes, another bolus was ordered, followed by a continuous infusion of diltiazem at 5 mg/hour. She was then transferred to an inpatient telemetry unit for further monitoring and clinical management.

This patient's symptoms are common indications of acute onset atrial fibrillation with rapid ventricular response. Her past medical history is positive for hypertension, which is a known risk factor for the development of atrial fibrillation, as is her increased age; however, she does not have evidence of known CAD or a prior myocardial infarction.

Women present with hypertension, valvular diseases, supraventricular arrhythmias, and preserved LV function more often than men. Men tend to be younger, with a history of smoking, CAD, or dilated cardiomyopathy. These sex-specific risk factors and concomitant disease entities reinforce the importance of personalized management of acute heart failure and arrhythmias.

Comprehensive echocardiographic evaluation provides prognostic information and guides therapy. This patient had a recent echocardiogram demonstrating valvular disease with preserved ejection fraction and no evidence of myocardial ischemia; her findings were consistent with diastolic heart failure. She presented to the ED with symptomatic atrial fibrillation. Women with AF tend to have higher mean heart rates, longer episodes of AF, and more prominent symptoms than men. The initial goal of treatment is to slow the patient's heart rate. It is beyond the scope of this chapter to discuss the many pharmacologic approaches and treatment strategies for atrial fibrillation and heart failure. Clinicians should consider the greater risk of prolonged QT and Torsades de Pointes in women when choosing anti-arrhythmic drugs.

Clinical Pearls

Atrial fibrillation is equally common in women and men, though women with AF tend to be older and have more comorbidities.

Valvular disease is a major risk factor for atrial fibrillation in women.

Treatment of atrial fibrillation is the same for women and men.

Women have increased risk of stroke compared to men when anticoagulation is not prescribed.

Women have increased rates of bleeding with anticoagulation therapy.

Section 4 Heart Disease in Pregnancy

Cardiovascular disorders in pregnant women pose challenges for diagnosis and management. The prevalence of CAD in women increases with age;[92] more women are currently delaying pregnancy, increasing the number of pregnant women who will be presenting with AMI. Risk factors for CAD in pregnancy include the traditional risk factors observed in the general population,[93] as well as additional risk factors such as gestational diabetes, gestational hypertension, and eclampsia. Surprisingly, pregnancy itself has been thought to increase the risk of AMI three- to fourfold.[94] The normal physiology of pregnancy can also exacerbate underlying CAD as well as increase the risk for coronary artery dissection and cardiomyopathy. The diagnosis of ischemic heart disease and AMI can be challenging in pregnant women and diagnostic testing can increase risk to the fetus.

Treatment is challenging in pregnancy as thrombolytics have controversial results. If coronary dissection has been diagnosed on angiography, thrombolysis can increase the risk of hemorrhage and further progression of the dissection.[95] According to the European Society of Cardiology and ACC/AHA guidelines, coronary angioplasty is the preferred reperfusion therapy for STEMI rather than thrombolysis during pregnancy.[96] Cardiac catheterization also carries risks, but pros and cons have to be weighed in relation to risk of MI compared with relative safety in pregnancy.

Pregnancy and the postpartum period increase the risk of arrhythmia, most commonly supraventricular tachycardia (SVT). The proposed mechanisms for this increased risk includes changes in hormone levels, changes in autonomic tone, and increased intravascular tone.[81] More fetal complications occur in women who develop arrhythmias during pregnancy. Current recommendations for treatment include medical management of tachyarrhythmias such as SVT, followed by postpartum radiofrequency ablation.

A diagnostic and treatment dilemma can arise when a previously healthy pregnant patient develops a particular life-threatening disease of uncertain etiology, which is known as peri-partum/postpartum cardiomyopathy (PPCM). At present, PPCM is considered to be a form of dilated cardiomyopathy (DCM) and is treated according to guidelines created for DCM without specific therapy or drug alterations tailored for pregnant or lactating women with PPCM.[93]

> **Clinical Pearls**
>
> Acute MI is rare in pregnancy.
>
> Pregnancy and the postpartum period increase the risk of arrhythmia in susceptible hosts.
>
> Peri-partum/postpartum cardiomyopathy is a form of dilated cardiomyopathy that can occur in previously healthy women.

Section 5 Gender Bias in Acute Care Cardiology

Studies have demonstrated that women who present with chest pain are treated less aggressively than men. Daly et al. examined the impact of gender on the investigation and management of stable angina and clinical outcome in 3,800 patients (42% female) and found lower rates of stress testing, angiography, coronary revascularization, and use of optimal medical therapy in women when compared to men.[43] They also found that adjusted one-year mortality rates in women were twice as great as those in men. Women were less likely to be discharged on aspirin or statin.[44] Women were also less likely to receive ASA or glycoprotineIIb/IIIa inhibitors. They were more likely to receive controlled substances and anxiolytics, whereas men were more likely to receive nitroglycerin, aspirin, heparin, and thrombolytic agents. On presentation, women are more likely to be taking anxiolytics, antidepressants, antibiotics, and pulmonary medications, potentially biasing physicians' calculations of pretest probability for determining appropriate approaches to diagnostic testing for heart disease in women. Awareness campaigns have helped reduce these biases and improper clinical choices.[44]

Section 6 Areas of Controversy and Directions for Further Research

Researchers must clarify the pathophysiological processes involved in sex differences in ACS and heart failure. They should develop a consensus defining the physiological entities that comprise microvascular dysfunction. Clinicians and patients would benefit from improved screening and diagnostic tools for microvascular disease that will improve management of this entity. Current approaches to diagnose and treat cardiovascular diseases are based on studies that preferentially included men. In the future, women must be included preferentially in clinical trials to bridge the gap in current knowledge and optimize treatment for all patients regardless of sex. A growing literature demonstrates pathophysiological differences in heart disease etiology and prognosis by sex, offering potential insights into novel treatment options with improved efficacy and outcomes for women when compared to older approaches that were developed solely for men.

References

1. Rosamond W, Flegal K, Furie K et al. Heart disease and stroke statistics – 2008 update: a report from the American Heart Association Statistics Committee and Stroke Statistics Subcommittee. *Circulation* 2008;**117**(4):e25–e146.

2. Towfighi A, Zheng L, Ovbiagele B. Sex-specific trends in midlife coronary heart disease risk and prevalence. *Archives of Internal Medicine* 2009;**169**(19):1762–6.

3. Anderson JL, Adams CD, Antman EM et al. 2012 ACCF/AHA focused update incorporated into the ACCF/AHA 2007 guidelines for the management of patients with unstable angina/non-ST-elevation myocardial infarction: a report of the American College of Cardiology Foundation/American Heart

Association Task Force on Practice Guidelines. *Circulation* 2013;**127**(23):e663–e828.

4. McSweeney JC, Cody M, O'Sullivan P, Elberson K, Moser DK, Garvin BJ. Women's early warning symptoms of acute myocardial infarction. *Circulation* 2003;**108**(21):2619–23.

5. Khan NA, Daskalopoulou SS, Karp I et al. Sex differences in acute coronary syndrome symptom presentation in young patients. *JAMA Internal Medicine* 2013;**173**(20):1863–71.

6. Ting HH, Chen AY, Roe MT et al. Delay from symptom onset to hospital presentation for patients with non-ST-segment elevation myocardial infarction. *Archives of Internal Medicine* 2010;**170**(20):1834–41.

7. Canto AJ, Kiefe CI, Goldberg RJ et al. Differences in symptom presentation and hospital mortality according to type of acute myocardial infarction. *American Heart Journal* 2012;**163**(4):572–79.

8. Almdal T, Scharling H, Jensen JS, Vestergaard H. The independent effect of type 2 diabetes mellitus on ischemic heart disease, stroke, and death: a population-based study of 13,000 men and women with 20 years of follow-up. *Archives of Internal Medicine* 2004;**164**(13):1422–26.

9. Huxley R, Barzi F, Woodward M. Excess risk of fatal coronary heart disease associated with diabetes in men and women: meta-analysis of 37 prospective cohort studies. *British Medical Journal (clinical research ed.)* 2006;**332**(7533):73–78.

10. Huxley RR, Woodward M. Cigarette smoking as a risk factor for coronary heart disease in women compared with men: a systematic review and meta-analysis of prospective cohort studies. *Lancet* 2011;**378**(9799):1297–1305.

11. Daugherty SL, Masoudi FA, Zeng C et al. Sex differences in cardiovascular outcomes in patients with incident hypertension. *Journal of Hypertension* 2013;**31**(2):271–77.

12. Rutledge T, Reis SE, Olson MB et al. Depression symptom severity and reported treatment history in the prediction of cardiac risk in women with suspected myocardial ischemia: the NHLBI-sponsored WISE study. *Archives of General Psychiatry* 2006;**63**(8):874–80.

13. Hak AE, Karlson EW, Feskanich D, Stampfer MJ, Costenbader KH. Systemic lupus erythematosus and the risk of cardiovascular disease: results from the nurses' health study. *Arthritis and Rheumatism* 2009;**61**(10):1396–1402.

14. Manzi S, Meilahn EN, Rairie JE et al. Age-specific incidence rates of myocardial infarction and angina in women with systemic lupus erythematosus: comparison with the Framingham Study. *American Journal of Epidemiology* 1997;**145**(5):408–15.

15. Frasure-Smith N, Lesperance F, Talajic M. The impact of negative emotions on prognosis following myocardial infarction: is it more than depression? *Health Psychology: Official Journal of the Division of Health Psychology, American Psychological Association* 1995;**14**(5):388–98.

16. Marroquin OC, Kip KE, Kelley DE et al. Metabolic syndrome modifies the cardiovascular risk associated with angiographic coronary artery disease in women: a report from the Women's Ischemia Syndrome Evaluation. *Circulation* 2004;**109**(6):714–21.

17. Kip KE, Marroquin OC, Kelley DE et al. Clinical importance of obesity versus the metabolic syndrome in cardiovascular risk in women: a report from the Women's Ischemia Syndrome Evaluation (WISE) study. *Circulation* 2004;**109**(6):706–13.

18. Han JH, Lindsell CJ, Hornung RW et al. The elder patient with suspected acute coronary syndromes in the emergency department. *Academic Emergency Medicine: Official Journal of the Society for Academic Emergency Medicine* 2007;**14**(8):732–39.

19. Choi J, Daskalopoulou SS, Thanassoulis G et al. Sex- and gender-related risk factor burden in patients with premature acute coronary syndrome. *The Canadian Journal of Cardiology* 2014;**30**(1):109–17.

20. Shaw LJ, Bugiardini R, Merz CN. Women and ischemic heart disease: evolving knowledge. *Journal of the American College of Cardiology* 2009;**54**(17):1561–75.

21. Cook NR, Paynter NP, Eaton CB et al. Comparison of the Framingham and Reynolds Risk scores for global cardiovascular risk prediction in the multiethnic Women's Health Initiative. *Circulation* 2012;**125**(14):1748–56 (S1741–s1711).

22. Than M, Flaws D, Sanders S et al. Development and validation of the Emergency Department Assessment of Chest Pain Score and 2 h accelerated diagnostic protocol. *Emergency Medicine Australasia: EMA* 2014;**26**(1):34–44.

23. Mieres JH, Shaw LJ, Arai A et al. Role of noninvasive testing in the clinical evaluation of women with suspected coronary artery disease: Consensus statement from the Cardiac Imaging Committee, Council on Clinical Cardiology, and the Cardiovascular Imaging and Intervention Committee, Council on Cardiovascular Radiology and Intervention, American Heart Association. *Circulation* 2005;**111**(5):682–96.

24. Achenbach S, Kramer CM, Zoghbi WA, Dilsizian V. The year in coronary artery disease. *Journal of the American College of Cardiology. Cardiovascular Imaging* 2010;**3**(10):1065–77.

25. Einstein AJ, Henzlova MJ, Rajagopalan S. Estimating risk of cancer associated with radiation exposure from 64-slice computed tomography coronary angiography. *Journal of the American Medical Association* 2007;**298**(3):317–23.

26. Vaccarino V, Badimon L, Corti R et al. Ischaemic heart disease in women: are there sex differences in pathophysiology and risk factors? Position paper from the working group on coronary pathophysiology and microcirculation of the European Society of Cardiology. *Cardiovascular Research* 2011;**90**(1):9–17.

27. Prinzmetal M, Kennamer R, Merliss R, Wada T, Bor N. Angina pectoris. I. A variant form of angina pectoris; preliminary report. *American Journal of Medicine* 1959;**27**:375–88.

28. Beltrame JF, Limaye SB, Horowitz JD. The coronary slow flow phenomenon – a new coronary microvascular disorder. *Cardiology* 2002;**97**(4):197–202.

29. Cannon RO, III, Epstein SE. "Microvascular angina" as a cause of chest pain with angiographically normal coronary arteries. *American Journal of Cardiology* 1988;**61**(15):1338–43.

30. Mohri M, Koyanagi M, Egashira K et al. Angina pectoris caused by coronary microvascular spasm. *Lancet* 1998;**351**(9110):1165–69.

31. Arbogast R, Bourassa MG. Myocardial function during atrial pacing in patients with angina pectoris and normal coronary arteriograms. Comparison with patients having significant coronary artery disease. *American Journal of Cardiology* 1973;**32**(3):257–63.

32. Di Fiore DP, Beltrame JF. Chest pain in patients with "normal angiography": could it be cardiac? *International Journal of Evidence-Based Healthcare* 2013;**11**(1):56–68.

33. Pepine CJ, Nichols WW, Pauly DF. Estrogen and different aspects of vascular disease in women and men. *Circulation Research* 2006;**99**(5):459–61.

34. Bugiardini R, Bairey Merz CN. Angina with "normal" coronary arteries: a changing philosophy. *Journal of the American Medical Association* 2005;**293**(4):477–84.

35. Likoff W, Segal BL, Kasparian H. Paradox of normal selective coronary arteriograms in patients considered to have unmistakable coronary heart disease. *New England Journal of Medicine* 1967;**276**(19):1063–66.

36. Dolor RJ, Melloni C, Chatterjee R et al. AHRQ Comparative Effectiveness Reviews, in *Treatment Strategies for Women with Coronary Artery Disease*. Rockville, MD: Agency for Healthcare Research and Quality (US); 2012.

37. Pedersen TR. Six-year follow-up of the Norwegian Multicenter Study on Timolol after Acute Myocardial Infarction. *New England Journal of Medicine* 1985;**313**(17):1055–58.

38. Randomized trial of intravenous streptokinase, oral aspirin, both, or neither among 17,187 cases of suspected acute myocardial infarction: ISIS-2.ISIS-2 (Second International Study of Infarct Survival) Collaborative Group. *Journal of the American College of Cardiology* 1988;**12**(6 Suppl A):3a–13a.

39. Duvernoy CS. Evolving strategies for the treatment of microvascular angina in women. *Expert Review of Cardiovascular Therapy* 2012;**10**(11):1413–19.

40. Vaccarino V, Parsons L, Every NR, Barron HV, Krumholz HM. Sex-based differences in early mortality after myocardial infarction. National Registry of Myocardial Infarction 2 Participants. *New England Journal of Medicine* 1999;**341**(4):217–25.

41. Vaccarino V, Krumholz HM, Yarzebski J, Gore JM, Goldberg RJ. Sex differences in 2-year mortality after hospital discharge for myocardial infarction. *Annals of Internal Medicine* 2001;**134**(3):173–81.

42. Vaccarino V. Ischemic heart disease in women: many questions, few facts. *Circulation. Cardiovascular Quality and Outcomes* 2010;**3**(2):111–15.

43. Daly C, Clemens F, Lopez Sendon JL et al. Gender differences in the management and clinical outcome of stable angina. *Circulation* 2006;**113**(4):490–98.

44. Akhter N, Milford-Beland S, Roe MT, Piana RN, Kao J, Shroff A. Gender differences among patients with acute coronary syndromes undergoing percutaneous coronary intervention in the American College of Cardiology – National Cardiovascular Data Registry (ACC-NCDR). *American Heart Journal* 2009;**157**(1):141–48.

45. Hendel RC. Myocardial infarction in women. *Cardiology* 1990;**77** (Suppl 2):41–57.

46. Dustan HP. Coronary artery disease in women. *Canadian Journal of Cardiology* 1990;**6** (Suppl B):19b–21b.

47. Bugiardini R. Women, "non-specific" chest pain, and normal or near-normal coronary angiograms are not synonymous with favourable

outcome. *European Heart Journal* 2006;**27**(12):1387–89.

48. Gulati M, Cooper-DeHoff RM, McClure C et al. Adverse cardiovascular outcomes in women with nonobstructive coronary artery disease: a report from the Women's Ischemia Syndrome Evaluation Study and the St James Women Take Heart Project. *Archives of Internal Medicine* 2009;**169**(9):843–50.

49. Shaw LJ, Min JK, Narula J et al. Sex differences in mortality associated with computed tomographic angiographic measurements of obstructive and nonobstructive coronary artery disease: an exploratory analysis. *Circulation. Cardiovascular Imaging* 2010;**3**(4):473–81.

50. Hemingway H, McCallum A, Shipley M, Manderbacka K, Martikainen P, Keskimaki I. Incidence and prognostic implications of stable angina pectoris among women and men. *Journal of the American Medical Association* 2006;**295**(12):1404–11.

51. Shaw LJ, Bairey Merz CN, Pepine CJ et al. Insights from the NHLBI-Sponsored Women's Ischemia Syndrome Evaluation (WISE) Study: Part I: gender differences in traditional and novel risk factors, symptom evaluation, and gender-optimized diagnostic strategies. *Journal of the American College of Cardiology* 2006;**47**(3 Suppl): s4–s20.

52. Bybee KA, Prasad A. Stress-related cardiomyopathy syndromes. *Circulation* 2008;**118**(4):397–409.

53. Bybee KA, Kara T, Prasad A et al. Systematic review: transient left ventricular apical ballooning: a syndrome that mimics ST-segment elevation myocardial infarction. *Annals of Internal Medicine* 2004;**141**(11):858–65.

54. Sharkey SW, Lesser JR, Zenovich AG et al. Acute and reversible cardiomyopathy provoked by stress in women from the United States. *Circulation* 2005;**111**(4):472–79.

55. Kurowski V, Kaiser A, von Hof K et al. Apical and midventricular transient left ventricular dysfunction syndrome (Tako-tsubo cardiomyopathy): frequency, mechanisms, and prognosis. *Chest* 2007;**132**(3):809–16.

56. Gianni M, Dentali F, Grandi AM, Sumner G, Hiralal R, Lonn E. Apical ballooning syndrome or Takotsubo cardiomyopathy: a systematic review. *European Heart Journal* 2006;**27**(13):1523–29.

57. Tsuchihashi K, Ueshima K, Uchida T et al. Transient left ventricular apical ballooning without coronary artery stenosis: a novel heart syndrome mimicking acute myocardial infarction. Angina Pectoris-Myocardial Infarction

Investigations in Japan. *Journal of the American College of Cardiology* 2001;**38**(1):11–18.

58. Prasad A. Apical ballooning syndrome: an important differential diagnosis of acute myocardial infarction. *Circulation* 2007;**115**(5):e56–e59.

59. Abe Y, Kondo M, Matsuoka R, Araki M, Dohyama K, Tanio H. Assessment of clinical features in transient left ventricular apical ballooning. *Journal of the American College of Cardiology* 2003;**41**(5):737–42.

60. Kneale BJ, Chowienczyk PJ, Brett SE, Coltart DJ, Ritter JM. Gender differences in sensitivity to adrenergic agonists of forearm resistance vasculature. *Journal of the American College of Cardiology* 2000;**36**(4):1233–38.

61. Mori H, Ishikawa S, Kojima S et al. Increased responsiveness of left ventricular apical myocardium to adrenergic stimuli. *Cardiovascular Research* 1993;**27**(2):192–98.

62. Donohue D, Movahed MR. Clinical characteristics, demographics and prognosis of transient left ventricular apical ballooning syndrome. *Heart Failure Reviews* 2005;**10**(4):311–16.

63. Elesber AA, Prasad A, Lennon RJ, Wright RS, Lerman A, Rihal CS. Four-year recurrence rate and prognosis of the apical ballooning syndrome. *Journal of the American College of Cardiology* 2007;**50**(5):448–52.

64. Leone F, Macchiusi A, Ricci R, Cerquetani E, Reynaud M. Acute myocardial infarction from spontaneous coronary artery dissection: a case report and review of the literature. *Cardiology in Review* 2004;**12**(1):3–9.

65. Tweet MS, Hayes SN, Pitta SR et al. Clinical features, management, and prognosis of spontaneous coronary artery dissection. *Circulation* 2012;**126**(5):579–88.

66. Alfonso F. Spontaneous coronary artery dissection: new insights from the tip of the iceberg? *Circulation* 2012;**126**(6):667–70.

67. Zupan I, Noc M, Trinkaus D, Popovic M. Double vessel extension of spontaneous left main coronary artery dissection in young women treated with thrombolytics. *Catheterization and Cardiovascular Interventions: Official Journal of the Society for Cardiac Angiography & Interventions* 2001;**52**(2):226–30.

68. Hugli O, Braun JE, Kim S, Pelletier AJ, Camargo CA, Jr. United States emergency department visits for acute decompensated heart failure, 1992 to 2001. *American Journal of Cardiology* 2005;**96**(11):1537–42.

69. Massie BM, Shah NB. Evolving trends in the epidemiologic factors of heart failure: rationale for

preventive strategies and comprehensive disease management. *American Heart Journal* 1997;**133**(6):703–12.

70. Redfield MM, Jacobsen SJ, Burnett JC, Jr., Mahoney DW, Bailey KR, Rodeheffer RJ. Burden of systolic and diastolic ventricular dysfunction in the community: appreciating the scope of the heart failure epidemic. *Journal of the American Medical Association* 2003;**289**(2):194–202.

71. Scantlebury DC, Borlaug BA. Why are women more likely than men to develop heart failure with preserved ejection fraction? *Current Opinion in Cardiology* 2011;**26**(6):562–68.

72. Heiat A, Gross CP, Krumholz HM. Representation of the elderly, women, and minorities in heart failure clinical trials. *Archives of Internal Medicine* 2002;**162**(15):1682–88.

73. Hsich EM, Pina IL. Heart failure in women: a need for prospective data. *Journal of the American College of Cardiology* 2009;**54**(6):491–98.

74. Ghali JK, Krause-Steinrauf HJ, Adams KF et al. Gender differences in advanced heart failure: insights from the BEST study. *Journal of the American College of Cardiology* 2003;**42**(12):2128–34.

75. Lee CS, Chien CV, Bidwell JT et al. Comorbidity profiles and inpatient outcomes during hospitalization for heart failure: an analysis of the U.S. nationwide inpatient sample. *BMC Cardiovascular Disorders* 2014;**14**:73.

76. Chung T, Sindone A, Foo F et al. Influence of history of heart failure on diagnostic performance and utility of B-type natriuretic peptide testing for acute dyspnea in the Emergency Department. *American Heart Journal* 2006;**152**(5):949–55.

77. Olivetti G, Giordano G, Corradi D et al. Gender differences and aging: effects on the human heart. *Journal of the American College of Cardiology* 1995;**26**(4):1068–79.

78. Shim CY, Park S, Choi D et al. Sex differences in central hemodynamics and their relationship to left ventricular diastolic function. *Journal of the American College of Cardiology* 2011;**57**(10):1226–33.

79. Mottram PM, Marwick TH. Assessment of diastolic function: what the general cardiologist needs to know. *Heart (British Cardiac Society)* 2005;**91**(5):681–95.

80. Piro M, Della Bona R, Abbate A, Biasucci LM, Crea F. Sex-related differences in myocardial remodeling. *Journal of the American College of Cardiology* 2010;**55**(11):1057–65.

81. Yarnoz MJ, Curtis AB. More reasons why men and women are not the same (gender differences in electrophysiology and arrhythmias). *American Journal of Cardiology* 2008;**101**(9):1291–96.

82. Braunwald E. Shattuck lecture – cardiovascular medicine at the turn of the millennium: triumphs, concerns, and opportunities. *New England Journal of Medicine* 1997;**337**(19):1360–69.

83. Go AS, Hylek EM, Phillips KA et al. Prevalence of diagnosed atrial fibrillation in adults: national implications for rhythm management and stroke prevention: the AnTicoagulation and Risk Factors in Atrial Fibrillation (ATRIA) Study. *Journal of the American Medical Association* 2001;**285**(18):2370–75.

84. Feinberg WM, Blackshear JL, Laupacis A, Kronmal R, Hart RG. Prevalence, age distribution, and gender of patients with atrial fibrillation. Analysis and implications. *Archives of Internal Medicine* 1995;**155**(5):469–73.

85. Benjamin EJ, Levy D, Vaziri SM, D'Agostino RB, Belanger AJ, Wolf PA. Independent risk factors for atrial fibrillation in a population-based cohort. The Framingham Heart Study. *Journal of the American Medical Association* 1994;**271**(11):840–44.

86. Dagres N, Nieuwlaat R, Vardas PE et al. Gender-related differences in presentation, treatment, and outcome of patients with atrial fibrillation in Europe: a report from the Euro Heart Survey on Atrial Fibrillation. *Journal of the American College of Cardiology* 2007;**49**(5):572–77.

87. Corley SD, Epstein AE, DiMarco JP et al. Relationships between sinus rhythm, treatment, and survival in the Atrial Fibrillation Follow-Up Investigation of Rhythm Management (AFFIRM) Study. *Circulation* 2004;**109**(12):1509–13.

88. Rienstra M, Van Veldhuisen DJ, Hagens VE et al. Gender-related differences in rhythm control treatment in persistent atrial fibrillation: data of the Rate Control Versus Electrical Cardioversion (RACE) study. *Journal of the American College of Cardiology* 2005;**46**(7):1298–1306.

89. Humphries KH, Kerr CR, Connolly SJ et al. New-onset atrial fibrillation: sex differences in presentation, treatment, and outcome. *Circulation* 2001;**103**(19):2365–70.

90. Poli D, Antonucci E, Grifoni E, Abbate R, Gensini GF, Prisco D. Gender differences in stroke risk of atrial fibrillation patients on oral anticoagulant treatment. *Thrombosis and Haemostasis* 2009;**101**(5):938–42.

91. Fang MC, Singer DE, Chang Y et al. Gender differences in the risk of ischemic stroke and peripheral embolism in atrial fibrillation: the

AnTicoagulation and Risk Factors in Atrial fibrillation (ATRIA) study. *Circulation* 2005;**112**(12):1687–91.

92. Elkayam U, Jalnapurkar S, Barakkat MN et al. Pregnancy-associated acute myocardial infarction: a review of contemporary experience in 150 cases between 2006 and 2011. *Circulation* 2014;**129**(16):1695–1702.

93. Sliwa K, Fett J, Elkayam U. Peripartum cardiomyopathy. *Lancet* 2006;**368**(9536):687–93.

94. Hilfiker-Kleiner D, Sliwa K, Drexler H. Peripartum cardiomyopathy: recent insights in its pathophysiology. *Trends in Cardiovascular Medicine* 2008;**18**(5):173–79.

95. Mielniczuk LM, Williams K, Davis DR et al. Frequency of peripartum cardiomyopathy. *American Journal of Cardiology* 2006;**97**(12):1765–68.

96. Brugger-Andersen T, Hetland O, Ponitz V, Grundt H, Nilsen DW. The effect of primary percutaneous coronary intervention as compared to tenecteplase on myeloperoxidase, pregnancy-associated plasma protein A, soluble fibrin and D-dimer in acute myocardial infarction. *Thrombosis Research* 2007;**119**(4):415–21.

Chapter 3

You've Come a Long Way, Baby: The Effects of Sex and Gender on Asthma, COPD, Smoking, and Smoking Cessation

Stacey Poznanski and Rita Cydulka

Opening Case

A 45-year-old female smoker presents to the Emergency Department with increased cough and wheezing for three days. She reports more copious sputum production that is unchanged in color from her baseline. She denies any fevers, chills, night sweats, or hemoptysis. At triage, her heart rate is 105, blood pressure is 125/85, respiratory rate is 21, O_2 saturation is 93% on room air, and temperature is 98.5 degrees Fahrenheit. Physical exam reveals no jugular venous distention, a tachycardic but regular rate, and a lung exam with diffuse tight wheezes. Pulses are symmetric and extremities have no clubbing, cyanosis, or edema. She has a history of asthma and uses an albuterol MDI and an inhaled corticosteroid daily. She has smoked 1.5 packs of cigarettes a day for the past 25 years and continues to smoke. This is her third "asthma attack" in two months.

Introduction

This chapter highlights the influence of sex and gender on three conditions: cigarette smoking as a form of tobacco abuse, asthma, and chronic obstructive pulmonary disease (COPD). This chapter addresses the role of sex and gender in the overall risk, natural history, presentation, diagnosis, acute management, clinical outcomes, and prevention for each of these disease processes, and it analyzes gaps in current knowledge and recommendations for future research.

Tobacco Abuse

Introduction

Tobacco abuse and the diseases associated with smoking have had a tremendous negative impact on the health of people in the United States and in every country of the world. The global economic costs of tobacco abuse including health care and lost workdays, and years of productive life are staggering. It is the leading cause of preventable morbidity and premature mortality in the United States. Smoking increases the risk of coronary artery disease, stroke, lung cancer, and COPD, accounting for one in five (443,000) deaths each year in the United States. According to World Health Organization (WHO) estimates, there are more than 1 billion smokers in the world with more than 15 billion cigarettes sold daily. The economic costs of smoking are astronomical. In 2004, tobacco abuse was estimated to cost the United States $193 billion, including $97 billion in lost productivity and $96 billion in direct health care expenditures (*Trends in Tobacco Use* 2011). Sex-specific data on economic impact are unfortunately lacking; however, sex-specific factors likely play a role in the morbidity and mortality suffered from tobacco-related illnesses. Tobacco use in and of itself is complex and is best understood with background knowledge of how gender and social norms shaped the patterns of use in this country (Bottorff et al. 2012).

Smoking in History

In the early 1900s, smoking was considered a male behavior; smoking by women, especially in public, challenged social convention and was interpreted as defiant and radical. However, for a new generation of women working hard to achieve equal rights socially, politically, and academically, the cigarette became a "symbol of emancipation, the temporary substitute for the ballot," as described by the *Atlantic Monthly* in 1916. Women demanded the public "privilege" of smoking and by the 1920s, cigarettes had become a "torch of freedom," associated with youth, independence, and the liberated, college-educated young woman in the workforce (Tanoue 2000).

The tobacco industry embraced this change in social mores and employed marketing campaigns specifically aimed at women. One of the more historically important was a campaign by Lucky Strikes that included testimonials of the beneficial dieting effects of smoking cigarettes by society women, actresses, and athletes: "Reach for a Lucky instead of a Sweet." With campaigns such as these, the cigarette was considered a glamorous status symbol of the American woman by the 1930s and 1940s, with women's smoking rates rising from approximately 6% in 1924 to 18.1% in 1935 (Tanoue 2000). Surprisingly, this mindset was so firmly inculcated by the media that it still can be seen among some women today.

Smoking prevalence peaked in the 1940s and 1950s for American men at approximately 67% (*Trends in Tobacco Use* 2011). The increase in prevalence among women peaked at approximately 44% around the time of the publication of the Surgeon General's Report on Smoking and Health in 1964 (*Trends in Tobacco Use* 2011). The report described cigarette smoking as a dose-related causal factor in lung cancer, as the basis for a 70% increase in age-specific death rates, as the most important cause of chronic bronchitis in the United States, and as the foundation for a higher death rate from coronary artery disease of males, as men were generally the subjects of most research at that time (Tanoue 2000; US Department of Health and Human Services 1964). Since this report, the rate of smoking has been declining for both sexes, although women's rates of smoking have been decreasing at a slower rate than men's rates.

The effects of cigarette smoking on women were underrepresented in the original Surgeon General's Report as the prevalence rates of women smoking were considerably lower than those of men (Tanoue 2000). In 1980, the Surgeon General's Report on the Health Consequences of Smoking for Women stated that women demonstrate the same dose-response relationship in the risk of developing lung cancer and COPD, with similar mortality rates, as men. Yet, the report also indicated that "the health consequences of the enhanced exposure to cigarette smoke among women are likely to be more prominent in the coming decades" (US Department of Health and Human Services 1980, Tanoue 2000). As predicted, the incidence of lung cancer in women increased at a steeper rate than in men (*Trends in Lung Cancer* 2014).

Clinical Manifestations

This gender-related trend in smoking rates has led to a shift in the sex-specific prevalence, morbidity, and mortality of tobacco-related illnesses, such as lung cancer and COPD (*Trends in Tobacco Use* 2011). Men and women who began smoking in the first half of the twentieth century have now reached the age at which insidious cigarette-related diseases are becoming clinically significant. Since 1950, lung cancer rates among women have increased by more than 500%, and lung cancer is the leading cause of cancer death in both men and women in the United States. Fortunately, the incidence and death rates for men have been steadily decreasing since the 1990s, likely secondary to the decline in cigarette use that began 50 years ago. Now, after several decades of increasing lung cancer mortality rates in women, these rates have finally plateaued (*Trends in Lung Cancer* 2014).

COPD mortality rates have followed similar trends. Historically, COPD was considered a disease of men, as evidenced by the classic drawings of the "blue bloater" and "pink puffer." More recently, the number of women with COPD has been rapidly increasing. For the past 10 years, the number of deaths from COPD has been higher in women than in men (Sorheim et al. 2010; Trends in COPD 2013). Women reached their current mortality rate from COPD faster when compared to men 20 to 30 years previously, suggesting that women may be more vulnerable to the effects of cigarette smoking than men (Tanoue 2000).

The difference in vulnerability to smoking-related illness between men and women is a matter of controversy. Some studies demonstrate an increased susceptibility to smoking in women with a greater decline in the forced expiratory volume in one second (FEV_1) in response to equal amounts of tobacco exposure, whereas other studies have suggested an opposite effect, an increase in men's susceptibility. Gan et al. published a systematic review and meta-analysis of longitudinal studies in 2006 examining decline in lung function and reported evidence of a faster decline in women smokers age >45–50 years compared to men who smoked (Gan et al. 2006; see also Sorheim et al. 2010). This discrepancy may be the result of sex differences in cigarette smoke metabolism (e.g., estrogen may affect the metabolism of various constituents of cigarette smoke through cytochrome P450 pathways) or may be reflective of the fact that each cigarette may represent a proportionally greater exposure in the anatomically smaller airways of women (Ben-Zaken Cohen et al. 2007; Han et al. 2007; Sorheim et al. 2010). Immunological and other hormonal determinants are additional biological explanations for this difference (Becklake & Kauffmann 1999; Sorheim et al. 2010; Kynyk et al. 2011).

Smoking Cessation

To mitigate the critical and costly impact that smoking has on health care, clinicians must intensify efforts to discourage smoking initiation and promote smoking cessation. Global data suggest that far fewer women than men use tobacco (10% vs. 48%, respectively); however, WHO reports that use among women is actually increasing in some countries and may double by the year 2025, historically mirroring the increased prevalence in the United States that occurred as women were "liberated" and became free to adopt men's social roles and habits. In the United States, the overall the rate of smoking for both sexes has continued to decline in the past 25 years, although men are quitting at a higher rate than women (World Health Organization 2010; *Trends in Tobacco Use* 2011; Bottorff et al. 2012)

The unrelenting attraction to smoking, and thus the inability to quit, is a complicated process and is not a reflection of pure physical dependence. Researchers must consider social changes and marketing campaigns from a historical perspective, taking into account the effect of gender, and the reasons women and men initiate smoking in the first place. Viewed with this broad and multifactorial lens, clinicians should not be surprised that there are sex differences in cessation rates and that these differences have been detectable for many years (Tanoue 2000; Piper et al. 2010).

In general, women have more difficulty quitting than men. Women often experience less

success than men on initial smoking cessation attempts, greater negative affective responses during withdrawal, and less successful cessation in relation to nicotine replacement therapy (Bottorff et al. 2012). This was reported in the 1980 Surgeon General's Report, which reviewed 39 studies on smoking cessation interventions, focusing on approaches that included education, physician advice, pharmacotherapy, psychotherapy, and behavioral modification (Tanoue 2000). The report concluded that "across all treatments, women have more difficulty giving up smoking than men, both at the end of treatment and at long-term points of measurement. No studies have been reported in which women do significantly better than men" (US Department of Health and Human Services 1980, p. 8411).

The Lung Health Study (LHS) was designed to evaluate the effects of smoking cessation and an inhaled bronchodilator on the annual rate of change of FEV_1 on participants who were required to enter a smoking cessation program. The LHS revealed that women had a higher rate of relapse to cigarette smoking, had histories of less frequent and shorter attempts at quitting, were more willing to use Nicorette® gum, and reported greater physical and emotional dependence on cigarettes. Although a higher level of education correlated with higher rates of sustained smoking cessation in both sexes, women with less than a high school education were significantly less likely to quit than men with equal educational background (Tanoue 2000).

Women are more likely to engage in cessation assistance programs and group treatments than men; however, lower expectations of their ability to be successful may affect attempts to quit (Tanoue 2000). There may be a link between phases of the menstrual cycle, the physiologic response to nicotine, and the presence of depressive symptoms. While more research is needed, the timing of the attempt to quit smoking in relation to the menstrual cycle may impact success, and consideration of this should influence how practitioners counsel their patients. (Allen et al. 2013). Research also indicates that women fail in situations involving negative emotions (e.g., conflict, financial stress), whereas men tend to fail in positive situations (e.g., social events). Finally, men – but not women – are more likely to be successful if they experience negative health events or experience pressure within social networks (e.g., spouse, family, friends) (Bottorff et al. 2012).

Fear of weight gain has been a barrier to cessation and a reason for relapse, especially for women (Bottorff et al. 2012). Women are more likely than men to acknowledge this concern as a negative influence on their motivation to quit. Their fears are valid, as several studies have shown that weight gain after smoking cessation is common. In the LHS study, despite efforts to minimize weight gain, which included monitoring participants' weight and providing nutritional counseling, weight gain after smoking cessation occurred in three-quarters of participants who quit smoking; a weight gain of 20% or more over baseline was reported in 7.6% of men and 19.1% of women. Although the health benefits of smoking cessation far outweigh the negative effects of weight gain, weight management should be incorporated in smoking cessation programs (Tanoue 2000; Bottorff et al. 2012).

Acute Management

The prevalence rate of smoking among patients treated in EDs in the United States tends to be higher than the general population; as high as 48% of ED patients in three US cities were current smokers, according to one prospective study (Lowenstein et al. 1998; Beaudoin et al. 2015). EDs are often the main source of medical care for patients who do not have health insurance or have limited access to medical services (Katz et al. 2012). While smoking cessation intervention has not historically been the purview of emergency medicine providers, the ED visit may be the ideal opportunity to provide interventions to this population. More than 79% of adult smokers in the ED are contemplating quitting or preparing to quit, indicating that most of these smokers are motivated to make a change. Research also demonstrates that these smokers are interested in receiving a cessation intervention during their visit, and when they do, patient satisfaction improves (Choo et al. 2012).

Bernstein and colleagues recommended that emergency physicians strongly advise their patients who use tobacco to quit and called for systems and practice policies to facilitate the delivery of smoking cessation counseling and pharmacotherapy (Table 3.1) (Bernstein et al. 2009). Although ED providers and administrators frequently balk at taking on this responsibility, citing the need to focus on acute care, the lack of an ongoing relationship with the patient, inadequate reimbursement, time pressures, and perceptions that counseling is ineffective, several studies report successful implementation of smoking cessation programs in the ED (Ersel et al. 2010; Katz et al. 2012). Katz et al. (2012) report success by integrating the cessation counseling into the role of ED nursing staff. Other studies report varying degrees of success using nonclinical personnel (Bock et al. 2008; Boudreaux et al. 2008; Neuner et al. 2009; Ersel et al. 2010).

An ED-based smoking cessation program requires good coordination, succinct yet personalized counseling that is gender sensitive and gender specific, trained ED personnel, and appropriately selected patients. Few resources are available to support providers wishing to address smoking in the ED. That is unfortunate as specific training on cessation counseling for providers can improve their confidence in being able to deliver the intervention. A pre-post study in eight EDs evaluated the effect of a one-hour didactic training session on use of the "ask–advise–refer" model coupled with quit-line referral cards; the study reported significant improvement in physicians' counseling and referral rates (Bernstein et al. 2009).

Given the differences between men and women in both the motivation to smoke and the ability to quit, studies have suggested that providing gender-sensitive interventions increases cessation rates. Several promising approaches to tobacco reduction and cessation interventions take into account gender influences. One such example is Smokefree Women, designed by the Tobacco Control Research Branch, Behavioral Research Program, Division of Cancer Control and Population Sciences of the National Cancer Institute. It is a comprehensive gender-specific and gender-sensitive program created specifically to help support the immediate and long-term needs of women who are trying to quit smoking. A free website (http://women.smokefree.gov) provides evidence-based information; professional assistance is provided to keep women connected, interested, involved, and motivated to quit (Bottorff et al. 2012). An example

Table 3.1 Cigarette-Smoking Treatment Options

Treatment	Example Regimen	Pearls
Pharmacotherapy		
Nicotine Replacement	*Patch* 5–10 cpd = 7–14 mg patch >10 cpd = 21 mg patch *Gum – 2 mg and 4 mg pieces* 1st cigarette >30 minutes after waking = 2 mg gum 1st cigarette <30 minutes after waking = 4 mg gum 1 piece every 2–4 hours *Others* Nasal spray, inhaler, lozenges	1 cigarette = 1 mg nicotine Providing multiple methods of nicotine replacement is more effective. Gums and sprays are absorbed rapidly and provide quick relief of withdrawal symptoms, while patches provide sustained release of nicotine. Multiple delivery systems safe and effective (patch + spray, patch + gum, synergistic with bupropion)
Bupropion SR 150	*Generic, Zyban, or Wellbutrin SR* Days 1–3: 150 mg each morning Days 4–end: 150 mg twice daily	Start 1–2 weeks before quit date; use 2–6 months Do not use if concurrently taking an MAOI or history of seizures or eating disorders
Varenicline	*Chantix* Days 1–3: 0.5 mg every morning Days 4–7: 0.5 mg twice daily Days 8–end: 1 mg twice daily	Start 1 week before quit date and use 3–6 months; alternatively begin medication then quit between days 8 and 35. Caution in patients with renal impairment, dialysis, or serious psychiatric illness
Counseling		
Group or Individual	*Professional Therapy Sessions* Check local resources *Online Support* Families Controlling & Eliminating Tobacco (FACET) http://facet.ubc.ca Smokefree Women http://women.smokefree.gov *Telephone (Quitline)* 1-800-QUIT-NOW	Cessation treatment comes in two forms: medication and counseling Smokers commonly need some combination of the two Providing gender-sensitive and gender-specific treatment interventions may increase cessation rates

Abbreviations: cpd = cigarettes per day; MAOI = monoamine oxidase inhibitor
Adapted from http://www.ctri.wisc.edu/HC.Providers/healthcare_FDA_Meds.htm
Clinical Practice Guideline 2008 Update: Treating Tobacco Use & Dependence, US Public Health Service, www.ctri.wisc.edu/HC.Providers/healthcare_CPGuideline.htm
New England Journal of Medicine 365:1222–1231 September 29, 2011, *www.ctri.wisc.edu/nejm*

of a gender-specific booklet targeting men is entitled *The Right Time, the Right Reasons: Dads Talk About Reducing and Quitting Smoking* (available at www.facet.ubc.ca). Rather than a "how to quit" guide, men are encouraged to consider the advantages to being a dad who does not smoke and are encouraged to be autonomous decision makers (Bottorff et al. 2012).

Prevention

In contrast to adults, cigarette-smoking rates among adolescents have been rising. In half of the 151 countries surveyed by WHO, equal numbers of boys and girls smoke (World Health Organization 2010). The cigarette, which served as a symbol of liberation and empowerment for women in the early 1900s, continues to be a symbol of independence for adolescents today, a display of their maturity, at once embracing and rejecting the adult world. Tobacco control strategies must recognize that decisions to start using tobacco are influenced by cultural, psychosocial, and socioeconomic factors, which are often different between the sexes.

Sociodemographic factors also affect smoking rates; lack of intent to pursue a college degree, low parental educational attainment, high school dropout status, and single-parent household all correlate with an increased risk for initiating smoking. For women, issues surrounding weight control also may play a role in smoking initiation, and girls who smoke may be vying for an appearance of self-confidence. Though counseling should occur for all adolescents, specific counseling could and should be provided to these high-risk groups (Tanoue 2000).

Conclusions

The relationship between gender, smoking, and lung function is complicated (Sorheim et al. 2010). Tobacco use is now the single leading preventable cause of death in the United States. Intensive public health efforts since the original Surgeon General's Report in 1964 have resulted in a declining prevalence of cigarette smoking in adults. Despite this, more than 20% of all Americans still smoke and, disturbingly, the prevalence of cigarette smoking among adolescents is rising. This trend portends another generation at high risk for cigarette-related disease (Tanoue 2000).

With the increasing incidence of lung cancer and COPD among women in this country, it is clear that public health efforts must target tobacco abuse by women. We need effective programs that prevent the initiation of smoking and target smoking cessation that are tailored specifically for men and for women (Tanoue 2000).

Asthma

Introduction

Asthma is a common serious disease that is increasing in prevalence, affecting an estimated 39.5 million Americans and more than 300 million people worldwide. In 2010 in the United States, there were 10.6 million physician office visits, 1.2 million hospital outpatient department visits, and 2.1 million Emergency Department visits because of asthma. In 2011, females were about 14% more likely than males to ever have been diagnosed with asthma, a trend that is consistent with respect to overall prevalence; however, there is variation by age. (*Trends in Asthma* 2012).

From 2002 to 2007, the annual economic cost of asthma in the United States was $56 billion; direct health care costs consisted of $50.1 billion with indirect costs (lost productivity) contributing an additional $5.9 billion. Since 1999, mortality and hospitalizations due to asthma have decreased; however, the prevalence of asthma in the United States, which had not changed since 2001, now appears to be increasing. In 2009, 3,388 people died of asthma. Approximately 64% were women, with a female age-adjusted death rate 50% greater than the rate seen in men (*Trends in Asthma* 2012). Recent research has revealed substantial differences between men and women in prevalence, morbidity, and health care utilization, although the underlying mechanisms have yet to be determined (Kynyk et al. 2011). In general, women consistently have higher rates of clinic visits, hospital admissions, and hospital readmissions for asthma compared to men (Clark et al. 2007).

Gender Risk

Studies consistently demonstrate that asthma prevalence rates by gender change with age. Prior to puberty, asthma prevalence is 16% greater in boys; in adulthood, prevalence is 62% greater in women, according to the most recent National Health Interview Survey (Kynyk et al. 2011). See Figure 3.1. After menopause, the prevalence in women begins to decrease (Kynyk et al. 2011; *Trends in Asthma* 2012; McCallister et al. 2013; Lin et al. 2013). These findings bring to light an interesting pattern: Asthma prevalence and severity appear to mirror transitions in the reproductive cycle of women. This phenomenon is further supported by the greater prevalence of asthma in women with early menarche, and by a peri-menstrual worsening of symptoms reported by 30% to 40% of asthmatic women. This suggests, and many researchers believe, that sex hormones play a role in asthma, although the exact mechanism has not yet been

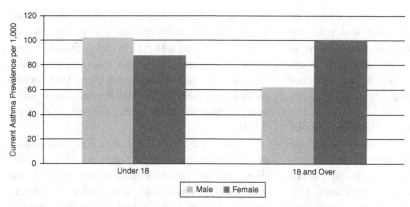

Figure 3.1 Asthma – current prevalence rate per 1,000 by sex and age, 2011
From *Trends in Asthma Morbidity & Mortality* 2012.

determined (Melgert & Postma 2009; Kynyk et al. 2011).

In general, studies on the role of sex hormones in asthma have been inconclusive. Theories include sex-related differences in immune cells, estrogen's involvement in signaling pathways directly related to organ function, and differing phenotypic expressions (Lin et al. 2013). Alternatively, testosterone may have a role in the relaxation of airway smooth muscle, or dehydroepiandrosterone (DHEA) may provide anti-inflammatory and immune-modulatory activity. This provides a possible explanation to the marked decrease in bronchial responsiveness observed in boys, but not in girls, older than age 11 in one study of a cohort of children with asthma (Melgert et al. 2007; Tantisira et al. 2008; Leynaert et al. 2012).

Asthma in pregnancy provides another layer of complication with regard to the role of sex hormones in this disease process. Asthma complicates approximately 4% of pregnancies, and data indicate that the course of asthma during pregnancy improves in one-third, worsens in one-third, and remains unchanged in one-third of asthmatic women (Cydulka 2006; Cydulka 2011). Asthma symptoms and exacerbations tend to peak during the second trimester. As many as 42% of pregnant asthmatics require hospitalization and an additional 11% to 18% have one or more visits to the ED for an asthma exacerbation (Cydulka 2006).

Research on how oral contraceptive pills mitigate the symptoms and prevalence of asthma has produced conflicting results. As reviewed by

Kynyk et al. 2011, two large prospective studies demonstrated that post-menopausal hormone replacement therapy was associated with an increased rate of newly diagnosed asthma (Troisi et al. 1995; Barr et al. 2004). In addition, postmenopausal women who do use hormone replacement therapy do not demonstrate the same postmenopausal decline in asthma prevalence as women who do not use hormone replacement therapy, further supporting the connection between asthma and a hormonal influence (Troisi et al. 1995; Barr et al. 2004; Melgert & Postma 2009).

Not only does asthma trend with the reproductive cycle, it is more common and more severe in women. Eight million women reported an asthma attack in 2011 compared to 5.1 million men, and the difference between men and women in the prevalence rates of asthma attacks has been significant each year since 1999 (*Trends in Asthma* 2012). The European Network for Understanding Mechanisms of Severe Asthma (ENFUMOSA) found that patients with severe asthma were more likely to be female, obese, and non-atopic (ENFUMOSA Study Group 2003; Lin et al. 2013).

Natural History

Asthma is generally a chronic illness with reversible exacerbations and a relatively good prognosis (Celli 2000). However, despite appropriate monitoring and treatment, asthma can lead to airway remodeling, a permanent decrease in lung function, and an increase in mortality (Fabbri et al. 1998; Lange et al. 1998). Gender-related issues and genetic, allergic, infectious, environmental, socioeconomic, and psychosocial factors contribute to the course of each individual's disease progression (Adams & Cydulka 2003).

Overall, mortality from asthma is an unlikely occurrence. The death rate per 1,000 persons with asthma declined from 2001 to 2009 and was 0.15 for the period from 2007 to 2009. Asthma death rates per 1,000 persons with asthma were more than 30% higher for women than for men from 2007 to 2009 (Akinbami et al. 2011); however, these rates do not adjust for women having a higher prevalence of asthma as adults and a higher death rate as adults when compared to children. As a result of these factors, data on the difference in mortality rates between men and women are conflicting and difficult to distinguish from purely age-related effects. While several studies report a higher mortality percentage in women compared with men, other data present a higher mortality in men younger than age 35, possibly resulting from the gender-based differences in symptom perception and reporting, as discussed in the next section. If men report severe symptoms less frequently, they may be treated less aggressively and suffer higher mortality (Kynyk et al. 2011).

Clinical Manifestations

Asthma is characterized by airway inflammation causing episodes of reversible airflow obstruction, variable degrees of wheezing, dyspnea, chest tightness, cough, and an increase in airway responsiveness to different stimuli (Celli 2000). The patient's ability to detect a change in airflow depends on his or her perception of those changes. Poor perceivers may not be able to recognize symptoms and identify deteriorating air flow. The literature suggests that women and men perceive and/or experience asthma symptoms differently (Cydulka et al. 2001; Kynyk et al. 2011).

Men tend to underrepresent their symptoms (Kynyk et al. 2011) and may have poorer perception of their disease severity than women (McCallister et al. 2013). In a study published in *Annals of Emergency Medicine* in 2001, men presenting to the ED tended to report less frequent and less distressful symptoms and less severe activity limitations than women, despite

a clinically similar but statistically worse airflow obstruction (Cydulka et al. 2001). Other authors have reported similar findings (Vollmer et al. 1993; Boezen et al. 1995; Osborne et al. 1998). Men's tendency to underrepresent the severity of their symptoms must be considered when men present to the ED with asthma.

Women perceive that they have a more difficult time controlling their asthma than men (Melgert & Postma 2009). They describe more frequent and more severe symptoms and a worse impact on their quality of life, despite using similar maintenance medications and having similar or better pulmonary function when compared to men (McCallister et al. 2013). In addition, they have a higher number of unscheduled physician visits, more frequent use of oral corticosteroids and rescue beta agonist inhalers, are 50% more likely to report continued symptoms after discharge (Kynyk et al. 2011), and have greater health care utilization than men (Osborne et al. 1998; Lee et al. 2006; Sinclair & Tolsma 2006; McCallister et al. 2013). Alternatively, men may report fewer symptoms because they find their symptoms less concerning or they practice denial (Cydulka et al. 2001). Many studies demonstrate an association between psychiatric disorders and asthma, specifically anxiety and depressive disorders; it is unclear whether these disorders precede or devolve from the asthma. In all likelihood, these comorbidities further contribute to the patient's perception of poorer quality of life.

Although researchers have not yet elucidated the underlying etiology for these sex-related variances in asthma morbidity and disease expression, potential hypotheses leading to the differences in perception of airflow obstruction probably result from the increased bronchial responsiveness seen in women (Paoletti et al. 1995; Leynaert et al. 1997; Osborne et al. 1998; Weiner et al. 2002; McCallister et al. 2013). Inspiratory muscle strength is significantly greater in men with asthma than in women and is inversely related to dyspnea (Weiner et al. 2002). Healthy female nonsmoking women demonstrate a lower cough reflex threshold associated with a greater urge to cough and a greater sense of dyspnea when compared to males (Gui 2010; McCallister et al. 2013). Increased susceptibility to cigarette smoke may also play a role in the increased prevalence of bronchial hyperresponsiveness seen in women, a phenomenon that has been demonstrated even in children (Leynaert et al. 1997). Exact mechanisms of the differences in symptom perception, psychosocial associations, airway responsiveness, and tobacco smoke susceptibility are unknown and warrant further research (Kynyk et al. 2011).

Diagnosis

The same diagnostic approach is used for asthmatic men and women. However, when taking a history from women with asthma, additional questioning should focus on changes in reproductive health to identify any sex-related triggers, such as timing of exacerbations with the menstrual cycle, use of oral contraceptives, or initiation of hormone replacement therapy. Other cultural or gender-related triggers may include symptoms related to housework or exposures through childcare. This additional information may assist in developing individualized strategies to improve control (Kynyk et al. 2011).

The hallmark presentation of asthma includes a medical history of episodic symptoms of cough, chest tightness, and dyspnea, with a physical examination that may reveal wheezes (Celli 2000). Although the physical exam can prove useful for eliminating other etiologies in the differential diagnosis, physical exam findings and vital signs are unfortunately often unreliable predictors of the degree of airway obstruction. Surprisingly, the many asthma scoring systems that have been developed to assist in triage and management have not performed better than good clinical judgment. Thus, clinical evaluation and diagnosis must truly depend on a quality history and pulmonary function testing (Adams & Cydulka 2003).

For the reasons mentioned, as well as the differences in symptom reporting between men and women, it is often difficult to assess the severity or predict the course of an asthma exacerbation at the bedside in the ED based purely on clinical assessment; consequently, the literature reports a 7% to 15% relapse rate after ED discharge, with no reported differences in relation to gender (Arnold et al. 2007). Spirometry is not available in most EDs, and patients experiencing clinically significant airflow obstruction are frequently unable to perform effective and accurate forced airway maneuvers (Arnold et al. 2007; Schneider et al. 2011). However, Piovesan et al. (2006) reported in their small prospective cohort study that measuring peak expiratory flow rate (PEFR) after 15 minutes of management in the emergency room may be a useful tool for predicting outcomes in cases of acute asthma. A PEFR $\geq$ 40% after 15 minutes of treatment showed significant power in predicting a favorable outcome (sensitivity = 0.74, specificity = 1.00, and positive predictive value = 1.00). A PEFR <30% after 15 minutes of treatment was predictive of a poor outcome (sensitivity = 0.54, specificity = 0.93, and positive predictive value = 0.87). The Expert Panel Report on Guidelines for the Diagnosis and Management of Asthma considers an exacerbation severe when FEV_1 or PEFR is <40% predicted and recommends that >70% predicted FEV_1 or PEFR is a goal for discharge from the emergency care setting (Busse et al. 2007). It is interesting that studies have suggested a gender difference in the use of peak flow meters; men learned the correct technique for using a peak flow meter and attained their best peak expiratory flow more quickly than women (Chafin et al. 2001; Self et al. 2005) This is important to note during the time-sensitive environment of the ED, as results may be affected and women may need additional instruction.

If objective measures are not used to assess the level of obstruction, patients, especially men, may be undertreated for severe obstruction. On the other hand, asthmatic women with a degree of air flow obstruction equal to men may perceive their symptoms as more severe, so objective measurements cannot be the sole factor directing disposition decisions. Some patients with asthma develop progressive airflow obstruction that may become irreversible and difficult to differentiate from COPD (Celli 2000). It is clinically essential to refer patients in the ED with a diagnosis of asthma that continues to worsen or is becoming less responsive to therapy for formal spirometry and further diagnostic testing to rule out underlying COPD. Women are more likely than men to be diagnosed with asthma than COPD. Without the use of formal diagnostic testing, this gender-based diagnostic bias could have important long-term treatment and outcome implications (Chapman 2001; Sorheim et al. 2010).

Acute Management

When evaluating a patient with asthma in the ED, stabilize the patient according to clinical guidelines, determine the precipitating factor for the current exacerbation if possible, and provide appropriate education and close follow-up if a discharge disposition is deemed appropriate.

Keep in mind that some asthmatics with significant airway obstruction tend to underestimate their symptoms. They may present with severe obstruction and little perception of any clinical change (Kikuchi et al. 1994). The mechanism for this is unclear and is an opportunity for sex-specific research. The FEV_1 and PEFR directly measure the degree of large airway obstruction. Sequential measurements can help assess severity and determine response to therapy. Knowledge of the patient's baseline PEFR can help determine the severity of the current exacerbation in relation to the patient's personal history, which may be the only clue to worsening asthma (Adams & Cydulka 2003).

The acceptance of inflammation as the primary mechanism for disease progression has resulted in the development of several effective pharmacotherapeutic agents capable of improving the overall outcome of men and women with asthma. Treatment of an acute exacerbation in the ED should correct tissue oxygenation, alleviate any reversible bronchospasm, remove underlying trigger(s), and respond to complications. Treatment in the ED may include the use of oxygen, adrenergic agents, anticholinergics, corticosteroids, and magnesium; for severe exacerbations, assisted ventilation may be needed. Table 3.2 provides a summary of the most current recommendations for management of acute exacerbations in the ED.

Once a patient's stabilization has begun, the provider should search for possible triggers. Recognized triggers of asthma include tobacco smoke, air pollution, occupational exposures, gastroesophageal reflux disease, exercise, medications (nonsteroidal anti-inflammatory drugs, aspirin, beta-blockers), viral upper respiratory infections, and hormone-related influences (Adams & Cydulka 2003). If triggers are identified, a plan should be made to limit the patient's exposure to those triggers. It is important to realize, though, that removing a susceptible individual from the offending environment may not totally reverse the symptomatology and altered pulmonary function, especially in asthma that is a so-called nonallergic type (Celli 2000).

While formal spirometry may not be feasible during the ED visit, expert consensus recommends that spirometric testing be completed as soon as possible, after treatment is initiated and symptoms have stabilized, and at least every one to two years after that initial evaluation. The measurement of PEFRs on a more regular basis is practical and is recommended for monitoring the patient who has received a diagnosis of moderate to severe asthma. Data from studies in which PEFR monitoring was one component of a comprehensive treatment program indicate favorable outcomes (Ignacio-Garcia & Gonzalez-Santos 1995). Providing a referral for spirometric testing and patient education about the importance of measuring peak flow rates is key to quality discharge planning from the ED and appropriate ongoing management aimed at decreasing relapse and re-hospitalization (Celli 2000).

Unfortunately, current asthma guidelines lack information about whether sex-specific approaches to asthma assessment or pharmacologic treatment should be considered (Celli 2000; Busse et al. 2007; Kynyk et al. 2011; McCallister et al. 2013). The potential of gender-specific guidelines demands future research, as gender-specific treatment approaches to asthma care have been developed and have shown benefit. Clark et al. (2007) conducted a randomized clinical trial of a self-regulation, telephone counseling intervention that emphasized women's concerns and sex and gender role factors in their management of asthma. A nurse health educator provided the intervention and the participants were educated on a self-regulatory, problem-solving process as well as sex and gender role–related problems in asthma, such as menstrual cycle, premenstrual symptoms, birth control pills, estrogen replacement therapy, and environmental exposures (e.g., cleaning products). Compared to control subjects, the women receiving the intervention had greater annual reductions in the average number of nights with asthma symptoms ($p = 0.04$), days of missed work/school ($p = 0.03$), emergency department visits ($p = 0.04$), unscheduled office visits ($p = 0.01$), and scheduled office visits ($p = 0.04$). They had greater recognition

Table 3.2 Asthma Exacerbation Treatment Options

Treatment	Example Regimen	Pearls
Short Acting B₂ Agonists (SABAs)		
Inhaled	*Albuterol Nebulizer Solution* 2.5–5 mg every 20 min for 3 doses, then 2.5–10 mg every 1–4 h, as needed, or 10–15 mg/h as continuous nebulization *Metered Dose Inhaler* 4–8 puffs every 20 min up to 4 h, then every 1–4 h as needed.	For optimal delivery, dilute aerosols to minimum of 3 mL at gas flow of 6–8 L/min. Use large-volume nebulizers for continuous administration. May mix with ipratropium nebulizer solution. In mild-to-moderate exacerbations, MDI plus valved holding chamber is as effective as nebulized therapy with appropriate administration technique and coaching by trained personnel.
Systemic	*Epinephrine* 1:1000 0.3–0.5 mg every 20 min for 3 doses SC *Terbutaline* 0.25 mg every 20 min for 3 doses SC	No proven advantage of systemic therapy over aerosol.
Anticholinergics		
In combination with SABA	*Ipratropium Bromide* 0.5 mg every 20 min for 3 doses, then as needed	Should not be used as first-line therapy; should be added to SABA therapy for severe exacerbations. The addition of ipratropium has not been shown to provide further benefit once the patient is hospitalized.
Systemic Corticosteroids		
Oral	*Prednisone* For inpatients: oral "burst," use 40–80 mg/d in 1 or 2 divided doses until PEF reaches 70% of predicted or personal best. For outpatients: oral "burst," use 40–60 mg in 1 or 2 divided doses for 5–10 d. *Prednisolone* 1–2 mg/kg/d for 5–10 d; may be divided twice daily.	No known advantage for higher doses of corticosteroids in severe asthma exacerbations. Inhaled corticosteroids can be started at any point in the treatment of an asthma exacerbation. Used in children due to increased palatably of available liquid formulations.
Systemic	*Methylprednisolone* IV: 1 mg/kg every 4–6 h.	Use IV therapy only when oral intake, GI transit time, or GI absorption is impaired.
Supplements in Severe Exacerbations (FEV₁ <25% predicted)		
Magnesium	1 to 2 grams IV over 30 minutes	Bronchodilating properties may be helpful in severe exacerbations. Should not be substituted for standard therapy regimens.
Heliox	Mixture of 80% helium and 20% oxygen	Insufficient data on whether this can avert tracheal intubation, change intensive care and hospital admission rates and duration, or mortality

Abbreviations: min = minutes, h = hour; d = day; PEF = peak expiratory flow
Adapted with permission from Cydulka 2011, p. 508; National Asthma Education and Prevention Program, Expert Panel Report 3: *Guidelines for the Diagnosis and Management of Asthma.* Publication No. 08-4051. Bethesda, MD, National Institutes of Health, 2007. Available at www.nhlbi.nih.gov/guidelines/asthma/asthgdln.pdf. Accessed March 30, 2014.

of asthma symptoms during the menstrual cycle (p = 0.0003) and greater improvement in quality of life (p = 0.0005), self-regulation (p = 0.03), and self-confidence to manage asthma (p = 0.001). At the two-year follow-up study, no significant health care use differences were evident; however, participants maintained improved health status and improved quality of life (Clark et al. 2010).

Prevention

While there is no known method of preventing the development of asthma or curing it, methods of controlling and preventing exacerbations are well established in evidence-based clinical guidelines (Akinbami et al. 2011). Increased exacerbation prevention efforts can have significant impacts on outcomes and cost. Referral to spirometry for patients with concerning respiratory symptoms or those at risk for the development of asthma and/or COPD could help detect cases at an early stage when intervention may prevent further deterioration (Celli 2000). Smoking cessation counseling is crucial for anyone with obstructive lung disease, as discussed earlier in the chapter. The use of sex-specific asthma education may result in improved outcomes, improved use of peak flow meters, reduction in use of short-acting beta-agonists, improved quality of life, and increased self-confidence in asthma management when compared to "unisex" guideline based care alone (Kynyk et al. 2011).

Obesity also appears to be a potential major risk factor for asthma development in women. Some studies suggest that obesity is a risk factor for asthma in women but not in men (e.g., Melgert et al. 2007). Obesity has been found to be more strongly associated with non-allergic asthma, also more common in women (Appleton et al. 2006). Although obesity alone seems unlikely to explain the higher risk of asthma in women, regulatory molecules secreted by the adipose tissues (such as leptin) might be involved in the sex differences in asthma (Melgert et al. 2007; Leynaert et al. 2012). Regardless of the mechanism, education about weight loss is prudent.

Clinical Outcomes

Sex differences exist that may affect overall clinical outcomes, specifically resource utilization and morbidity. It is not clear whether disparities in asthma management between men and women currently contribute significantly to these disparities in outcome, thus highlighting further questions about mechanisms (Kynyk et al. 2011). Women adhere more closely to management guidelines and are more likely to use peak flow meters regularly, to follow a written action plan, and to have a primary physician with regularly scheduled clinic visits (Kynyk et al. 2011). Despite these choices, women are more frequently hospitalized for asthma exacerbations in spite of having better pulmonary function, less hypoxia, less hypercapnia, similar maintenance medication regimens, and similar ED treatment when compared to their male counterparts (Cydulka et al. 2001; Kynyk et al. 2011). Hospitalization usage like prevalence rates mirrors transitions in reproductive life: Patients younger than age 15 admitted with asthma are twice as likely to be male whereas asthmatics older than age 15 who are admitted are three times more likely to be female. Lin et al. (2013) demonstrated that the disparity between female and male asthma hospitalization rates in adults appears to peak in the fifth and sixth decades of life, independent of many known comorbidities, including smoking and obesity. While the difference in prevalence certainly plays a role in the difference in hospitalization rates, additional factors such as differences in the perception of airflow obstruction and dyspnea may also contribute (Kynyk et al. 2011). Data on length of hospital stay are conflicting, although at this point African American women appear to have longer lengths of stays and more frequent ICU admissions.

Conclusion

Asthma is more prevalent in women and follows a pattern that appears to be influenced by sex hormones. Differences in symptom manifestation and reporting are likely multifactorial with both sex and gender influences. Treatment should continue to be guideline-based with attention to identifying aspects or triggers of the disease that may be sex or gender specific (Kynyk et al. 2011). Education about symptom perception and reporting as well as links to the reproductive cycle may provide huge benefits to both patients and providers in the diagnosis and acute and chronic management of asthma.

Chronic Obstructive Pulmonary Disease

Introduction

Chronic obstructive pulmonary disease (COPD) is projected to become the fourth leading cause of death worldwide by the year 2030 (GOLD 2014). In the United States, COPD is now the third leading cause of death, and the only one that continues to increase in prevalence. Acute exacerbations of COPD in the United States account for more than 1.5 million ED visits annually and more than 125,000 deaths (Mannino et al. 2002; Brulotte & Lang 2012). As reported by the National Heart Lung and Blood Institute, the national projected annual cost for COPD in 2010 was $49.9 billion, including $29.5 billion in direct health care expenditures, $8 billion in indirect morbidity costs, and $12.4 billion in indirect mortality costs (*Trends in COPD* 2013). While COPD was historically considered a disease of men, this is no longer the case. In recent years, that gender disparity has reversed, with women surpassing men in the prevalence, hospitalization rates, and mortality from COPD (Brulotte & Lang 2012).

Gender Risk

From 1980 to 2000, COPD mortality rates tripled for women in the United States. By the year 2000, for the first time, more women than men died from COPD (Figure 3.2). Unfortunately, the trend has continued, reflecting the morbid outcome set in motion years before as the prevalence of women smoking began to increase (Han et al. 2007; Kamil et al. 2013; Mannino et al. 2002). Globally, the prevalence of smoking in men still far exceeds that of women, as does the mortality rates from COPD; nevertheless, both of these numbers are rising in parallel as they are ineluctably linked. Among women, the annual number of deaths increased 11% from 2000 to 2005, compared to 5% in men (Brown et al. 2008). The rising rates of smoking in the United States undoubtedly play a major role in the increasing morbidity and mortality from COPD among women. There are likely several underlying causes for the new prominence of COPD in women, including a difference in susceptibility and expression of the COPD disease process itself and increased susceptibility to the negative effects of tobacco smoke compared to men (Kamil et al. 2013). In addition, women in developing countries who cook in poorly ventilated homes and have exposure to noxious gases have a disturbing prevalence of COPD unrelated to smoking (Brulotte & Lang 2012; GOLD 2014).

Exposure to noxious particulate gas is the greatest risk factor for the development of COPD: Tobacco smoke is the particulate and etiologic agent most commonly implicated in developed countries (Brulotte & Lang 2012). At a particular level of tobacco exposure, women appear to be at greater risk of lung function impairment than men. Gan et al. (2006) performed a systematic review and meta-analysis of studies examining the longitudinal loss of lung function, concluding that current women smokers had a significantly faster

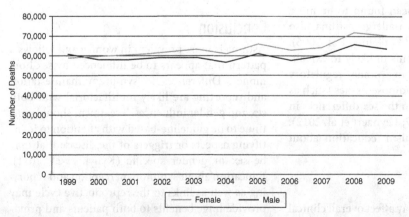

Figure 3.2 COPD – Number of deaths by sex, 1999–2009
From *Trends in COPD: Morbidity & Mortality* 2013.

annual decline in FEV_1 percentage predicted than their male counterparts who smoked equivalently (see also Han et al. 2007; Kamil et al. 2013). A study of 84 families with early-onset COPD not only revealed a high prevalence of affected women (71.4%), it also demonstrated that female first-degree relatives who had a history of smoking had significantly greater bronchodilator responsiveness and greater risk of reduced FEV_1 than male first-degree relatives. These differences were only seen among current or ex-smokers, implying a genetic predisposition to smoking-related lung damage that is sex specific (Silverman et al. 2000; Han et al. 2007). This increased risk is seen even in children with respect to lung development. Gold and colleagues (1996) found that girls in the United States ages 10–18 who smoked at least five cigarettes per day had 1.09% slower growth in FEV_1 per year compared to never-smokers. This value was only 0.20% in age-matched boys (see also Camp et al. 2009).

Women also appear to have an increased susceptibility to the development of COPD. There is an interaction between sex and gender, and many of the known risk factors for COPD, such as genetics, inhalational exposure, lung growth and development, oxidative stress, infections, socioeconomic status, nutrition, and asthma, although exact mechanisms of influence remain undetermined (GOLD 2014; Ohar et al. 2011). Even in health, women have a relatively reduced maximum ventilatory reserve when compared with age-matched men, reflecting natural anatomic differences in the size of the lungs, airways, and respiratory musculature. In men, relatively less effort needs to be expended to drive ventilation during exercise, given men's naturally larger lungs and stronger respiratory muscles. This likely also plays a role in the increased sensation of breathlessness experienced by women (Camp et al. 2009), as well as a dose-dependent effect of tobacco smoke. Women receive a proportionately greater exposure to dangerous inhaled particulate matter from a single cigarette because of their anatomically smaller airways (Han et al. 2007). Furthermore, researchers have theorized that sex hormones impact lung growth and maturation, airway hyperresponsiveness, detoxification of tobacco smoke, and the manifestation of chronic lung diseases, in a manner similar to the pubertal

change in asthma prevalence discussed in the "Asthma" section (Townsend et al. 2012). Menopause has been cited as an important cause of lung function decline and accelerated alveolar loss; studies have demonstrated that women using hormone replacement therapy have had less inflammation and decline with increase in forced vital capacity and FEV_1 (e.g., Kamil et al. 2013).

Natural History

COPD is an umbrella term that is used to describe a heterogeneous group of progressive chronic respiratory diseases consisting of mucous production (obstructive) and parenchymal destruction (emphysema), the relative contributions of which vary from person to person. *Emphysema* is the destruction of the gas exchange surfaces of the lungs, and *chronic bronchitis* is the clinical presence of cough and sputum production for at least three months of two consecutive years. These terms are not part of the current definition of the Global Initiative for Chronic Obstructive Lung Disease (GOLD), as their clinical utility is often limited. Rather, the GOLD definition stresses flexibility, acknowledging that most patients have a combination of different diseases: chronic bronchitis, emphysema, bronchiectasis, and, to a lesser extent, asthma (Brulotte & Lang 2012; GOLD 2014; Bates & Cydulka 2011). As stated by Brulotte and Lang (2012, 223–24).

The GOLD consensus definition for COPD consists of three key points:

> 1. The pulmonary component of COPD is characterized by a limitation in airflow that is not fully reversible. It is usually progressive and is associated with an abnormal inflammatory response of the lung to noxious particles or gases. 2. COPD has significant extra-pulmonary effects that contribute to disease severity. 3. COPD is common and often preventable and treatable.

The evolution of COPD can be insidious and clinically undetectable for decades. Objectively, progression can be measured by small changes in peripheral airway resistance or lung compliance. Over time, irritants such as tobacco smoke and air pollution trigger an increase in inflammatory cells in the airways, lung interstitium, and alveoli, which in turn leads to a slow destruction of the lung parenchyma and an increase in mucus secretion. Ultimately, loss of elastic recoil and narrowing of the smaller airways occur, resulting in clinically significant dyspnea, hypersecretion, bronchospasm, and bronchoconstriction with decreased total minute ventilation, increased respiratory work, and progressive hypoxia and hypercapnia. Continued destruction, especially in emphysematous-dominant types, leads to alveolar hypoventilation and ventilatory-perfusion mismatch with a resulting increase in pulmonary hypertension, right ventricular hypertrophy, and ultimately right heart failure as the disease worsens in severity. The progression of pathology and symptoms is evident in the GOLD classification of COPD by severity (Table 3.3) (Bates & Cydulka 2011).

Increasing evidence supports these phenotypic expressions of COPD and suggests that this divergence may be the result of underlying gender- and sex-based variations in pulmonary structure and function. Women with COPD tend to have thicker airway walls and more airway disease, while men have more emphysematous destructive changes. These distinctions may have important therapeutic implications. For instance, the increased responsiveness of women's immune systems may be a factor in the development of thicker bronchiole walls and smaller airway lumens in response to the chronic inflammatory process and progressive infiltration of inflammatory leukocytes. Some of the lung destruction seen in COPD results from autoimmune processes. Autoimmune diseases tend to be more prevalent in women and may contribute to the greater prevalence of COPD in women among nonsmokers (Han et al. 2007).

Table 3.3 GOLD Classification of COPD by Severity

Stage	Characteristics: For All Stages FEV$_1$/Forced Vital Capacity <0.7
I. Mild COPD	FEV$_1$ ≥ 80% predicted With or without chronic symptoms (cough, sputum production)
II. Moderate COPD	FEV$_1$ between 50% and 79% predicted
III. Severe COPD	FEV$_1$ between 30% and 49% predicted With or without chronic symptoms (cough, sputum production)
IV. Very Severe COPD	FEV$_1$ <30% predicted Or FEV$_1$ <50% predicted *plus* respiratory failure Or FEV$_1$ <50% predicted *plus* clinical signs of right heart failure

Note: Respiratory failure = PaO$_2$ <60 mm Hg (8.0 kPa) with or without PaCO2 >50 mm Hg (6.7 kPa) while breathing air at sea level.
Abbreviations: GOLD = Global Initiative for Chronic Obstructive Lung Disease; COPD = chronic obstructive pulmonary disease; FEV$_1$ = forced expiratory volume in 1 second.
Reproduced with permission from Bates and Cydulka 2011, p. 512.

Clinical Manifestations

One of the hallmarks of COPD is exertional dyspnea. The degree of lung dysfunction is only one of several components that determine a patient's overall experience of dyspnea. In addition to the physical element, there are affective and cognitive elements. The patient's emotional response and cognitive interpretation of the sensation of dyspnea have a significant impact on his or her functioning. Patients may be more disturbed by exercise limitations than by the sensation of dyspnea itself. Neurobiologic and neuroimaging studies demonstrate that women have a higher intrinsic sensitivity to noxious stimuli, including noxious somatic sensations, with an overall greater awareness of these stimuli compared to men. This sensitivity may be a major factor in the sex and gender differences in patients' awareness, concern, and sense of medical urgency in response to clinical manifestations in both asthma and COPD (Han et al. 2007).

As delineated for patients with asthma, symptoms, frequency of exacerbations, quality of life, and associated comorbidities are different between men and women with COPD (Han et al. 2007; Ohar et al. 2011). Research consistently reports that female patients with similar levels of pulmonary physiologic impairment and significantly fewer pack-years of smoking report more dyspnea and more frequent exacerbations than men (Watson et al. 2004; Cydulka 2005; Watson

2006; Celli et al. 2011). The literature reports that women with COPD note higher levels of anxiety and depression and declarations of worse quality of life (Di Marco et al. 2006; Ohar et al. 2011; Naberan et al. 2012; Kamil et al. 2013). The frequency of cough and sputum production is less consistent, although women tend to report less sputum production than their male counterparts. This may be a manifestation of a gender more than a sex influence, as sputum production may be considered "less feminine" in some cultures (Watson 2006; Camp et al. 2009; Ohar et al. 2011). The presence of symptoms may be a good predictor of disease status and underlying disease activity in men; a prospective study of symptoms in male and female patients with mild to moderate COPD demonstrated that the FEV_1 and its fluctuation over time correlated more closely with the prevalence, remission, and incidence of symptoms in men with COPD than in women (Watson 2006; Han et al. 2007).

Diagnosis

COPD is currently defined and classified by clinical history (symptoms of dyspnea, chronic cough or sputum production, and a history of exposure to risk factors for the disease) and confirmed by spirometry (the presence of a post-bronchodilator $FEV_1/FVC < 0.70$, which confirms the presence of persistent airflow limitation and thus of COPD) as recommended by the GOLD report (GOLD 2014). Once the disease progresses, the percentage of predicted FEV_1 is a better measure of disease severity than clinical signs and symptoms (Bates & Cydulka 2011).

Without confirmatory testing, there is significant potential for gender bias if the diagnosis is based on clinical presentation alone. Research has consistently demonstrated that regardless of clinical presentation, women are more likely to be diagnosed with asthma and men with COPD (Chapman 2001; Watson et al. 2004; Miravitlles et al. 2006; Han et al. 2007; Ohar et al. 2011). Another study found that women more commonly than men report that they are given a mixed diagnosis of asthma and COPD (48% vs. 39%) when presenting with an exacerbation of obstructive lung disease (Cydulka 2005). This bias among health care providers may be the result of the historically higher prevalence of COPD in men and is quite

concerning as data from the Confronting COPD International Survey confirm that only 34% of women and 39% of men report ever having received a spirometry test as part of their work-up and diagnosis of COPD (Watson et al. 2004). This was similar to a 2006 study reporting that only 31% of patients discharged with a COPD diagnosis had had spirometry (Damarla et al. 2006). The increasing prevalence of COPD in women and the difference in disease expression between men and women underscore the importance of referral for formal outpatient spirometry for patients presenting with symptoms suggestive of COPD.

Acute Management

Acute exacerbations of COPD are usually triggered by an infection or respiratory irritant. Evidence of infection appears in more than 75% of acute exacerbations, half of which are bacterial. A thorough history and physical may help identify important triggers, including hypoxia, cold weather, beta-blockers, narcotics, and sedative-hypnotic agents. The symptom of dyspnea, which compels the patient to seek medical care for an exacerbation, is the result of ventilation-perfusion mismatching as opposed to the expiratory airflow limitation seen in asthma exacerbations. Patients will present with hypoxemia, increased work of breathing, CO_2 retention, and respiratory acidosis. Supplemental oxygen increases blood oxygen concentration; however, reversing pulmonary vasoconstriction and increasing blood flow to inadequately ventilated regions of the lung can increase V/Q mismatch and worsen dyspnea. Exogenous oxygen can also blunt the respiratory drive of patients who chronically retain CO_2, leading to hypoventilation, hypercapnea, decreasing level of consciousness, and respiratory arrest. An arterial blood gas may be useful in light of the differences in symptom reporting and is currently recommended as part of the GOLD strategy for severe exacerbations (Bates & Cydulka 2011; GOLD 2014).

Physical examination and pulmonary function estimates by both the patient and the physician are highly inaccurate (Emerman et al. 1994; Bates & Cydulka 2011). In addition, spirometry is often difficult to obtain and perform and is inaccurate in severely dyspneic patients with exacerbations of COPD (Brulotte & Lang 2012).

If the patient is able to cooperate, a PEFR of <100 L per minute or an FEV_1 of <1.00 L in a patient without chronic severe obstruction indicates a severe exacerbation. Sequential measurements can then be used to determine the patient's response to therapy. Measurement of FEV_1 is preferred to PEFR, because FEV_1 allows comparison with baseline studies and published guidelines; however, FEV_1 is not readily available in all EDs (Bates & Cydulka 2011).

Treatment of an acute exacerbation in the ED should be aimed at correcting tissue oxygenation, alleviating reversible bronchospasm, and treating underlying trigger(s) or complications.

Treatment in the ED may include the use of oxygen, B2-adrenergic agonists, anticholinergics, corticosteroids, antibiotics, and assisted ventilation in severe exacerbations. Table 3.4 provides a summary of the most current recommendations. As for asthma, guidelines for the acute care of COPD exacerbations do not include any gender-specific recommendations, as research into this important issue awaits future investigations (Bates & Cydulka 2011).

Smoking cessation, as discussed in the section on "Tobacco Abise," is the most effective preventive intervention for patients with COPD. Although smoking interventions are not a

Table 3.4 COPD Exacerbation Treatment Options

Treatment	Example Regimen	Pearls
Bronchodilators		
B$_2$ Adrenergic Agonists	*Albuterol Nebulizer Solution* 2.5–5 mg every 20 min for 3 doses (if side effects are tolerated), then 2.5–10 mg every 1–4 h, as needed, or 10–15 mg/h as continuous nebulization *Metered Dose Inhaler* 4–8 puffs every 20 min up to 4 h, then every 1–4 h as needed.	For optimal delivery, dilute aerosols to minimum of 3 mL at gas flow of 6–8 L/min. Use large-volume nebulizers for continuous administration. May mix with ipratropium nebulizer solution. In patients with cardiac disease, consider continuous cardiac monitoring in frequent dosing.
Anticholinergic Agents	*Ipratropium Bromide* 0.5 mg every 20 min for 3 doses, then as needed	Use in combination with B$_2$ agonist leads to improved clinical outcomes and shorter ED lengths of stay.
Antibiotics		
Most common pathogens: *Streptococcus pneumoniae*, *Haemophilus influenzae*, and *Moraxella catarrhalis*	No specific agent is superior. Duration of treatment ranges 3–14 days.	Add if increased sputum volume, change in sputum color, fever, or suspicion of infectious etiology.
Systemic Corticosteroids		
Oral	*Prednisone* Short course of 40–60 mg/d in 1 or 2 divided doses for 7–14 days. Consider taper if >7 days.	No known advantage for higher doses of corticosteroids. Use in the ED does not affect rate of hospitalization; however, it does decrease rate of return visits.
Systemic	*Methylprednisolone* IV: 1 mg/kg every 4–6 h.	Use IV therapy only when oral intake, GI transit time, or GI absorption are impaired.

Table 3.4 (cont.)

Treatment	Example Regimen	Pearls
Assisted Ventilation		
Noninvasive positive pressure ventilation (NPPV)	*Selection Criteria* Moderate to severe dyspnea with use of accessory muscles and paradoxical abdominal motion Moderate to severe acidosis (pH ≥7.35) and/or hypercapnia (PaCO₂ >45 mm Hg or 6.0 kPa) Respiratory frequency >25 breaths/min	*Exclusion Criteria* Respiratory arrest Cardiovascular instability Change in mental status High aspiration risk Viscous or copious secretions Recent facial or gastroesophageal surgery Craniofacial trauma Fixed nasopharyngeal abnormalities Burns Extreme obesity
Invasive Mechanical Ventilation	Severe respiratory muscle fatigue RR >35 breaths/min PaO₂ <50 mm Hg (<5.3 kPa) or PaO₂/FiO₂ <200 mmHg pH <7.25 and/or PaCO₂ >60 mmHg or >8.0 kPa Respiratory arrest Somnolence, agitation Cardiovascular complications NPPV failure	Indicated in evidence of respiratory muscle fatigue, worsening respiratory acidosis, deteriorating mental status, or hypoxia refractory to supplemental oxygen by usual techniques Main goals of assisted ventilation are to rest ventilatory muscles and to restore gas exchange to a stable baseline

Adapted with permission from Cydulka 2011, p. 508; Bates and Cydulka 2011, pp. 515–516.
Abbreviations: COPD = chronic obstructive pulmonary disease.

treatment for the acute exacerbation seen in the ED, gender-sensitive and gender-specific counseling can and should be part of the ED visit, as this visit is a teachable moment for the patient and is often the first, and may be the only, opportunity. In the Confronting COPD International Survey, only 37% of women and 28% of men reported ever receiving any anti-smoking advice. Further data from the LHS demonstrated that women who became sustained quitters had an average improvement in FEV₁ percentage predicted during the first year that was 2.5 times greater than the improvement in men (Scanlon et al. 2000; Han et al. 2007). Some studies have demonstrated that men have greater symptomatic improvement in COPD symptoms after quitting smoking than women, which may further explain the difficulties women with COPD have with quitting and staying quit (e.g., Han et al. 2007).

Disposition decisions for these patients should take into account both the acute presentation and their COPD history. Among patients discharged to home after ED treatment of a COPD exacerbation, one in five will experience an urgent/emergent relapse event during the next two weeks. Evidence has shown that ≥ five clinic or ED visits in the previous year, elevated respiratory rate on presentation (for each 5 breaths/min over 16 breaths/min), current oral steroid use, and a history of significantly limited activity from dyspnea are all associated with a high risk for relapse within two weeks after ED discharge (Bates & Cydulka 2011). Further research should address these high-risk patients and determine how sex and gender influence hospitalization and relapse rates.

Prevention

As defined in GOLD, COPD is a preventable disease. Although tobacco smoke is the major cause of COPD, occupational dust, chemical exposure, and air pollution are other significant risk factors for COPD. α1-Antitrypsin deficiency is rare and accounts for <1% of COPD patients (Bates & Cydulka 2011). Limiting these exposures, especially smoking, is essential to mitigating COPD, which is a rising cause of health care utilization, morbidity and mortality, and financial burden. In developing countries where women are exposed to noxious gases while cooking in their homes and working in toxic, poorly ventilated factories, educational programs and public health initiatives to increase awareness of the dangers of such exposures and programs to decrease occupational exposure may be beneficial. Nevertheless, the most important health initiative to decrease the ravages of COPD in women and men is smoking cessation, an initiative that can and should begin in the Emergency Department.

Clinical Outcomes

While there appears to be some agreement among experts on the difference in expression of COPD between men and women, differences in overall outcome and mortality are less conclusive. Population-based reports indicate that more women than men are dying from COPD. Studies have been conducted to confirm this, with conflicting results; one investigation reported a higher mortality in women, whereas three studies found that men have a higher mortality rate. These studies focused on similar populations, enrolling mostly men and, in general, patients with advanced disease. More recent studies have included similar numbers of men and women and taken into account other factors that contribute to outcomes, such as obesity, comorbidities, and disease severity. De Torres et al. (2009) reported a lower mortality rate in women than in men. In the larger three-year "Toward a Revolution in COPD Health (TORCH)" study, Celli and colleagues initially found a higher mortality rate in men; however, this was statistically insignificant after adjusting for important confounding baseline variables (Celli et al. 2011).

The TORCH study also confirmed that women with worse dyspnea and quality of life scores, a shorter time to first exacerbation, and a higher number of exacerbations than men had a heightened perception of dyspnea (Celli et al. 2011). The root cause of the difference in symptom reporting and quality of life is unknown, and

it is unclear if difference in management plays a role. It appears that hospitalization and emergency room visits are not significantly different between men and women, nor is the likelihood of being treated with an inhaled corticosteroid or being trained to use an inhaler (Watson et al. 2004). Unfortunately, few studies have been designed to assess sex and gender differences in the acute pharmacologic treatment of COPD; therefore, data are inconclusive and minimal. It has been suggested that in a general COPD population, the probability of respiratory deterioration after stopping inhaled steroids is higher in women than men. This deterioration may play a role in COPD exacerbations in women seen in the ED (Schermer 2004; Han et al. 2007). Future COPD research must increase the number of women included in therapeutic trials to allow adequate power to examine sex-stratified analyses. At this point, acute treatment should be guideline based for both sexes (Han et al. 2007).

Conclusions

There are complex interactions between biological sex, the varying exposures influenced by gender, and the development and manifestation of a chronic disease such as COPD. Women who smoke tend to develop COPD at younger ages with less tobacco exposure and experience poorer quality of life. Many opportunities are available to explore these interactions, their consequences, and the common message that women may be more susceptible to the effects of smoking and the development of COPD. COPD and asthma evidence a difference in disease expression between men and women, with an increase in report of dyspnea, frequency of exacerbations, and association with anxiety and depression in women compared to men, likely influenced by the intrinsic differences in how men and women sense and respond to noxious stimuli and the sensation of dyspnea. Gender biases exist in diagnosing COPD and in the counseling clinicians provide regarding smoking cessation. COPD is the only common cause of mortality that is increasing around the world. Women are the principal population suffering these premature deaths. Therefore, efforts to accurately diagnose, treat, and counsel patients with COPD must increase in Emergency Departments and all other clinical settings.

Gaps in Knowledge and Research Questions

Smoking

The catastrophic morbidity, mortality, and cost associated with tobacco use in this country and around the world must prompt smoking cessation and lung cancer prevention programs for populations at risk. Controversy still exists surrounding women's susceptibility to the carcinogenic effects of cigarette smoke; nevertheless, the influence of gender should impact the ways in which health care providers evaluate and screen patients in the ED and emphasize the need to direct future research to target women specifically (Tanoue 2000).

The ED may be an ideal place to help individuals quit tobacco use; however, further work is needed to increase systems support for the development and implementation of effective and feasible ED-based smoking cessation interventions. The broad range in preferences for interventions and counseling types supports the developing, testing, and disseminating a wide range of treatment options that can be tailored to individual patient needs and characteristics, as well as the demands and capacities of the clinical setting (Choo et al. 2012).

Asthma

Furthering understanding of this common disease demands continued research to determine the underlying mechanisms unique to men and women. There are multiple avenues for further study, although two of the most important are the link to sex hormones and the reproductive cycle and the difference in symptom reporting with resulting increases in hospital utilization.

There are potential implications for treatment devolving from the proposed link between a woman's menstrual cycle and asthma exacerbations, such as the use of leukotriene receptor antagonists, intramuscular progesterone, or premenstrual long-acting B_2 agonists. While there is no solid evidence yet, this research focus, if successful, has the potential to improve patient morbidity and mortality (Kynyk et al. 2011). The tendency of women in their fifth and sixth decades of life to be admitted for asthma suggests that efforts for better asthma control in this subgroup may improve morbidity and mortality and lead to national cost savings (Lin et al. 2013).

The difference in symptom perception and reporting supports the use of objective measurements of airway obstruction, such as PEFR, when managing patients with asthma. While spirometry in the ED may not be feasible, improving the ED's use of PEFRs for management of asthma exacerbations and developing a program for quick and seamless referral to spirometry and pulmonary follow-up would be beneficial. Tailored educational programs for men and women, as well as health care providers, may lead to patients' more accurate perception and reporting of symptoms (Cydulka et al. 2001). In addition, development of a sex-specific questionnaire that a patient can complete while undergoing evaluation and management in the ED may assist with identifying sex- or gender-related triggers and symptoms and prompt improved self-management strategies (Kynyk et al. 2011).

Chronic Obstructive Pulmonary Disease

An estimated 12.7 to 14.7 million adults have been diagnosed with COPD in their lifetime (*Trends in COPD* 2013). In general, women and men with COPD present differently and have a different disease course; women have demonstrated increased susceptibility in response to inhaled particulates, faster rate of FEV_1 decline, and higher morbidity and mortality (Ohar et al. 2011). The true cause of these disparities is unknown. Future studies are needed to address the relationship between sex and gender and physiologic differences in lung development, function, and decline; COPD phenotypic characterization; inflammatory mechanisms; the immunologic and hormonal determinants of airway obstruction; and treatment response (Han et al. 2007; Camp et al. 2009).

Case Resolution

A female smoker presenting with cough and wheezing represents a typical scenario for an acute care physician. She was treated with oral steroids and a combination of inhaled albuterol and ipratropium bromide with improvement in her exam and vital signs; however, she continued

Table 3.5 Sex and Gender Pearls for Pulmonary Disease

Disease	Practice Pearls
Tobacco Abuse	• When evaluating patients, consider that the gender-related trend in smoking rates has led to a shift in the gender-specific prevalence, morbidity, and mortality of tobacco-related illnesses. • Women may be more vulnerable to the effects of cigarette smoking than men, thus expressing disease states earlier and more severely. • Women tend to have more difficulty with smoking cessation. Consider gender-specific counseling, which may include attention to timing with the menstrual cycle, weight gain, and positive reinforcement. • Successful smoking cessation counseling programs can occur in the ED and should target both prevention and cessation.
Asthma	• There is a greater prevalence of asthma in women during reproductive years, suggesting hormonal influence; exacerbations can be linked to menstrual cycles and pregnancy. • Differences in symptoms reporting between men and women may affect acute presentation. • Use objective measurements of lung function when available, while recognizing that women may take longer to learn how to use tools effectively. • Consider gender-specific treatment interventions, such as telephone counseling to address gender- and sex-specific triggers, in addition to standard treatment.
COPD	• When evaluating patients, recognize that COPD is no longer a disease of men; women are surpassing men in prevalence, hospitalization rates, and mortality. • Women appear to have increased susceptibility to COPD and may develop the disease at a younger age. Avoid misdiagnosis with asthma by referring patients for pulmonary function testing. • Women may experience more dyspnea and sense of medical urgency with similar lung function; consider this when making dispositions. • Smoking cessation is the most effective intervention.

to be quite symptomatic. She was admitted to the hospital where she underwent further spirometry, revealing a new diagnosis of COPD. She received gender-specific counseling for smoking cessation and was referred to a pulmonologist for further evaluation and care.

Take-Away Points

• The increasing incidence of COPD and lung cancer in women mirrors the increased prevalence in cigarette smoking.
• Smoking cessation efforts must continue to address gender-specific triggers and reasons to quit.
• Asthma control and exacerbation may be related to cyclical hormonal changes.

Treatment may need to be adjusted to reflect these changes.
• Asthma in pregnancy is variable: One-third of women improve, one-third experience no change, and one-third worsen.
• Women may experience a more accelerated course of COPD than men.
• Women with COPD are often misdiagnosed as having asthma.

References

Adams, B.K. & Cydulka, R.K. 2003. Asthma evaluation and management. *Emergency Medicine Clinics of North America*, 21(2), 315–330.

Akinbami, L.J., Moorman, J.E. & Liu, X. 2011. Asthma Prevalence, Health Care Use, and Mortality: United

States, 2005–2009. *National Health Statistics Reports* (**32**), 1–15.

Allen, S.S. et al. 2013. Menstrual phase and depressive symptoms differences in physiological response to nicotine following acute smoking abstinence. *Nicotine & Tobacco Research*, **15**(6), 1091–1098.

Appleton, S. et al. 2006. Central obesity is associated with nonatopic but not atopic asthma in a representative population sample. *Journal of Allergy and Clinical Immunology*, **118**(6), 1284–1291.

Arnold, D.H. et al. 2007. Clinical measures associated with FEV_1 in persons with asthma requiring hospital admission. *The American Journal of Emergency Medicine*, **25**(4), 425–429.

Barr, R.G. et al. 2004. Prospective study of postmenopausal hormone use and newly diagnosed asthma and chronic obstructive pulmonary disease. *Archives of Internal Medicine*, **164**(4), 379–386.

Bates, C. & Cydulka, R. 2011. Chronic Obstructive Pulmonary Disease. In J. Tintinalli et al., eds. *Tintinalli's Emergency Medicine: A Comprehensive Study Guide*, 7th ed. New York: McGraw Hill Professional.

Beaudoin, F.L. et al. 2015. Sex differences in substance use among adult emergency department patients: Prevalence, severity, and need for intervention. *Academic Emergency Medicine*, **22**(11), 1307–1315.

Becklake, M.R. & Kauffmann, F. 1999. Gender differences in airway behaviour over the human life span. *Thorax*, **54**(12), 1119–1138.

Ben-Zaken Cohen, S. et al. 2007. The growing burden of chronic obstructive pulmonary disease and lung cancer in women: Examining sex differences in cigarette smoke metabolism. *American Journal of Respiratory and Critical Care Medicine*, **176**(2), 113–120.

Bernstein, S.L. et al. 2009. Efficacy of a brief intervention to improve emergency physicians' smoking cessation counseling skills, knowledge, and attitudes. *Substance Abuse*, **30**(2), 158–181.

Bock, B. et al. 2008. Smoking cessation among patients in an emergency chest pain observation unit: Outcomes of the Chest Pain Smoking Study (CPSS). *Nicotine & Tobacco Research*, **10**(10), 1523–1531.

Boezen, H.M. et al. 1995. Relation between respiratory symptoms, pulmonary function and peak flow variability in adults. *Thorax*, **50**(2), 121–126.

Bottorff, J.L. et al. 2012. Gender influences in tobacco use and cessation interventions. *Nursing Clinics of NA*, **47**(1), 55–70.

Boudreaux, E.D. et al. 2008. Emergency Department Initiated Treatments for Tobacco (EDITT): A pilot study. *Annals of Behavioral Medicine*, **36**(3), 314–325.

Brown, D. et al. 2008. Deaths from chronic obstructive pulmonary disease – United States, 2000–2005. *MMWR. Morbidity and Mortality Weekly Report*, **57**(45), 1229–1232.

Brulotte, C.A. & Lang, E.S. 2012. Acute exacerbations of chronic obstructive pulmonary disease in the emergency department. *Emergency Medicine Clinics of North America*, **30**(2), 223–247.

Busse, W. et al., 2007. Expert Panel Report 3 (EPR-3): Guidelines for the Diagnosis and Management of Asthma – Summary Report 2007. *Journal of Allergy and Clinical Immunology*, **120**(5), S94–S138.

Camp, P.G., O'Donnell, D.E. & Postma, D.S. 2009. Chronic obstructive pulmonary disease in men and women: Myths and reality. *Proceedings of the American Thoracic Society*, **6**(6), 535–538.

Celli, B. et al. 2011. Sex differences in mortality and clinical expressions of patients with chronic obstructive pulmonary disease. *American Journal of Respiratory and Critical Care Medicine*, **183**(3), 317–322.

Celli, B.R., 2000. The importance of spirometry in copd and asthma: Effect on approach to management. *Chest*, **117**(90020), 15S–19.

Chafin, C.C. et al. 2001. Are there gender differences in the use of peak flow meters? *Journal of Asthma*, **38**(7), 541–543.

Chapman, K.R. 2001. Gender bias in the diagnosis of COPD. *Chest*, **119**(6), 1691–1695.

Choo, E.K. et al. 2012. Patient preferences for emergency department-initiated tobacco interventions: A multicenter cross-sectional study of current smokers. *Addiction Science & Clinical Practice*, **7**(1), 4.

Clark, N.M. 2007. A randomized trial of a self-regulation intervention for women with asthma. *Chest*, **132**(1), 88.

Clark, N.M. et al. 2010. From the female perspective: Long-term effects on quality of life of a program for women with asthma. *Gender Medicine*, **7**(2), 125–136.

Cydulka, R.K. 2011. Acute Asthma in Adults. In J. Tintinalli et al., eds. *Tintinalli's Emergency Medicine: A Comprehensive Study Guide, Seventh Edition*. New York: McGraw Hill Professional.

Cydulka, R.K. 2006. Acute asthma during pregnancy. *Immunology and Allergy Clinics of North America*, **26**(1), 103–117.

Cydulka, R.K. 2005. Gender differences in emergency department patients with chronic obstructive pulmonary disease exacerbation. *Academic Emergency Medicine*, **12**(12), 1173–1179.

Cydulka, R.K. et al. 2001. Differences between men and women in reporting of symptoms during an asthma exacerbation. *Annals of Emergency Medicine*, **38**(2), 123–128.

Damarla, M. et al. 2006. Discrepancy in the use of confirmatory tests in patients hospitalized with the diagnosis of chronic obstructive pulmonary disease or congestive heart failure. *Respiratory Care*, 51(10), 1120–1124.

de Torres, J.P. et al. 2009. Sex differences in mortality in patients with COPD. *European Respiratory Journal*, 33(3), 528–535.

Di Marco, F. et al. 2006. Anxiety and depression in COPD patients: The roles of gender and disease severity. *Respiratory Medicine*, 100(10), 1767–1774.

Emerman, C.L., Lukens, T.W. & Effron, D. 1994. Physician estimation of FEV1 in acute exacerbation of COPD. *Chest*, 105(6), 1709–1712.

ENFUMOSA Study Group. 2003. The ENFUMOSA cross-sectional European multicentre study of the clinical phenotype of chronic severe asthma. *European Respiratory Journal*, 22(3), 470–477.

Ersel, M. et al. 2010. Are emergency department visits really a teachable moment? Smoking cessation promotion in emergency department. *European Journal of Emergency Medicine: Official Journal of the European Society for Emergency Medicine*, 17(2), 73–79.

Fabbri, L.M. et al. 1998. Physiologic consequences of long-term inflammation. *American Journal of Respiratory and Critical Care Medicine*, 157(5 Pt 2), S195–S198.

Gan, W.Q. et al. 2006. Female smokers beyond the perimenopausal period are at increased risk of chronic obstructive pulmonary disease: A systematic review and meta-analysis. *Respiratory Research*, 7, 52.

Global Strategy for the Diagnosis, Management, and Prevention of Chronic Obstructive Pulmonary Disease, Global Initiative for Chronic Obstructive Lung Disease (GOLD) 2014. Available at www.goldcopd.org/. Accessed March 30, 2014.

Gold, D.R. et al. 1996. Effects of cigarette smoking on lung function in adolescent boys and girls. *The New England Journal of Medicine*, 335(13), 931–937.

Gui, P. 2010. Gender differences in perceptions of urge to cough and dyspnea induced by citric acid in healthy never smokers. *Chest*, 138(5), 1166.

Han, M.K. et al. 2007. Gender and chronic obstructive pulmonary disease. *American Journal of Respiratory and Critical Care Medicine*, 176(12), 1179–1184.

Ignacio-Garcia, J.M. & Gonzalez-Santos, P. 1995. Asthma self-management education program by home monitoring of peak expiratory flow. *American Journal of Respiratory and Critical Care Medicine*, 151(2 Pt 1), 353–359.

Kamil, F., Pinzon, I. & Foreman, M.G. 2013. Sex and race factors in early-onset COPD. *Current Opinion in Pulmonary Medicine*, 19(2), 140–144.

Katz, D.A. et al. 2012. The Emergency Department Action in Smoking Cessation (EDASC) Trial: Impact on Delivery of Smoking Cessation Counseling. *Academic Emergency Medicine*, 19(4), 409–420.

Kikuchi, Y. et al. 1994. Chemosensitivity and perception of dyspnea in patients with a history of near-fatal asthma. *The New England Journal of Medicine*, 330(19), 1329–1334.

Kim, S. et al. 2004. Prospective multicenter study of relapse following emergency department treatment of COPD exacerbation. *Chest*, 125(2), 473–481.

Kynyk, J.A., Mastronarde, J.G. & McCallister, J.W. 2011. Asthma, the sex difference. *Current Opinion in Pulmonary Medicine*, 17(1), 6–11.

Lange, P. et al. 1998. A 15-year follow-up study of ventilatory function in adults with asthma. *The New England Journal of Medicine*, 339(17), 1194–1200.

Lee, J.H. et al. 2006. Gender Differences in IgE-Mediated Allergic Asthma in the Epidemiology and Natural History of Asthma: Outcomes and Treatment Regimens (TENOR) Study. *Journal of Asthma*, 43(3), 179–184.

Leynaert, B. et al. 2012. Gender differences in prevalence, diagnosis and incidence of allergic and non-allergic asthma: A population-based cohort. *Thorax*, 67(7), 625–631.

Leynaert, B. et al. 1997. Is bronchial hyperresponsiveness more frequent in women than in men? A population-based study. *American Journal of Respiratory and Critical Care Medicine*, 156(5), 1413–1420.

Lin, R.Y.-W., Ji, R. & Liao, W. 2013. Age dependent sex disproportion in US asthma hospitalization rates, 2000–2010. *Annals of Allergy, Asthma & Immunology*, 111(3), 176–181.

Lowenstein, S.R. et al. 1998. Behavioral risk factors in emergency department patients: A multisite survey. *Academic Emergency Medicine: Official Journal of the Society for Academic Emergency Medicine*, 5(8), 781–787.

Mannino, D.M. et al. 2002. Chronic obstructive pulmonary disease surveillance – United States, 1971–2000. *Morbidity and Mortality Weekly Report. Surveillance Summaries*, 51(6), 1–16.

McCallister, J.W. et al. 2013. Sex differences in asthma symptom profiles and control in the American Lung Association Asthma Clinical Research Centers. *Respiratory Medicine*, 107(10), 1491–1500.

Melgert, B.N. et al. 2007. Are there reasons why adult asthma is more common in females? *Current Allergy and Asthma Reports*, 7(2), 143–150.

Melgert, B.N. & Postma, D.S. 2009. All men are created equal?: New leads in explaining sex differences in adult asthma. *Proceedings of the American Thoracic Society*, 6(8), 724–727.

Miravitlles, M. et al. 2006. [Attitudes toward the diagnosis of chronic obstructive pulmonary disease in primary care]. *Archivos de bronconeumología*, 42(1), 3–8.

Naberan, K. et al. 2012. Impairment of quality of life in women with chronic obstructive pulmonary disease. *Respiratory Medicine*, 106(3), 367–373.

National Asthma Education and Prevention Program, Expert Panel Report 3: *Guidelines for the Diagnosis and Management of Asthma*. Publication No. 08–4051. Bethesda, MD: National Institutes of Health, 2007. Available at http://www.nhlbi.nih.gov/guidelines/asthma/asthgdln.pdf. Accessed March 30, 2014.

Neuner, B. et al. 2009. Emergency department-initiated tobacco control: A randomised controlled trial in an inner city university hospital. *Tobacco Control*, 18(4), 283–293.

Ohar, J., Fromer, L. & Donohue, J.F. 2011. Reconsidering sex-based stereotypes of COPD. *Primary Care Respiratory Journal*, 20(4), 370.

Osborne, M.L. et al. 1998. Characteristics of patients with asthma within a large HMO: A comparison by age and gender. *American Journal of Respiratory and Critical Care Medicine*, 157(1), 123–128.

Paoletti, P. et al. 1995. Distribution of bronchial responsiveness in a general population: Effect of sex, age, smoking, and level of pulmonary function. *American Journal of Respiratory and Critical Care Medicine*, 151(6), 1770–1777.

Patil, S.P. et al. 2003. In-hospital mortality following acute exacerbations of chronic obstructive pulmonary disease. *Archives of Internal Medicine*, 163(10), 1180–1186.

Piovesan, D.M. et al. 2006. [Early prognosis of acute asthma in the emergency room.] *Jornal brasileiro de pneumologia: publicação oficial da Sociedade Brasileira de Pneumologia e Tisilogia*, 32(1), 1–9.

Piper, M.E. et al. 2010. Gender, race, and education differences in abstinence rates among participants in two randomized smoking cessation trials. *Nicotine & Tobacco Research*, 12(6), 647–657.

Scanlon, P.D. et al. 2000. Smoking cessation and lung function in mild-to-moderate chronic obstructive pulmonary disease. The Lung Health Study. *American Journal of Respiratory and Critical Care Medicine*, 161(2 Pt 1), 381–390.

Schermer, T. 2004. Probability and determinants of relapse after discontinuation of inhaled corticosteroids in patients with COPD treated in general practice. *Primary Care Respiratory Journal*, 13(1), 48–55.

Schneider, W.V. et al. 2011. Utility of Portable Spirometry in a Pediatric Emergency Department in Children with Acute Exacerbation of Asthma. *Journal of Asthma*, 48(3), 248–252.

Self, T.H. et al. 2005. Gender differences in the use of peak flow meters and their effect on peak expiratory flow. *Pharmacotherapy*, 25(4), 526–530.

Silverman, E.K. et al. 2000. Gender-related differences in severe, early-onset chronic obstructive pulmonary disease. *American Journal of Respiratory and Critical Care Medicine*, 162(6), 2152–2158.

Sinclair, A.H. & Tolsma, D.D. 2006. Gender differences in asthma experience and disease care in a managed care organization. *Journal of Asthma*, 43(5), 363–367.

Sorheim, I.C. et al., 2010. Gender differences in COPD: are women more susceptible to smoking effects than men? *Thorax*, 65(6), 480–485.

Tanoue, L.T. 2000. Cigarette smoking and women's respiratory health. *Clinics in Chest Medicine*, 21(1), 47–65, viii.

Tantisira, K.G. et al. 2008. Airway responsiveness in mild to moderate childhood asthma. *American Journal of Respiratory and Critical Care Medicine*, 178(4), 325–331.

Townsend, E.A., Miller, V.M. & Prakash, Y.S. 2012. Sex differences and sex steroids in lung health and disease. *Endocrine Reviews*, 33(1), 1–47.

Trends in Asthma Morbidity and Mortality, American Lung Association Epidemiology and Statistics Unit. 2012. Available at www.lung.org/finding-cures/our-research/trend-reports/asthma-trend-report.pdf. Accessed March 30, 2014.

Trends in COPD (Chronic Bronchitis and Emphysema): Morbidity and Mortality, American Lung Association Epidemiology and Statistics Unit Research and Health Education Division. 2013. Available at www.lung.org/finding-cures/our-research/trend-reports/copd-trend-report.pdf. Accessed March 30, 2014.

Trends in Lung Cancer: Morbidity and Mortality, American Lung Association Epidemiology and Statistics Unit Research and Health Education Division. 2014. Available at www.lung.org/assets/documents/research/lc-trend-report.pdf. Accessed November 27, 2015.

Trends in Tobacco Use, American Lung Association Research and Program Services Epidemiology and Statistics Unit. 2011. Available at www.lung.org/finding-cures/our-research/trend-reports/Tobacco-Trend-Report.pdf. Accessed March 30, 2014.

Troisi, R.J. et al. 1995. Menopause, postmenopausal estrogen preparations, and the risk of adult-onset asthma. A prospective cohort study. *American Journal of Respiratory and Critical Care Medicine*, 152(4 Pt 1), 1183–1188.

US Department of Health and Human Services. *The Health Consequences of Smoking – 50 Years of Progress:*

A Report of the Surgeon General. Atlanta, GA: US Department of Health and Human Services, Centers for Disease Control and Prevention, National Center for Chronic Disease Prevention and Health Promotion, Office on Smoking and Health, 2014.

US Department of Health and Human Services. *The Health Consequences of Smoking for Women: A Report of the Surgeon General.* Atlanta, GA: US Department of Health and Human Services, Centers for Disease Control and Prevention, National Center for Chronic Disease Prevention and Health Promotion, Office on Smoking and Health, 1980.

US Department of Health and Human Services. *Smoking and Health: Report of the Advisory Committee of the Surgeon General of the Public Health Service.* Atlanta, GA: US Department of Health and Human Services, Centers for Disease Control and Prevention, National Center for Chronic Disease Prevention and Health Promotion, Office on Smoking and Health, 1964.

Vollmer, W.M., Osborne, M.L. & Buist, A.S. 1993. Temporal trends in hospital-based episodes of asthma care in a health maintenance organization. *The American Review of Respiratory Disease,* 147(2), 347–353.

Watson, L. 2006. Predictors of COPD symptoms: Does the sex of the patient matter? *European Respiratory Journal,* 28(2), 311–318.

Watson, L. et al., 2004. Gender differences in the management and experience of chronic obstructive pulmonary disease. *Respiratory Medicine,* 98(12), 1207–1213.

Weiner, P. et al. 2002. Influence of gender and inspiratory muscle training on the perception of dyspnea in patients with asthma. *Chest,* 122(1), 197–201.

World Health Organization, 2010. 10 Facts on Gender and Tobacco. Available at: http://www.who.int/fea tures/factfiles/gender_tobacco/en/index.html. Accessed March 30, 2014.

Sex and Gender-Specific Differences in Alcohol and Drug use Among Patients Seeking Treatment in the Acute Care Setting

Esther K. Choo, Marna Greenberg and Grace Chang

Clinical Case

A 34-year-old intoxicated female patient presents to the emergency department (ED) on a busy Friday evening. She receives a brief screening physical exam, which reveals no obvious medical problems or injuries. Her vital signs are normal and her blood glucose is 96 mg/dL. She is clinically intoxicated and cannot identify a sober caretaker, so she is moved to the ED observation area for the remainder of the evening. Several hours after arrival, a urine sample is sent and reveals the patient is pregnant; she recalls that her last menstrual period was about six weeks earlier. After change of shift in the morning, the nurses notify the incoming clinical team that the patient is now clinically sober and requests discharge. She reports drinking two or three beers each evening to "take the edge off," and as much as four drinks on the weekends. She expresses an interest in decreasing her alcohol use but declines referrals to substance use treatment centers.

Introduction

Alcohol and drug use are highly prevalent among individuals presenting to the ED: 24% to 45% report high-risk drinking, and 5% dependent drinking. Drug use prevalence in the ED setting is higher than the national average with 30% reporting drug use in the past year and 17% having a moderate to severe drug problem.[1] These behaviors are closely associated with injury – the leading cause of ED visits – and many other acute health problems. Alcohol is an established risk factor for sexual assault, drownings, homicides, fatal falls, burns, and motor vehicle accidents.[2–4] However, substance misuse also leads to many other health

care costs because of the many associated health outcomes, including neurologic, cardiac, and liver disease; it is also associated with high-risk sexual behaviors, violence involvement, and mental health conditions, including depression, anxiety, and suicidality. In this chapter, we explore the vulnerability of women, in particular, to the health sequelae of drug and alcohol use.

Substance use places a high burden on public health and health care expenditures, both as a primary cause of visits to the ED and the trauma and other health problems that are a direct result of alcohol and drug use. The treatment needs of those with substance misuse account for an estimated average of $1,500 excess cost per hospital visit.[5] Motor vehicle collision (MVC) ED patients with positive alcohol tests have median hospital costs four times higher than MVC patients who were negative for alcohol tests.[6,7] Dischinger et al. famously followed trauma patients presenting to one center over a 14-year period and found that 35% of those who tested positive for alcohol or drugs subsequently died from a traumatic injury, compared to 15% of those who tested negative.[8]

The hope that patients will receive substance use interventions or referrals to treatment on their own or through primary care is overly optimistic: Rockett et al. found that 27% of patients in the ED had unmet substance use treatment needs.[5] Given the high utilization of the ED for health care in the United States and the lack of availability of primary care, the visit represents an opportunity to reach a large proportion of the population to intervene in these high-risk health behaviors. The most opportune moments for screening and interventions for substance use disorders may well be within the scope of emergency medicine practice. Whether gender-specific interventions may increase their effectiveness is an important questions for emerging research.

Screening and Brief Interventions and Referral to Treatment in the ED

ED screening, brief intervention, and referral to treatment (SBIRT) have been studied for more than 25 years and have been implemented in ED practice in a few institutions.[9,10] Evidence of effectiveness for reducing primary outcomes of substance use has been mixed, with both positive and negative results and modest effect sizes.[11] There are many potential explanations for this finding, including the possibility that the observed effect is blunted by the improvement in the control arms of alcohol and drug brief intervention studies, a phenomenon known as "assessment reactivity."[12] However, ED alcohol and drug interventions have inherent limitations: They are performed on patients who have no preexisting relationship with their providers and with little opportunity for clinical follow-up or longitudinal care to assist in maintenance of abstinence from alcohol or drug use. Only very brief, single-session interventions are possible, and these typically occur in the context of other acute health problems. The ED population faces many barriers to timely follow-up for substance use treatment, including lack of availability of substance use treatment services and their cost. Researchers have sought to augment the success of SBIRT within these confines. For example, some researchers have added a telephone "booster" session that occurs one or two weeks after the initial ED visit that reinforces change goals and provides additional counseling and support.[13–15]

Another possible explanation for the limited success of SBIRT is that the one-size-fits-all approach taken in these brief interventions to date may be improved by tailoring based on important, basic patient characteristics, including demographic factors or comorbidities. Could gender-specific screening and interventions improve the effectiveness of ED SBIRT programs? Given the many ways in which substance use differs between men and women, greater gender specificity could be another avenue for increasing engagement and effectiveness within the

limitations inherent to the emergency practice setting. In this chapter, we discuss how substance use differs between men and women, how this might lead to differential presentations to the ED, and the gender clinical considerations that may be relevant to acute care practice and future interventions.

Gender-Specific Substance Use Prevalence and Factors Related to Use

Alcohol Use

While a higher proportion of men than women have substance use problems in the general population, recent trends suggest that this gender gap is narrowing for all types of risky drinking, including binge drinking, abuse, and dependence.[16] Also concerning is the prevalence of alcohol use among pregnant women: In the 2011–2012 National Study on Drug Use and Health, 8.5% of pregnant women reported current alcohol use, 2.7% reported binge drinking, and 0.3% reported heavy drinking.[17]

Research in non-ED settings suggests gender differences in almost every aspect of substance use, from initiation to progression to addiction to development of health sequelae to reasons for cessation. Men are more likely than women to report drinking to escape or to cope with stress. Men also have higher "positive expectancies" about alcohol, meaning that they attribute positive qualities to ingestion of alcohol, including that it will reduce tension, increase social or physical pleasure, and facilitate social interactions.[18] In contrast to these positive expectancies, women have been described as having concerns that alcohol will interfere with their ability to handle difficult situations well and, therefore, may avoid alcohol when dealing with stressful situations. Women also tend to feel more concerned about their own problem drinking[19] and to drink less as a result of social norms and stigmas around heavy alcohol use.[20] Women are more likely than men to abuse prescription drugs to improve their appearance (e.g., to help them lose weight), to use drugs or alcohol to self-treat mental health disorders, particularly depression and post-traumatic stress disorder.[21]

Another marked gender difference in substance use is the phenomenon of "telescoping," or rapid progression from initiation to dependence. Some studies suggest that women are more prone than men to telescoping;[21] if true, the ED visit may be a particularly critical opportunity to identify and intervene with female high-risk drinkers, and specific, short-term follow-up with substance use treatment resources or primary care may be most appropriate.

Drug Use

The sociocultural factors that contribute to drug use in women are different from those for men. Strong correlates of drug use for women include history of physical and sexual abuse and depression. Women also are sensitive about stigmas related to drug use, fear that they will lose their children if they divulge drug use, and are often in abusive relationships that prevent them from seeking help or changing their substance use.[22] As with alcohol, some studies have shown that females may be at increased risk of abuse of both licit and illicit substances compared to males, demonstrate telescoping to addiction, and have higher risk of relapse following abstinence.[23] Female drug users face similar specific barriers to seeking substance use treatment services that can reduce the practical utility of referrals from the ED.

In certain subgroups of drug users, gender differences are more marked. For example, among prisoners, women use drugs more frequently, tend to use harder drugs, and use them for different reasons than men.[24–26] Women prisoners with substance use problems are more often poor, uninsured, and have multiple children, and they face complex mental and physical health problems, have unstable housing, and have had little education and fewer employment opportunities.[27,28] While male prisoners are more likely to enter substance use treatment programs, they are also more likely to reenter the criminal justice system and more likely to have antisocial personality disorders.

Although nonmedical use of prescription opioids is still more common among men, the recent rise in fatal prescription opioid overdoses in women has been alarming: Deaths among women have increased by 400% since 1999, compared to 265% among men. Furthermore, rates of presentation to the ED involving opioids are high

and similar between men and women.[29] Multiple studies have described differences between men and women in reasons for using and patterns of opioids use.[30] Men report using opioids more often for recreational reasons, whereas women tend to describe using them to help them cope with negative affective states or personal stressors and are also more likely to use other prescription medications (including hallucinogens), potentially to enhance the therapeutic effect of prescription opioids.[30–32] Prescribing biases may also be playing a role in the gender disparities: Women are more likely than men to be prescribed prescription pain medications, are given higher doses, and use them for longer time periods than men,[33] factors that may be responsible for the rapid rise of opioid-related deaths among women.

Alcohol and Drug Metabolism and Clinical Consequences of Substance Use

Alcohol

The definition of at-risk alcohol use is different based on gender: For men, at-risk alcohol use is defined as more than 4 drinks at one time or 14 drinks within a week; for women and those over age 65, at-risk drinking is defined as more than 3 drinks at one time or 7 drinks within a week.[34] These gender-specific criteria reflect the impact of gender on susceptibility to negative health consequences of alcohol: At equivalent amounts of consumption, women reach higher serum concentrations of alcohol and are more vulnerable to liver disease, cognitive impairment, and relative risk of fatality in motor vehicle collisions;[35] therefore, evaluating patients based on their consumption can underestimate their risk for morbidity and mortality, particularly in women. Women also demonstrate higher-risk sexual activities during binge drinking.[36]

Regular alcohol use increases women's risk of certain medical conditions including breast cancer.[37] Prenatal alcohol exposure leads to a range of neurodevelopmental problems, including fetal alcohol spectrum disorders (FASD). Nearly 1 in 10 children born in the United States have some form of FASD.[38] Other risks include low birth weight and early term labor. Less well recognized is the effect of alcohol on male fertility: Alcohol leads to poor sperm quality and quantity and lower fertilization rates, likely through direct effects on the testicles and a central effect on male hormones.[39]

Drug Use

Sex-related differences have been identified at every step of drug ingestion and metabolism, including gastric absorption, plasma blood levels (for given amount of use), hepatic and renal excretion, drug sensitivity, drug toxicity, and side effects.[40] Overall, these parameters conspire to make female patients more susceptible to the adverse effects of drugs. For example, women have a higher incidence of drug-induced hepatic failure[41] and experience two-thirds of all cases of drug-induced torsades de pointes.[42,43]

Although some of the differences in patterns of use mentioned earlier are likely related to cultural and societal norms, neuroendocrine differences likely play a role as well.[44,45] For example, dopamine neurotransmission, intimately involved in reinforcing behaviors and drug craving, is different between genders and may be partially explained by hormonal differences: Estrogen mediates enhancement of dopaminergic transmission, whereas progestins have been shown to block reinforcing and other behavioral effects of cocaine in animal models.

Differences in Screening, Response to Treatment, and Clinical Outcomes

Provider biases may affect the identification of substance use problems among women: Beasley et al. found that women trauma patients were less likely than male patients to receive blood alcohol or drug screening.[46] Women are more sensitive to social perceptions and stigma against problem drinking; this may translate into reduced reporting during screening by gender.

Gender also affects treatment for substance use disorders.[19–21] Women are less likely than men to seek substance abuse treatment, tend to seek treatment later, have more severe problems on entry, and have lower rates of completion of substance use treatments.[22] They report specific barriers to accessing and completing treatments, including negative stereotypes about those seeking services, lack of awareness of treatment options, concerns about childcare, fears of the time and financial costs of residential treatment, and concerns about the confrontational models used by some treatment services. A substance user at home is a risk factor for resuming substance use for women.[47] Other barriers include lack of available treatment spots, transportation, and services for pregnant women.[48] Single-gender programs and those with childcare services have demonstrated dramatic improvements in treatment retention for women, but these have limited availability.[49]

Specific factors appear to impact men's success in completing treatments and entering and maintaining recovery. Men are more likely than women to transition from recovery to using and to change status in the recovery cycle in general; they are more likely to have criminal justice involvement in the years following substance use treatment; and they are more likely to transition to recovery based on the amount of treatment received yet are less responsive than women to self-help treatments.[47,50]

There is some evidence that women and men respond differently to existing brief intervention protocols, which are most directly relevant to acute care and emergency medicine. For example, one large multicenter trial of SBIRT for drugs and alcohol in both primary care and hospital settings demonstrated increased abstinence across sites and substance types; however, in one of the two sites that included EDs, only men reduced cocaine use after the intervention.[51] Among adolescents in the ED, SBIRT has demonstrated efficacy for decreasing drug use; in two studies, that effect was greater in males compared to females.[14,52] However, gender differences have not been the stated purpose of most ED drug intervention studies, meaning they are usually underpowered to examine differences between genders or to examine potential interaction effects involving gender. Furthermore, it remains unclear what effect abstinence or reduced consumption has on patient-centered outcomes by gender.

Interventions have been designed for specific subpopulations within gender (e.g., pregnant women, those with PTSD). However, these have not been studied in the ED setting. Many models for incorporating gender-specific approaches have been suggested, including addressing intimate partner violence (IPV), PTSD, or eating disorders along with substance use interventions for women or using gender-specific approaches to address sexual risk behaviors or HIV testing with substance use interventions. How to prioritize and address high-risk behaviors or conditions associated with substance use by gender remains unanswered. However, many gender-sensitive interventions almost universally share certain qualities. These include (a) an acknowledgment of the high prevalence of violence involvement among those who use alcohol or drugs (in particular, peer violence for men and intimate partner violence for women; partner abuse among women), and the fact that partner abuse victimization may serve as a barrier to accessing services and making behavior change; (b) consideration of mental health problems common among women with alcohol and drug use, including PTSD and depression, and concurrent needs for general mental health services; (c) consideration of pregnancy and dependent children, which may prevent women from divulging drug use, accessing treatment services, and successfully completing treatments. For now, common sense dictates that clinicians take special care to screen for substance use problems among vulnerable populations, including those involved in violence, pregnant women, and those with mental health disorders.

Limited evidence supports gender-specific approaches to substance use. Houry et al. provided community resources to African American women based on results of a screening survey conducted in the triage area of an urban ED that covered a wide range of health topics, including IPV and alcohol and drug use, and found greater use of resources and reduced risk behaviors.[53] Choo et al. developed a Web-based intervention for women with drug use incorporating content related to coexisting IPV that demonstrated acceptability and feasibility in the ED.[54] Among adolescents, there is evidence that interventions should be tailored by gender, as well as by substance use and violence involvement.[55]

Although women have increased susceptibility to alcohol-related medical conditions, this also is likely to translate to meaningful gender-specific differences in patient-centered outcomes. Peters et al. found that women alcohol misusers reported decreased scores on nearly all parameters of quality of life.[56] These clinical consequences of alcohol and drug use can guide clinical care for the emergency provider, including guidance on counseling patients on specific, relevant health risks of substance use within a structured brief bedside intervention.

Gender and ED Health Services Utilization

Motor Vehicle Collisions

Both alcohol and drug use confer high risk for motor vehicle–related mortality. Men are much more likely to drive under the influence of alcohol,[57] which is explained by increased risk taking by men and different gender perceptions of social acceptability; men are more accepting of driving after drinking alcohol.[58] However, for a given level of alcohol use, women are at higher risk for injury from motor vehicle collisions.[57]

Few studies have examined the risk of MVC conferred by individual drugs. One study of statewide California data found that all types of drug use – amphetamines, cocaine, marijuana, opioids, and polydrug use –led to elevated risk of MVC deaths. However, the risk for death was highest among males for all drug categories; in the cannabis group, the standardized mortality risk for males was more than twice that of females.[59] Young male drivers have been observed to increase risk-taking behaviors,[60] and male drivers more often report being injured while driving under the influence of drugs.[61] Men are also at high risk of riding with an intoxicated driver, a behavior that is mediated by greater sensation seeking, perceived peer pressure, and frequent harmful drinking.[62]

Violence

Those with involvement in violence are more likely to present to the ED with a positive blood alcohol level, to report drinking prior to the event, to report heavy drinking more often, and to report more alcohol-related problems than patients with injuries not related to alcohol.[63] The relationship between alcohol and drug use and violence appears to differ between genders.[64–66] Among men, alcohol use has an association with perpetration of several types of violence, including violence in pursuit of profit-based goals, violence in pursuit of social dominance goals, and violence as a response to perceived threat.[67] In men, alcohol use often precipitates injury from fights or assault,[68] and this is a consistent finding across many different cultures and geographic locations.[65]

While intimate partner abuse affects both men and women of all ages, females have a higher incidence and are more likely to be injured from the abuse.[69] Alcohol and drug use is virtually inseparable from partner abuse among women presenting to the ED. Studies in this setting have consistently reported rates of substance use among partner abuse victims that far exceed those of the general population, ranging from 19% to 64% for alcohol use.[11,15] In women, it is likely that this relationship is bidirectional, with violence leading to increased alcohol use, and alcohol use a predisposing factor for the occurrence of violence. Drug use is also closely associated with partner abuse: Rhodes et al. reported that 13% of partner abuse victims in an urban hospital used illicit drugs in the past month[70]; Grisso et al. found cocaine use in 26% of partner abuse victims.[71] In substance abuse treatment programs, histories of lifetime IPV are so common[16–18] that the Substance Abuse and Mental Health Services Administration (SAMHSA) has recommended that women with substance use problems uniformly receive trauma-informed care.[19] Such interventions have demonstrated effectiveness but have not yet been implemented in the context of a single, brief intervention or in the emergency care setting.

There is a paucity of literature describing the relationship between substance use and non-partner violence among women, although it is important to note that in ED populations, women, as well as men, report a high prevalence of involvement in non-partner violence,[72,73] that both men and women report victimization and perpetration[74–77], and that substance abuse is associated with partner violence for both men and women.[74]

Sexual Assault

The incidence of sexual assault that involves alcohol or drugs (whether intentionally taken by the victim or surreptitiously administered) is difficult to determine accurately, because sexual assault is often unreported, victims who do present are not always tested for the presence of drug or alcohol, substance use is underreported, and information on the perpetrator is rarely available.[78] However, the data that are available have long implicated a strong role for alcohol and other drugs in the occurrence of sexual assault. Depending on the sample studied and the measures used, estimates for alcohol use among perpetrators are as high as 74% among perpetrators and as high as 30% to 79% among victims.[78,79] Illicit drug use, whether alone or in combination with alcohol, has been detected in 19% to 34% of victims.[80–83] Female binge drinkers are three times more likely than female non-binge drinkers to be victims of sexual assault; 50% of adolescent girls reporting sexual assault are under the influence of alcohol or another psychotropic substance at the time of the event.[84,85]

Substance Use Contributing to Falls in the Elderly

The U.S. census projects a doubling of the population of elders, age 65 and older between 2012 and 2060, from 43.1 million to 92.0 million.[86] As the U.S. population ages, fall-related injuries will increase,[87,88] and these injuries will be associated with significant health consequences and health care costs.[89] Sex and gender have a role in fall morbidity and mortality: Controlling for age, the death rate attributed to falls is 34% higher in men than women;[90] however, women are more likely to sustain serious injury that is debilitating, leads to medical care and loss of function and independence, and is complicated by other health conditions.[91,92] As with injury in the general population, injury and fatality from falls among the elderly is increased by alcohol consumption.[93] The current National Institute on Alcohol Abuse and Alcoholism (NIAAA) definition of high-risk drinking acknowledges that advanced age confers risk for alcohol-related health consequences, defining risky drinking in both men and women over age 65 at the same level as for women younger than age 65: greater than seven drinks/week or greater three drinks per occasion.[34] It is not clear whether this is a sufficiently safe parameter or if parameters for the elderly should be further stratified by gender. Fall risk in the elderly is also increased by medications, particularly psychoactive drugs, even when taken as prescribed.[94,95]

Some elderly patients presenting after injuries from falls will have undetected elder abuse. The group at highest risk for elder abuse are those with psychiatric and substance abuse problems, and those whose caregivers also have either psychiatric disease or abuse substances or both.[96] EDs are just beginning to ask routinely about smoking and alcohol and drug use by the patient; it is less common to ask about the behavioral characteristics of the caregivers of the elderly. The precise relationship that exists between high-risk alcohol drinking in the elderly, the presence of mental health problems, and the occurrence of elder abuse is poorly defined; however, all of these interactions potentiate fall risk.

Mental Health Comorbidities

Mental health problems are common and related to drug and alcohol use in both men and women, although depression is more strongly associated with high-risk drinking in women. However, some theorize that men are more likely to engage in heavy drinking as part of avoidant coping behaviors, and that heavy drinking masks depression in men, who may be more reluctant than women to report depressive symptoms (creating the appearance of greater depression in women).[19]

Gender differences in ED Patients Who Are Chronically Intoxicated

The vast majority of chronic inebriates, who are frequent users of the ED and other medical resources, are men, suggesting a gender component to the health risk factors, progression of substance use and mental illness, and social service needs of this population.[97] The most common injuries found (often incidentally) are intracranial and facial injuries; the most frequent illnesses requiring therapy are gastritis, mild dehydration, and hypothermia.[98] Relatively little is known about this population, but care for these "superutilizers" with complex health care needs complicated by chronic substance abuse is gaining attention in the context of the need for health care cost-containment strategies.[99]

Treatment Implications

A gender-specific approach may increase the specificity of interventions for alcohol and drug use and allow the ED to better acknowledge and address different experiences of negative consequences, different motivations to use, and different factors contributing to success of treatments. What does gender-specific substance use treatment mean? For women, a gender-specific approach would mean inclusion of childcare or other caretaking needs, incorporation of risks and resource needs related to intimate partner abuse, acknowledgment of trauma from childhood or past abuse, and treatment for co-occurring mental health disorders. For men, such an approach might mean gender-sensitive screening for specific types of violence involvement or HIV risk behaviors. Such gender-specific treatments have been emerging in the outpatient setting.[25] For example, National Institute on Drug Abuse (NIDA)'s National Drug Abuse Clinical Trials Network (CTN)'s gender-specific research group reviewed CTN studies that addressed gender: Thus far, the network has examined gender-specific needs around substance use and eating disorders, PTSD, sexual risk behaviors, and pregnancy.[100] Outcomes in these studies have largely been positive. Additional research is needed to determine the applicability, feasibility, and effectiveness of such approaches in the ED setting.

Among pregnant patients, clinicians should not assume abstinence and fail to perform substance use screening; this is a time when it is more crucial than ever to capture and treat substance use. Pregnant women with substance use problems generally have less prenatal care[101] and will require specialized clinical services – often high-risk obstetric services and high-intensity substance use treatments – throughout their pregnancy. Because an ED visit may indicate that patients do not have a primary obstetrician – for example, because they may be in transition between geographic locations, have unstable housing, or limited access to routine health care, this is a particularly important population in which to identify substance use and supply active referrals that will increase the chance of a healthy pregnancy and newborn. Clinicians should also be aware that some states have mandatory reporting of substance use during pregnancy.[102]

Until gender-specific programs are readily available, however, clinicians may focus on a practical approach to substance use that takes into account key gender differences:

1. Determination of high-risk drinking should use age-correlated gender-specific thresholds.

2. Men and women with drug or alcohol use problems should be screened for partner abuse, elder abuse, and mental health problems requiring immediate intervention or expedited follow-up.
3. All pregnant women should be screened for alcohol and drug use.
4. Clinicians should consider gender-specific factors that may influence likelihood of successful follow-up with treatment services.

A positive screen should prompt appropriate resources (such as counseling by social workers) in accordance with the institutional practice, and referral of patients to inpatient or outpatient substance use treatment. Clinicians should consider if provided referrals are feasible or if the patient has any barriers to accessing services. Whenever possible, facilities that offer single-gender treatment and childcare services should be offered.

Conclusion

There is strong evidence for gender differences in every aspect of substance use, including motivations for use, clinical consequences of use, motivations for changing drug and alcohol use, treatment needs, and barriers to treatment (Table 4.1). However, much remains to be learned about the relationship between gender and substance use, particularly in subgroups of age and specific high-risk behaviors. Researchers are just beginning to understand the impact of gender on substance use and its sequelae among patients in the emergency care setting and to use this knowledge toward meaningful improvements in clinical care. Emerging investigations on the efficacy of brief interventions for substance use disorders with content tailored by gender may mean these will be available to address the existing gaps in knowledge to better guide clinical practice in the future. In the meantime, clinicians must be aware of gender-specific differences in screening guidelines, vulnerability to the adverse consequences of drugs and alcohol, and barriers to follow-up.

Clinical Case Follow-Up

The treating provider recognized high-risk alcohol use, based on both her female gender and her pregnancy status; a full assessment of her drinking patterns did not suggest alcohol dependence. Further discussion with the patient identified that she was motivated to stop drinking, particularly given the news of her pregnancy, but she

Table 4.1 Example of Gender Differences in Substance Use Disorders

Definitions of High-Risk Alcohol Use	Men: >4 drinks at one time = binge drinking, 14 drinks within 1 week Women (& those > 65): >3 drinks at one time = binge drinking, 7 drinks within 1 week
Adverse Effects of Drug and Alcohol Use	Men: Alcohol impairs male fertility through effect on sperm and testosterone. Women: Alcohol confers risk on developing fetus. Higher incidence of drug-induced hepatic failure and drug-induced torsades de pointes.
Prevalence / Patterns of Use	Men: Prevalence higher for alcohol and most drugs. Women: Fatal prescription opioid overdoses increasing rapidly. Telescoping more evident in women.
Motivations / Deterrents of Use	Men: More positive expectancies around alcohol and drug use. Women: More negative expectances; more sensitivity to social stigma.
High-Risk Behaviors	Men: More likely to drive under the influence of alcohol or drugs; risk of MVC fatality while intoxicated higher. Women: More likely to exhibit high-risk sexual behaviors when under the influence.
Screening Issues	Men: May be less likely to report associated mental health illness. Women: Provider biases likely underestimate prevalence of drug and alcohol use.
Barriers to Treatment	Men: More likely to interact with the criminal justice system; less responsive to self-help programs. Women: Lack of childcare and mixed-gender facilities adversely affect treatment completion.

feared losing her job if she needed to go into inpatient treatment. She expressed anxiety over the reaction from her live-in boyfriend if she decided to stop drinking alcohol, as this was their nightly activity together and he was controlling and frequently verbally abusive. Although she did not wish to leave her boyfriend, she was receptive to contacting domestic violence community organizations to receive counseling. The ED nurse identified a substance use treatment clinic at an adjoining hospital that provided free programs for pregnant women with drug or alcohol problems during daytime hours. The patient expressed interest in attending and was relieved that she would not have to be admitted.

References

1. Sanjuan PM, Rice SL, Witkiewitz K, Mandler RN, Crandall C, Bogenschutz MP. Alcohol, tobacco, and drug use among emergency department patients. *Drug Alcohol Dependence.* 2014. doi:10.1016/j.drugalcdep.2014.01.025.

2. Levy DT, Mallonee S, Miller TR et al. Alcohol involvement in burn, submersion, spinal cord, and brain injuries. *Medical Science Monitor* 2004; 10(1):CR17–24. Available at www.ncbi.nlm.nih.gov/pubmed/14704631. Accessed July 3, 2014.

3. Hingson R, Howland J. Alcohol and non-traffic unintended injuries. *Addiction* 1993; 88(7):877–83. Available at www.ncbi.nlm.nih.gov/pubmed/8358259. Accessed July 3, 2014.

4. Smith GS, Branas CC, Miller TR. Fatal nontraffic injuries involving alcohol: A metaanalysis. *Annals of Emergency Medicine* 1999; 33(6):659–68. Available at www.ncbi.nlm.nih.gov/pubmed/10339681. Accessed July 3, 2014.

5. Rockett IRH, Putnam SL, Jia H, Chang CF, Smith GS. Unmet substance abuse treatment need, health services utilization, and cost: A population-based emergency department study. *Annals of Emergency Medicine* 2005; 45(2):118–27. doi:10.1016/j.annemergmed.2004.08.003.

6. Maio RF, Waller PF, Blow FC, Hill EM, Singer KM. Alcohol abuse/dependence in motor vehicle crash victims presenting to the emergency department. *Academy of Emergency Medicine* 1997; 4(4):256–62. Available at www.ncbi.nlm.nih.gov/pubmed/9107322. Accessed February 19, 2014.

7. Lee MH, Mello MJ, Reinert S. Emergency department charges for evaluating minimally injured alcohol-impaired drivers. *Annals of Emergency Medicine* 2009; 54(4):593–99. doi:10.1016/j.annemergmed.2009.05.018.

8. Dischinger PC, Mitchell KA, Kufera JA, Soderstrom CA, Lowenfels AB. A longitudinal study of former trauma center patients: The association between toxicology status and subsequent injury mortality. *Journal of Trauma* 2001; 51(5):877–84; discussion 884–86. Available at www.ncbi.nlm.nih.gov/pubmed/11706334. Accessed February 19, 2014.

9. D'Onofrio G, Degutis LC. Integrating Project ASSERT: A screening, intervention, and referral to treatment program for unhealthy alcohol and drug use into an urban emergency department. *Academy of Emergency Medicine* 2010; 17(8):903–11. doi:10.1111/j.1553-2712.2010.00824.x.

10. Bernstein E, Bernstein J, Levenson S. Project ASSERT: An ED-based intervention to increase access to primary care, preventive services, and the substance abuse treatment system. *Annals of Emergency Medicine* 1997; 30(2):181–89. Available at www.ncbi.nlm.nih.gov/pubmed/9250643. Accessed November 14, 2012.

11. Bernstein E, Bernstein JA, Stein JB, Saitz R. SBIRT in emergency care settings: Are we ready to take it to scale? *Academy of Emergency Medicine* 2009; 16(11):1072–77. doi:10.1111/j.1553-2712.2009.00549.x.

12. Walters ST, Vader AM, Harris TR, Jouriles EN. Reactivity to alcohol assessment measures: An experimental test. *Addiction* 2009; 104(8):1305–10. doi:10.1111/j.1360-0443.2009.02632.x.

13. Mello MJ, Longabaugh R, Baird J, Nirenberg T, Woolard R. DIAL: A telephone brief intervention for high-risk alcohol use with injured emergency department patients. *Annals of Emergency Medicine* 2008; 51(6):755–64. doi:10.1016/j.annemergmed.2007.11.034.

14. Bernstein E, Edwards E, Dorfman D, Heeren T, Bliss C, Bernstein J. Screening and brief intervention to reduce marijuana use among youth and young adults in a pediatric emergency department. *Academy of Emergency Medicine* 2009; 16(11):1174–85. doi:10.1111/j.1553-2712.2009.00490.x.

15. D'Onofrio G, Fiellin DA, Pantalon MV et al. A brief intervention reduces hazardous and harmful drinking in emergency department patients. *Annals of Emergency Medicine* 2012. doi:10.1016/j.annemergmed.2012.02.006.

16. Keyes KM, Grant BF, Hasin DS. Evidence for a closing gender gap in alcohol use, abuse, and dependence in the United States population. *Drug and Alcohol Dependence Journal* 2008; 93(1–2):21–29. doi:10.1016/j.drugalcdep.2007.08.017.

17. Substance Abuse and Mental Health Services Administration. *Results from the 2012 National Survey on Drug Use and Health: Summary of National Findings, NSDUH Series H-46, HHS Publication No. (SMA) 13-4795*. Rockville, MD: Author, 2013.

18. Nolen-Hoeksema S, Hilt L. Possible contributors to the gender differences in alcohol use and problems. *Journal of General Psychology* 2006; **133**(4):357–74. doi:10.3200/GENP.133.4.357-374.

19. Nolen-Hoeksema S. Gender differences in risk factors and consequences for alcohol use and problems. *Clinical Psychology Rev* 2004; **24**(8):981–1010. doi:10.1016/j.cpr.2004.08.003.

20. DeVisser RO, McDonnell EJ. "That's OK. He's a guy": A mixed-methods study of gender double-standards for alcohol use. *Psychological Health* 2012; **27**(5):618–39. doi:10.1080/08870446.2011 .617444.

21. Brady KT, Randall CL. Gender differences in substance use disorders. *Psychiatric Clinics of North America* 1999; **22**(2):241–52. Available at www.ncbi.nlm.nih.gov/pubmed/10385931. Accessed January 24, 2012.

22. Coletti S. *Service Providers and Treatment Access Issues. Drug Addiction Research and the Health of Women. NIH Publication No. 98-4290*. Rockville, MD; 1998:236–44.

23. Becker JB, Hu M. Sex differences in drug abuse. *Frontiers in Neuroendocrinology* 2008; **29**(1):36–47. doi:10.1016/j.yfrne.2007.07.003.

24. Kissin WB, Tang Z, Campbell KM, Claus RE, Orwin RG. Gender-sensitive substance abuse treatment and arrest outcomes for women. *Journal of Substance Abuse Treatment* 2014; **46**(3):332–39. doi:10.1016/j.jsat.2013.09.005.

25. Langan NP, Pelissier BM. Gender differences among prisoners in drug treatment. *Journal of Substance Abuse* 2001; **13**(3):291–301. Available at www.ncbi.nlm.nih.gov/pubmed/11693453. Accessed March 10, 2014.

26. Messina N, Burdon W, Hagopian G, Prendergast M. Predictors of prison-based treatment outcomes: A comparison of men and women participants. *American Journal of Drug and Alcohol Abuse* 2006; **32**(1):7–28. Available at www.ncbi.nlm.nih.gov/pubmed/16450640. Accessed March 10, 2014.

27. O'Brien P. *Making It a Free World: Women in Transition from Prison*. Albany: State University of New York Press; 2001:220.

28. Binswanger IA, Merrill JO, Krueger PM, White MC, Booth RE, Elmore JG. Gender differences in chronic medical, psychiatric, and substance-dependence disorders among jail inmates. *American Journal of Public Health* 2010; **100**(3):476–82. doi:10.2105/AJPH.2008.149591.

29. Choo E, Douriez C, Green T. Gender and Prescription Opioid Misuse in the Emergency Department. *Academy of Emergency Medicine* 2014; **21**(12):1493–98.

30. Back SE, Payne RL, Simpson AN, Brady KT. Gender and prescription opioids: Findings from the National Survey on Drug Use and Health. *Addictive Behaviors* 2010; **35**(11):1001–7. doi:10.1016/j.addbeh.2010.06.018.

31. Jamison RN, Butler SF, Budman SH, Edwards RR, Wasan AD. Gender differences in risk factors for aberrant prescription opioid use. *The Journal of Pain* 2010; **11**(4):312–20. doi:10.1016/j.jpain .2009.07.016.

32. Green TC, Grimes Serrano JM, Licari A, Budman SH, Butler SF. Women who abuse prescription opioids: Findings from the Addiction Severity Index – Multimedia Version Connect prescription opioid database. *Drug and Alcohol Dependence* 2009; **103**(1–2):65–73. doi:10.1016/j. drugalcdep.2009.03.014.

33. CDC. Vital signs: Overdoses of prescription opioid pain relievers – United States, 1999–2008. *Morbidity and Mortality Weekly Report* 2011:1–6.

34. National Institute on Alcohol Abuse and Alcoholism (NIAAA). Moderate and binge drinking. n.d. Available at www.niaaa.nih.gov/alc ohol-health/overview-alcohol-consumption/mod erate-binge-drinking. Accessed June 5, 2013.

35. NIAAA. Alcohol Alert: Are women more vulnerable to alcohol's effects? 1999. Available at http://pubs.niaaa.nih.gov/publications/aa46.htm. Accessed May 5, 2012.

36. Hutton HE, McCaul ME, Santora PB, Erbelding EJ. The relationship between recent alcohol use and sexual behaviors: Gender differences among sexually transmitted disease clinic patients. *Alcoholism: Clinical and Experimental Research* 2008; **32**(11):2008–15. doi:10.1111/j.1530-0277.2008.00788.x.

37. Longnecker M. Alcoholic beverage consumption in relation to risk of breast cancer: Meta-analysis and review. *Cancer Causes Control* 1994; **5**:73–82.

38. Bailey BA, Sokol RJ. Pregnancy and alcohol use: Evidence and recommendations for prenatal care. *Clinical Obstetrics and Gynecology* 2008; **51**(2):436–44. doi:10.1097/GRF.0b013e31816fea3d.

39. La Vignera S, Condorelli RA, Balercia G, Vicari E, Calogero AE. Does alcohol have any effect on male reproductive function? A review of literature.

Asian Journal of Andrology 2013; **15**(2):221–25. doi:10.1038/aja.2012.118.

40. Marazziti D, Baroni S, Picchetti M et al. Pharmacokinetics and pharmacodynamics of psychotropic drugs: Effect of sex. *CNS Spectrums* 2013; **18**(3):118–27. doi:10.1017/S109285291 2001010.

41. Amacher DE. Female gender as a susceptibility factor for drug-induced liver injury. *Human and Experimental Toxicology* 2013; **33**(9):928–39. doi:10.1177/0960327113512860.

42. Fanoe S, Jensen GB, Sjøgren P, Korsgaard MPG, Grunnet M. Oxycodone is associated with dose-dependent QTc prolongation in patients and low-affinity inhibiting of hERG activity in vitro. *British Journal of Clinical Pharmacology* 2009; **67**(2):172–79. doi:10.1111/j.1365–2125.2008 .03327.x.

43. Coker SJ. Drugs for men and women – how important is gender as a risk factor for TdP? *Pharmacology and Therapeutics* 2008; **119**(2):186–94. doi:10.1016/j.pharmthera.2008.03 .005.

44. Carroll ME, Lynch WJ, Roth ME, Morgan AD, Cosgrove KP. Sex and estrogen influence drug abuse. *Trends in Pharmacolical Sciences* 2004; **25**(5):273–79. doi:10.1016/j.tips.2004.03.011.

45. Roth ME, Cosgrove KP, Carroll ME. Sex differences in the vulnerability to drug abuse: A review of preclinical studies. *Neuroscience and Biobehavioral Reviews* 2004; **28**(6):533–46. doi:10.1016/j.neubiorev.2004.08.001.

46. Beasley GM, Ostbye T, Muhlbaier LH et al. Age and gender differences in substance screening may underestimate injury severity: A study of 9793 patients at level 1 trauma center from 2006 to 2010. *Journal of Surgical Research* 2013; **188**:190–97. doi:10.1016/j.jss.2013.11.1103.

47. Grella CE, Scott CK, Foss MA, Dennis ML. Gender similarities and differences in the treatment, relapse, and recovery cycle. *Evaluation Review* 2008; **32**(1):113–37. doi:10.1177/0193841X 07307318.

48. Gehshan S. *A Step Toward Recovery: Improving Access to Substance Abuse Treatment for Pregnant Women. Southern Regional Project on Infant Mortality*. Washington, DC; Abuse and Mental Health Services Admin (SAMHSA), US Dept of Health and Human Services, 1993.

49. Grella CE, Greenwell L. Treatment needs and completion of community-based aftercare among substance-abusing women offenders. *Womens Health Issues*; **17**(4):244–55. doi:10.1016/j.whi .2006.11.005.

50. Grella CE, Scott CK, Foss MA. Gender differences in long-term drug treatment outcomes in Chicago PETS. *Journal of Substance Abuse Treatment* 2005; **28** Suppl 1:S3–12. doi:10.1016/j.jsat.2004.08.008.

51. Madras BK, Compton WM, Avula D, Stegbauer T, Stein JB, Clark HW. Screening, brief interventions, referral to treatment (SBIRT) for illicit drug and alcohol use at multiple healthcare sites: Comparison at intake and 6 months later. *Drug and Alcohol Dependence* 2009; **99**(1–3):280–95. doi:10.1016/j.drugalcdep.2008.08.003.

52. Tait RJ, Hulse GK, Robertson SI, Sprivulis PC. Emergency department-based intervention with adolescent substance users: 12-month outcomes. *Drug and Alcohol Dependence* 2005; **79**(3):359–63. doi:10.1016/j.drugalcdep.2005.03.015.

53. Houry D, Hankin A, Daugherty J, Smith LS, Kaslow N. Effect of a targeted women's health intervention in an inner-city emergency department. *Emergency Medicine International* 2011:543493. doi:10.1155/2011/543493.

54. Choo EK, Zlotnick C, Strong DR, Squires DD, Tapé C, Mello MJ. *B-SAFER: A Web-Based Intervention for Drug Use and Intimate Partner Violence Demonstrates Feasibility and Acceptability Among Women in the Emergency Department.* Accepted by Substance Abuse, November 2015, in press.

55. Epstein-Ngo QM, Walton MA, Chermack ST, Blow FC, Zimmerman MA, Cunningham RM. Event-level analysis of antecedents for youth violence: Comparison of dating violence with non-dating violence. *Addictive Behaviors* 2014; **39**(1):350–53. doi:10.1016/j.addbeh.2013.10.015.

56. Peters EN, Khondkaryan E, Sullivan TP. Associations between expectancies of alcohol and drug use, severity of partner violence, and posttraumatic stress among women. *Journal of Interpersonal Violence* 2012. doi:10.1177/ 0886260511432151.

57. Zador PL. Alcohol-related relative risk of fatal driver injuries in relation to driver age and sex. *Journal of Studies on Alcohol and Drugs* 1991; **52**(4):302–10. Available at www.ncbi.nlm.nih.gov/ pubmed/1875701. Accessed March 26, 2014.

58. Greenfield TK, Room R. Situational norms for drinking and drunkenness: Trends in the US adult population, 1979–1990. *Addiction* 1997; **92**(1):33–47. Available at www.ncbi.nlm.nih.gov/ pubmed/9060196. Accessed March 26, 2014.

59. Callaghan RC, Gatley JM, Veldhuizen S, Lev-Ran S, Mann R, Asbridge M. Alcohol- or drug-use disorders and motor vehicle accident mortality: A retrospective cohort study. *Accident Analysis &*

Prevention 2013; **53**:149–55. doi:10.1016/j.aap.2013.01.008.

60. Turner C, McClure R. Age and gender differences in risk-taking behaviour as an explanation for high incidence of motor vehicle crashes as a driver in young males. *International Journal of Injury Control and Safety Promotion* 2003; **10**(3):123–30. doi:10.1076/icsp.10.3.123.14560.

61. Darke S, Kelly E, Ross J. Drug driving among injecting drug users in Sydney, Australia: Prevalence, risk factors and risk perceptions. *Addiction* 2004; **99**(2):175–85. Available at www.ncbi.nlm.nih.gov/pubmed/14756710. Accessed March 26, 2014.

62. Kim J-H, Kim KS. The role of sensation seeking, perceived peer pressure, and harmful alcohol use in riding with an alcohol-impaired driver. *Accident Analysis & Prevention* 2012; **48**:326–34. doi:10.1016/j.aap.2012.01.033.

63. Weinsheimer RL, Schermer CR, Malcoe LH, Balduf LM, Bloomfield LA. Severe intimate partner violence and alcohol use among female trauma patients. *Journal of Trauma* 2005; **58**:22–29. doi:10.1097/01.TA.0000151180.77168.A6.

64. Walton MA, Cunningham RM, Chermack ST, Maio R, Blow FC, Weber J. Correlates of violence history among injured patients in an urban emergency department: Gender, substance use, and depression. *Journal of Addictive Diseases* 2007; **26**(3):61–75. doi:10.1300/J069v26n03_07.

65. Wells S, Thompson JM, Cherpitel C, Macdonald S, Marais S, Borges G. Gender differences in the relationship between alcohol and violent injury: An analysis of cross-national emergency department data. *Journal of Studies on Alcohol and Drugs* 2007; **68**(6):824–33. Available at www.ncbi.nlm.nih.gov/pubmed/17960300. Accessed April 8, 2012.

66. Kellermann AL, Mercy JA. Men, women, and murder: Gender-specific differences in rates of fatal violence and victimization. *Journal of Trauma* 1992; **33**(1):1–5. Available at www.ncbi.nlm.nih.gov/pubmed/1635092. Accessed April 8, 2012.

67. McMurran M, Jinks M, Howells K, Howard RC. Alcohol-related violence defined by ultimate goals: A qualitative analysis of the features of three different types of violence by intoxicated young male offenders. *Aggressive Behavior* 2010; **36**(1):67–79. doi:10.1002/ab.20331.

68. Borges G, Cherpitel CJ, Rosovsky H. Male drinking and violence-related injury in the emergency room. *Addiction* 1998; **93**(1):103–12. Available at www.ncbi.nlm.nih.gov/pubmed/9624715. Accessed April 22, 2012.

69. Breiding MJ, Black MC, Ryan GW. Prevalence and risk factors of intimate partner violence in eighteen U.S. states/territories, 2005. *American Journal of Preventive Medicine* 2008; **34**:112–18. doi:10.1016/j.amepre.2007.10.001.

70. Rhodes KV, Lauderdale DS, He T, Howes DS, Levinson W. "Between me and the computer": Increased detection of intimate partner violence using a computer questionnaire. *Annals of Emergency Medicine* 2002; **40**(5):476–84. Available at www.ncbi.nlm.nih.gov/pubmed/12399790. Accessed January 10, 2012.

71. Grisso JA, Schwarz DF, Hirschinger N et al. Violent injuries among women in an urban area. *New England Journal of Medicine* 1999; **341**(25):1899–905. doi:10.1056/NEJM199912163412506.

72. Walton M, Cunningham R, Goldstein A et al. Rates and correlates of violent behaviors among adolescents treated in an urban emergency department. *Journal of Adolescent Health* 2009; **45**(1):77–83.

73. Cunningham R, Walton MA, Maio RF, Blow FC, Weber JE, Mirel L. Violence and substance use among an injured emergency department population. *Academic Emergency Medicine* 2003; **10**(7):764–75. Available at www.ncbi.nlm.nih.gov/pubmed/12837651. Accessed March 20, 2014.

74. Walton MA, Murray R, Cunningham RM et al. Correlates of intimate partner violence among men and women in an inner city emergency department. *Journal of Addictive Diseases* 2009; **28**(4):366–81. doi:10.1080/10550880903183018.

75. Cunningham RM, Murray R, Walton MA et al. Prevalence of past year assault among inner-city emergency department patients. *Annals of Emergency Medicine* 2009; **53**(6):814–23.e15. doi:10.1016/j.annemergmed.2009.01.016.

76. Houry D, Rhodes KV, Kemball RS et al. Differences in female and male victims and perpetrators of partner violence with respect to WEB scores. *Journal of Interpersonal Violence* 2008; **23**(8):1041–55. doi:10.1177/0886260507313969.

77. Lipsky S, Caetano R. Intimate partner violence perpetration among men and emergency department use. *Journal of Emergency Medicine* 2011; **40**(6):696–703. doi:10.1016/j.jemermed.2008.04.043.

78. Abbey A, Zawacki T, Buck P, Clinton A, McAuslan P. NIAAA: Alcohol and Sexual Assault. n.d. Available at http://pubs.niaaa.nih.gov/publications/arh25-1/43–51.htm. Accessed April 14, 2014.

79. Abbey A, Ross L, McDuffie D. Alcohol's Role in Sexual Assault. In: Watson R, ed. *Drug and Alcohol Abuse Reviews. Volume 5: Addictive Behaviors in Women.* Totowa, NJ: Humana Press; 1994:97–123.

80. Hagemann CT, Helland A, Spigset O, Espnes KA, Ormstad K, Schei B. Ethanol and drug findings in women consulting a sexual assault center – associations with clinical characteristics and suspicions of drug-facilitated sexual assault. *Journal of Forensic and Legal Medicine* 2013; 20(6):777–84. doi:10.1016/j.jflm.2013.05.005.

81. Juhascik MP, Negrusz A, Faugno D et al. An estimate of the proportion of drug-facilitation of sexual assault in four U.S. localities. *Journal of Forensic Sciences* 2007; 52(6):1396–400. doi:10.1111/j.1556–4029.2007.00583.x.

82. Scott-Ham M, Burton FC. Toxicological findings in cases of alleged drug-facilitated sexual assault in the United Kingdom over a 3-year period. *Journal of Clinical Forensic Medicine* 2005; 12(4):175–86. doi:10.1016/j.jcfm.2005.03.009.

83. McGregor MJ, Lipowska M, Shah S, Du Mont J, De Siato C. An exploratory analysis of suspected drug-facilitated sexual assault seen in a hospital emergency department. *Women Health* 2003; 37(3):71–80. Available at www.ncbi.nlm.nih.gov/pubmed/12839308. Accessed July 3, 2014.

84. Stolle M, Sack P-M, Thomasius R. Binge drinking in childhood and adolescence: Epidemiology, consequences, and interventions. *Deutsches Arzteblatt International* 2009; 106(19):323–28. doi:10.3238/arztebl.2009.0323.

85. Mouilso ER, Fischer S, Calhoun KS. A prospective study of sexual assault and alcohol use among first-year college women. *Violence and Victims* 2012; 27(1):78–94. Available at www.ncbi.nlm.nih.gov/pubmed/22455186. Accessed July 3, 2014.

86. Bureau of the Census (US). Population Projections Program, Population Division, 2010 2012.

87. Englander F, Hodson TJ, Terregrossa RA. Economic dimensions of slip and fall injuries. *Journal of Forensic Science* 1996; 41(5):733–46. Available at www.ncbi.nlm.nih.gov/pubmed/8789837. Accessed July 3, 2014.

88. Peel NM, Kassulke DJ, McClure RJ. Population based study of hospitalised fall related injuries in older people. *Injury Prevention* 2002; 8(4):280–83. Available at www.pubmedcentral.nih.gov/articler ender.fcgi?artid=1756575&tool=pmcentrez&ren dertype=abstract. Accessed July 3, 2014.

89. Sterling DA, O'Connor JA, Bonadies J. Geriatric falls: Injury severity is high and disproportionate to mechanism. *Journal of Trauma* 2001; 50(1):116–19. Available at www.ncbi.nlm.nih.gov/pubmed/11231681. Accessed June 24, 2014.

90. Hornbrook MC, Stevens VJ, Wingfield DJ, Hollis JF, Greenlick MR, Ory MG. Preventing falls among community-dwelling older persons: Results from a randomized trial. *Gerontologist* 1994; 34(1):16–23. Available at www.ncbi.nlm.nih.gov/pubmed/8150304. Accessed July 8, 2014.

91. Centers for Disease Control and Prevention, National Center for Injury Prevention and Control. Web–based Injury Statistics Query and Reporting System (WISQARS). 2013. Available at www.cdc.gov/injury/wisqars/nonfatal.html. Accessed June 3, 2014.

92. Stevens JA, Sogolow ED. Gender differences for non-fatal unintentional fall related injuries among older adults. *Injury Prevention* 2005; 11(2):115–19. doi:10.1136/ip.2004.005835.

93. Sorock GS, Chen L-H, Gonzalgo SR, Baker SP. Alcohol-drinking history and fatal injury in older adults. *Alcohol* 2006; 40(3):193–99. doi:10.1016/j.alcohol.2007.01.002.

94. Gaxatte C, Faraj E, Lathuillerie O et al. Alcohol and psychotropic drugs: Risk factors for orthostatic hypotension in elderly fallers. *Journal of Human Hypertension* 2013. doi:10.1038/jhh.2013.82.

95. Onder G, Landi F, Fusco D et al. Recommendations to prescribe in complex older adults: Results of the CRIteria to assess appropriate medication use among elderly complex patients (CRIME) project. *Drugs & Aging* 2014; 31(1):33–45. doi:10.1007/s40266-013-0134-4.

96. Nelson H, Bougatsos C, Blazina I. *Screening Women for Intimate Partner Violence and Elderly and Vulnerable Adults for Abuse: Systematic Review to Update the 2004 U.S. Preventive Services Task Force Recommendation.* Rockville, MD; Agency for Healthcare Research and Quality. 2012. Available at www.ncbi.nlm.nih.gov/books/NBK97299/.

97. Thornquist L, Biros M, Olander R, Sterner S. Health care utilization of chronic inebriates. *Academic Emergency Medicine* 2002; 9(4):300–8. Available at www.ncbi.nlm.nih.gov/pubmed/11927454. Accessed March 24, 2014.

98. Biros MH. The frequency of unsuspected minor illness or injury in intoxicated patients. *Academic Emergency Medicine* 1996; 3(9):853–58. Available at www.ncbi.nlm.nih.gov/pubmed/8870757. Accessed July 3, 2014.

99. Bodenheimer T, Berry-Millett R. *Care Management for Patients with Complex Healthcare Needs* 2009. Available at http://www.rwjf.org/en/library/research/2009/12/care-management-of-patients-with-complex-health-care-needs.html.

100. Greenfield SF, Rosa C, Putnins SI et al. Gender research in the National Institute on Drug Abuse National Treatment Clinical Trials Network: A summary of findings. *The American Journal of Drug and Alcohol Abuse* 2011; **37**(5):301–12. doi:10.3109/00952990.2011.596875.

101. Funkhouser AW, Butz AM, Feng TI, McCaul ME, Rosenstein BJ. Prenatal care and drug use in pregnant women. *Drug and Alcohol Dependence* 1993; **33**(1):1–9. Available at www.ncbi.nlm.nih.gov/pubmed/8396528. Accessed February 19, 2014.

102. Jimerson SD, Musick S. Screening for substance abuse in pregnancy. *Journal of the Oklahoma State Medical Association* 2013; **106**(4):133–34. Available at www.ncbi.nlm.nih.gov/pubmed/23795524. Accessed February 19, 2014.

Sex and Gender; Pharmacology, Efficacy, Toxicity, and Toxicology

Annette Lopez and Robert G. Hendrickson

Opening Case

A 30-year-old female presents via emergency medical transport after being involved in a single-vehicle crash at 0730. She was found by police restrained, resting her head on the steering wheel while her car rested in a ditch. When awoken, she appeared to be in a dreamlike state.

On arrival to the Emergency Department, she was noted to have normal vital signs. Evaluation revealed a sleeping, well-appearing female who was difficult to arouse. Examination revealed no signs of trauma and was only remarkable for somnolence. On arousal, she was questioned about the circumstances leading to the collision. She had no recollection of the events leading to the collision; she remembered waking up, getting ready, and being on her way to work. On probing her activities the previous night, she denied any alcohol or drug consumption (confirmed by negative blood alcohol concentrations and negative urine studies for benzodiazepines, opiates, cannabis, cocaine, and amphetamines). Prescription drug history was significant for use of zolpidem 10 mg at bedtime.

In January 2013, the Food and Drug Administration (FDA) notified the public regarding concerns for next morning impairment with the use of zolpidem. The agency was particularly concerned regarding increased susceptibility by women because of their slower elimination of the drug when compared to males. Given the risks for impaired alertness, dosing recommendations were lowered for women (FDA 2013a). This notice was followed in May 2013 by label changes to zolpidem dosing, as well as recommendations to avoid driving after using controlled-release zolpidem. The new label dosing reduced the initial starting doses of the immediate-release formulation to 5 mg from 10 mg, while the controlled-release formulation was lowered from 12.5 mg to 6.25 mg (FDA 2013b).

Introduction

As in every other part of medicine, sex and gender have a great deal of influence on the effects that pharmaceuticals have on an individual. Sex and gender can determine drug dosing; the rate of drug–drug interactions; the body's ability to absorb, distribute, metabolize, and excrete medications; and differences in the time course and intensity of adverse effects. It is well known that women account for the majority of acute overdose ingestions, and they have a higher rate of adverse effects from medications. Sex is also responsible for the generation of unique populations – pregnant and breastfeeding women – in which drug effects have unique consequences to the patient as well as their progeny. Finally, unique effects have been noted for women when exposed to particular medications related to chronic conditions such as human immunodeficiency infections and cancer.

Women and men may differ in many aspects of their health and in how they respond to pharmacotherapy. Unfortunately, research on these differences has only recently become a priority. The FDA issued the first guideline for the evaluation of gender differences during drug trials in 1993. It allowed more women to be included in clinical trials, with further enforcements in 1998 demanding equal male and female participation. Further expansion occurred in 2004 when the FDA produced a draft guideline addressing pharmacokinetics in pregnancy. Reviews of participation after these guidelines were published revealed increasing involvement of women but with continued underrepresentation in early phases of clinical trials (McGilvera, 2011; Nicolson et al. 2010). Concerns of teratogenicity are likely responsible for the noted underrepresentation, since most agree that it is unnecessary to expose women of reproductive age and their potential fetuses to the risks associated with phase I clinical trials

(McGilveray 2011; Beierle et al. 1999; Franconi and Campesi 2014). However, this underrepresentation goes against the current FDA recommendation for representative inclusion of both males and females for drugs intended to be used by both sexes.

A Note on Terminology

Sex and gender are commonly interchangeable terms. However, "sex" refers to the physiological differences between males and females that are most heavily influenced by hormones and anatomy. In contrast, "gender" is a societally ascribed term that reflects environmental, cultural, and behavioral differences (Franconi et al. 2012). In this chapter, we will be using the term "sex differences" given that the available pharmacologic data reflects mostly hormonal influences, rather than environmental and behavioral differences.

Pharmacology

Sexual hormones can lead to direct and indirect effects on the pharmacology of medications as a result of direct effects on drug response or by leading to modifications in the intrinsic hormonal sequences (Franconi et al. 2007; Spoletini et al. 2012; Franconi and Campesi 2014).

Differential Drug Dosing

Although individuals vary, men and women differ significantly in body size and composition, with women, in general, having a higher percentage of body fat and lower total mass. Recommended drug dosages for medications are currently calculated for the "average" 70-kilogram healthy male. With significant differences noted between men and women in regard to size and composition, the single-dosing approach leads to the potential for higher concentrations and more adverse effects occurring in women (Franconi et al. 2012).

Drug–Drug Interactions

Drug–drug interactions are an increasing focus of pharmacology and a major cause of morbidity. Perhaps the most common interaction for which the patient's sex is a factor involves oral contraceptive pills (OCPs).

OCPs are the most commonly prescribed medication for women of reproductive age (Services 2013). These medications undergo both absorption and metabolism within the gastrointestinal tract via gastric CYP3A4, followed by hepatic metabolism through oxidation by hepatic CYP3A4 and hepatobiliary cycling. Studies researching drug metabolism of OCPs have generated mixed results with the metabolism of some drugs being inhibited, unaffected, or even enhanced (Schwartz 2003).

The combined use of anticonvulsants (e.g., phenytoin, primidone, and carbamezipine) or antituberculars (e.g., rifampin) with OCPs increases drug clearance and leads to decreased OCP serum concentrations with decreased efficacy. Conversely, the coadministration of antifungals (e.g., ketoconazole, fluconazole, itraconazole, and griseofulvin) or warfarin with OCPs may lead to decreased OCP clearance and increased OCP concentrations. OCP concentrations are also increased in the presence of antibacterials such as penicillin, ampicillin, tetracyclines, and cephalosporins because of inhibited enterohepatic recirculation (Schwartz 2003).

OCPs may lead to alterations in the concentrations of coadministered drugs as well. In the presence of OCPs, benzodiazepines, clofibric acid, cyclosporine, phenytoin, rifampin, and warfarin demonstrate increased drug clearance, thus, lower serum concentrations and decreased efficacy. Conversely, OCPs lead to decreased drug clearance of imipramine, amitriptyline, caffeine, corticosteroids, selegiline, and theophylline and result in increased concentration as well as effect.

Placebo Effect

The placebo effect may play an important role in therapeutic management (Franconi 2013) and its effect may vary with sex. Studies on the efficacy of placebo have found women to be either less responsive (Franconi et al. 2007; Compton et al. 2003; Wilcox et al. 1992) or more responsive (Franconi et al. 2007; Pud et al. 2006; Saxon et al. 2001) than men. However, women report more side effects to medications than men with either active or inactive drugs, while men only reported adverse effects with the active pharmaceutical (Rickels 1965; Franconi et al. 2007).

Pharmacokinetics

Absorption

Pharmaceutical absorption may be somewhat slower in women than men, although this effect is not consistently reported (McGilveray 2011; Schwartz 2003). The absorption of medications is dependent on multiple variables; some of which are dependent on the drug's characteristics, while others are due to the route of administration (Marazziti et al. 2013). Absorption depends on the pH differences between the lumen and the mucosal, surface area of the pharmaceutical, perfusion to the absorptive villi, available digestive enzymes within bile, and the integrity of the gastrointestinal epithelium.

Women tend to have higher gastric pH levels, leading to rapid absorption of basic medications (e.g., benzodiazepines and tricyclic antidepressants) and with subsequently higher peak concentrations (Hamilton 1996; Franconi and Campesi 2014; Grossman et al. 1963; Marazziti et al. 2013; Pollock 1997). Women have less active gastric enzymes in general, which may lead to higher drug concentrations. For example, women have lower concentrations of gastric alcohol dehydrogenase than men, which leads to higher alcohol concentrations even after equivalent weight-based dosing. Men and women differ in regard to the composition of bile acids, which may explain the differential absorption of several medications. Chenodeoxycholic acid, found in higher concentration in women when compared to men, inhibits CYP450 enzymes involved in the metabolism of aniline, benzo (a) pyrene, 7-ethoxy-coumarin, p-nitroanisole, aminopyrine, and testosterone (Kawalek 1979; Marazziti et al. 2013). Women also have slower gastric as well as intestinal transit times than men (Franconi and Campesi 2014; Frezza et al. 1990; Hamilton 1996; Marazziti et al. 2013; Rao et al. 1987). Many of these noted differences may be accounted for by progesterone and estrogen effects, as reflected by changes occurring in relation to the menstrual cycle as well as pregnancy (Franconi and Campesi 2014).

Absorption Differences in Women
Increased gastric pH
- Higher absorption of basic medications
- Higher peaks
Decreased activity of gastric enzymes
- Increased drug concentrations
Increased concentrations chenodeoxycholic acid
- Inhibition of some cytochrome P450 activities
Slower gastric times
- Increased concentrations

These effects are supported by a review of bioequivalence studies submitted to the FDA between 1977 and 1995. In these studies with equivalent per kilogram dosing, the maximum concentration (Cmax) of medication in women was higher than in men 87% of the time, while the area under the curve (AUC) for women was higher 71% of the time (Chen et al. 2000; Marazziti et al. 2013; McGilveray 2011).

Respiratory tract delivery of medications has also been found to be affected by sex differences. Limited studies have noted that both ribavirin and cyclosporine have decreased absorption via the inhaled route when administered to women. This may potentially lead to alterations in management of medical conditions treated in this manner such as asthma, chronic obstructive pulmonary disease, and pulmonary infections (Schwartz 2003).

Ethanol

Since antiquity, it has been known that women are more sensitive to the clinical effects of ethanol ingestion. These effects are in part due to a lower body mass leading to higher blood concentrations with equivalent doses (McGilveray 2011). Clinical evaluation of male and female subjects has found that the AUC after equivalent weight-based doses was 28% higher in women compared to men (Ammon et al. 1996; McGilveray 2011). Body mass is not the only factor; a study conducted in 2001 revealed that lower gastric alcohol dehydrogenase (ADH) activity plays a dominant role in the noted sex difference in alcohol metabolism (Baraona et al. 2001; McGilveray 2011). Other contributors to the observed sex difference include lean body mass and gastric emptying as well as hepatic oxidation, all of which are influenced by sex hormones, liver volume, ethnicity, and genetic polymorphisms of both ADH and aldehyde dehydrogenase (McGilveray 2011; Ramchandani et al. 2001).

Distribution

Distribution of a medication after absorption is best described by the volume of distribution, the theoretical body volume that would be occupied by the drug given the measured serum concentration. The volume of distribution for medications is dependent on several factors: body mass, body fat composition, local perfusion, and protein binding, all of which differ between men and women (Marazziti et al. 2013).

Women tend to have a lower body mass and lower blood volume when compared to men. Given that adult drug dosing is generally not weight based, the average woman when compared to the average man will have higher drug concentrations. The higher percentage of body fat found in women may lead to initially lower drug concentrations of lipid soluble compounds, but it places them at risk for bioaccumulation within fatty tissue, leading to prolonged half-lives of elimination. For example, women who receive propofol infusions have lower serum concentrations and wake up faster than men given the same weight-based dose (Ward et al. 2002). Elderly women are at an increased risk of accumulation and therefore higher elimination half-lives because of body fat percentage increases with age (Marazziti et al. 2013).

Plasma protein binding is important in the determination of drug effects. Non-protein-bound ("free") drugs are responsible for clinical effects, whereas medications that are bound to protein cannot penetrate tissues or bind to receptor sites. Women have lower protein-binding

capacity and, therefore, higher concentrations of free drug, which may contribute to their increased rate of adverse effects (Marazziti et al. 2013).

Metabolism

Medication metabolism involves many enzymatic processes. Sex differences are responsible for slower rates of both glucuronidation and hydro-lyzation in women when compared to men. These slower rates result in higher concentrations of active substances in women, thus, the potential for greater clinical effects as well as the potential for more adverse effects (Marazziti et al. 2013).

CYP450

The majority of hepatic metabolism occurs via the CYP450 system, which is composed of more than 30 isoenzymes (Marazziti et al. 2013; Preskorn 1997; Wilson 1984). It has been theorized that sex-related pharmacokinetic differences may be due to hormonal influences causing differential expression as well as altered activity of the multiple isoforms (Kalra 2007; Marazziti et al. 2013; Nicolas et al. 2009; Zhou et al. 2005).

Table 5.1 CYP System and Gender Effects

CYP	Drugs		
	F>M Activity	**M>F Activity**	**No Reported Effect**
1A2	Theophylline	Caffeine, Thiothixene, Olanzapine, Clozapine, Riluzole, Acetaminophen, Ronipirole, Clopidogrel	
3A4	Cyclosporine, Erythromycin, Tirilazad, Verapamil, Nifedipine, Diazepam, Alfentanil, Dapsone, Bromazepam, Chlordiazepoxide, Prednisolone, Methylprednisolone		Midazolam
2D6		Dextrometorphan, Dextrorphan, Metoprolol, Sertraline, Desipramine, Clomipramine, Mirtazapine, Propanolol	Debrisoquine, Sparteine
2C9		Naproxen	S-mephenytoin
2C19	Clomipramine, Imipramine, Citalopram, Diazepam	R-mephobarbital, Propanolol, Mephenytoin*, Omeprazole*	Piroxicam, Irbersartan
2E1		Chlorzoxazone, Benzene, Toluene	

* OCP influence

There is conflicting evidence for many of these agents. These are consensus data from various sources (Franconi et al. 2007, 2012; Franconi and Campesi 2014; Marazziti et al. 2013; Meibohm et al. 2002; Schwartz 2003; Spoletini et al. 2012; Tanaka 1999).

CYP3A4 accounts for about 60% of all metabolic activities due to the CYP450 enzyme system. It also accounts for the most important sex-related differences noted in medication metabolism (Marazziti et al. 2013; Nemeroff et al. 1996). This particular isozyme is influenced by sex as well as age, with 20%–40% higher CYP3A4 activity in young women when compared to both men and elderly women (Krecic-Shepard et al. 2000a; Marazziti et al. 2013; Pollock, 1997; Spoletini et al. 2012). Thus, young women will metabolize certain medications more quickly, leading to lower concentrations of the medication and less efficacy (Marazziti et al. 2013).

Women have greater CYP2C19 activity than men, leading to faster metabolism and lower drug concentrations, although this enzyme's activity may fluctuate in the presence of other medications (Brosen 1993; Ketter et al. 1995; Marazziti et al. 2013; Pollock 1997; Pollock et al. 1992; Preskorn 1997). Studies in both the Netherlands and Sweden found CYP2C19 activity to be 40% greater in men and 61% lower in women taking OCPs (Hagg et al. 2001; Marazziti et al. 2013; Tamminga et al. 1999).

The CYP2D6 isoform metabolizes many pharmaceuticals. It is commonly implicated in drug-drug interactions and its inhibition is responsible for increases in drug concentrations. Men tend to have higher enzyme expression when compared to females, likely explaining the higher risk of adverse events found in women when they use medications cleared by this enzyme system (Marazziti et al. 2013; Pollock 1997; Pollock et al. 1992; Schwartz 2003; Spoletini et al. 2012). Pregnancy increases the activity of CYP2D6. Thus, it may be under the influence of sex steroids, although so far there has been no supporting data of their role in changing drug concentrations (Kashuba et al. 1998; Labbe et al. 2000; Marazziti et al. 2013; McCune et al. 2001; Wadelius et al. 1997).

CYP1A2, whose common substrates include the clearance of caffeine and theophylline, appears to have sex differences unique to each pharmaceutical. Caffeine is metabolized more slowly in women compared to men in some ethnic groups (e.g., Chinese). Olanzapine and clozapine also have decreased clearance in women when compared to men. In contrast, theophylline has higher clearances in women. Interestingly, the use of oral contraceptives eliminates these sex differences for caffeine, acetaminophen. and ronipirole (Ford et al. 1993; Franconi et al. 2007; Hartter et al. 1993; Kalow and Tang 1991; Kaye and Nicholls 2000; Marazziti et al. 2013; Miners et al. 1983).

CYP2C9 is responsible for approximately 20% of all CYP enzyme activity. It is involved in the metabolism of phenytoin, warfarin, naproxen, and tolbutamide. Although it has been found that older women have higher serum concentrations of naproxen, sex has not been found to lead to clinically significant differences in metabolism (Tanaka 1999).

Elimination

Drug elimination takes place for the most part via hepatic, renal, and pulmonary routes, with minor contributions through exocrine secretion into sweat, tears, and breast milk (Marazziti et al. 2013).

Hepatic clearance of medications depends on both blood flow as well as intrinsic hepatic enzyme activity. Women have lower hepatic blood flow; thus, they have less medication made available for elimination by the liver. As previously discussed, sex differences in hepatic enzymes also put women at risk of differential drug effects compared to men (Marazziti et al. 2013). Of particular concern is the role of hormones in the expression of P-glycoprotein. These proteins regulate the biliary excretion of drugs and have been found to be 2.4-fold lower in women when compared to men (Marazziti et al. 2013; Nicolas et al. 2009; Schuetz et al. 1995).

Renal clearance accounts for the majority of excretion of both the parent drug as well as metabolites. Women have lower rates of glomerular filtration (10% lower) (Anderson 2002) passive diffusion and active secretion and therefore lower elimination than men (Marazziti et al. 2013). Thus, adjustments for renal clearance may reduce the amount of adverse effects of drugs that are renally excreted.

Drug Transporters

Molecular drug transporters have been found to alter pharmacokinetics by influencing absorption, distribution, and excretion of pharmaceuticals. The most commonly recognized drug transporter is P-glycoprotein. This transporter is the gene product of human multidrug resistance gene 1. Studies looking at sex differences have found that women express one-third to one-half of the hepatic protein concentrations that men express (Meibohm et al. 2002; Schuetz et al. 1995). The implications of reduced expression affect several steps in medication metabolism. Low levels of P-glycoprotein have been found to affect absorption by leading to reduced gastrointestinal transit time, thus decreased intestinal wall metabolism via CYP3A4 and increased concentration and effect. Decreased P-glycoprotein levels within the liver lead to increased CYP3A4 metabolism (Benet et al. 1999; Lown et al. 1997; Meibohm et al. 2002), as noted by the metabolism of both alfentanil and nifedipine, which are substrates of CYP3A4 and are found in lower concentration in women because of their more extensive metabolism (Franconi et al. 2007; Krecic-Shepard et al. 2000b; Lemmens et al. 1990).

Pharmacodynamics

Pharmacodynamics refers to the effects that a medication has on the individual and involves both the clinical effect as well as adverse effects. Unfortunately, there is limited data on sex-related effects on pharmacodynamics

Women are more likely to take medications, in particular hormonal contraceptives and replacement, but also psychotropics and opioids, when compared to men. Available data indicate that this may be due to sex-related differences in drug responses. Antipsychotics have been reported to lead to a more pronounced response in women (Marazziti et al. 2013). This effect may be due to hormonal influences leading to higher dopamine uptake in the striatum (Cohen et al. 1999; Franconi et al. 2007). In regard to antidepressants, women are more likely to respond to selective serotonin reuptake inhibitors (SSRI), while men are more likely to respond to tricyclic antidepressants (Brose 1993; Kornstein et al. 2000; Marazziti et al. 2013; Parker et al. 2003). This response has been

attributed to women's ability to increase tryptophan, while at the same time reducing cortisol in the setting of SSRI exposure (Bano et al. 2004; Marazziti et al. 2013).

Illicit drugs also appear to have sex-related differences. Women are more responsive to both cocaine and methylphenidate (Dafny and Yang 2006; Franconi et al. 2007; Kosten et al. 1996), but they are less responsive to amphetamines because of the release of lower amounts of dopamine from the striatum (Franconi et al. 2007; Munro et al, 2006). In addition, the subjective effects of cocaine and amphetamine are reduced by hormonal influences during the luteal phase of the menstrual cycle. Women are less susceptible to toxicity resulting from methamphetamine and have even demonstrated fewer electroencephalographic (EEG) changes when compared to men (Dluzen et al. 2003; Franconi et al. 2007; King et al. 2000).

It is clear that women have a higher rate and more severe adverse drug reactions (Baggio et al. 2013; Franconi and Campesi 2014; Franconi et al. 2012; Patel et al. 2007; Pirmohamed et al. 2004), but whether these are primarily pharmacokinetic or pharmacodynamic effects or a combination is not yet clear.

Site of Action Effects

Although limited data are available, some site of action effects that appeared to be enhanced in women include

Hemorrhagic consequences with anticoagulation and thrombolytics

Diuretic-induced electrolyte abnormalities

Myopathy in the setting of statins

Cough from angiotensin converting enzyme (ACE) inhibitor therapy

QTc effects

Prolongation of the QT interval has been shown to increase the risk of sudden tachydysrhythmias, specifically polymorphic ventricular tachycardia (torsades de pointes), leading to increasing morbidity and even mortality (Nicolson et al. 2010). Women account for more than 70% of all cases of drug-induced polymorphic ventricular tachycardia (Makkar et al. 1993; Nicolson et al. 2010).

Multiple medications have been shown to prolong the QT interval of the heart. The length of the QT interval is directly proportional to the flow of potassium through potassium channels and therefore the number of potassium channels available. The cellular production of potassium channels is enhanced by testosterone. Prepubertal children have similar testosterone concentrations and density of cardiac potassium channels and, thus, have equivalent QT_c (rate corrected QT) durations. When boys' testosterone concentration increases at puberty, the QT_c shortens in men because of increased production of potassium channels, as it gradually increases in women (Kurokawa et al. 2009; Spoletini et al. 2012). As a result of aging, as testosterone concentrations decrease in men after age 50, QT_c durations in men and women become similar. Furthermore, treatment with exogenous testosterone results in decreases in QT_c duration as well as a decrease in the risk of dysrhythmia. Decreased testosterone in women not only increases baseline QT_c length but also enhances the effect of QT-prolonging medications. This is best exemplified by women developing a proportionally longer increase in their QT when compared to men when they are given an identical per weight dose of some QT-prolonging medications.

Female sexual hormones may also affect QT_c duration and dysrhythmia risk. The QT_c increases and dysrhythmia risk increases with high estrogen concentrations, and the risk lowers in the setting of high progesterone concentrations (Franconi and Campesi 2014; James et al. 2007; Janse de Jonge et al. 2001; Nakagawa et al. 2006). These changes may be explained by sex hormone effects leading to ion channel blockade of calcium and/or potassium in myocytes (Hreiche et al. 2009; Johnson et al. 1997; Moller and Netzer 2006; Nicolson et al. 2010; Spoletini et al. 2012).

Adverse Effects

All of the previously described pharmacodynamic changes help explain the higher risk (50%–70%) of adverse effects experienced by women (Spoletini et al. 2012). Adverse reactions commonly experienced by women include rashes, immune reactions, and drug-induced liver injury (Anderson 2008).

Acute Overdoses
General Concepts

Although men and women attempt suicide at similar rates (Crosby et al. 2011b), men are more likely to complete suicide by more immediate and violent methods (Crosby et al. 2011a; Henderson et al. 2005), while women are significantly more likely to use medication overdose as their method of suicide (Henderson et al. 2005). There is little comprehensive literature on sex differences in acute overdoses; however, some patterns are evident in overdoses of acetaminophen and opioids.

Acetaminophen

Acetaminophen-induced liver failure and liver injury are more common in men after overdose, and men have a longer duration of hospital stay. The cause of this inequity may be that men ingest larger doses of acetaminophen and present later to health care (Zyoud et al. 2010), although animal data suggests that hepatic glutathione handling may be a contributing factor (Dai et al. 2006; Masubuchi et al. 2011).

Opioids

In the past two decades, opioid use, abuse, and dependence have increased significantly with several interesting sex differences emerging. While the rate of substance abuse disorders is higher in men for most drugs, the rate of opioid abuse is roughly equivalent among men and women (Parsells Kelly et al. 2008). Several factors may contribute to this: women are more likely than men to be prescribed opioid pain medication (Parsells Kelly et al. 2008), women more commonly treat negative affective and somatic complaints with opioids (McHugh et al. 2013), and women are more likely to have depression (McHugh et al. 2013). In regard to accidental deaths from prescription opioids in the United States, deaths are 1.5 times more common in men (McHugh et al. 2013).

Antidotes
Intravenous Lipid Emulsion

Intravenous lipid emulsion is being used in the treatment of severe toxicity of lipid-soluble medications. Its use is currently standard therapy for local anesthetic toxicity, but animal data suggest that it may also be effective for other lipid-soluble medications, such as propranolol and verapamil.

Data are limited regarding sex differences in the use of intravenous lipid emulsion therapy. Animal research shows differences in lipid metabolism. When rats received a bolus of 0.2 g/kg of 10% fat emulsion, females have faster clearance rates when compared to males, likely because of greater activity of postheparin lipoprotein lipase. Increases in females' metabolism may lead to potentially faster rebound of pharmaceutical concentrations because of dissociation of the agent from the lipid or might lead to lower concentrations because of enhanced liver delivery (Jesmok et al. 1981).

Special Topics

HIV

Infection with the human immunodeficiency virus is a unique situation in which there appear to be significant sex-related differences. Women are more vulnerable to infections than males because of higher surface area and trauma during intercourse (Floridia et al. 2008). Once infected, hormones are influential, with estrogen inhibiting the action of tumor necrosis factors responsible for viral replication, leading to lower viral loads (Athreya et al. 1993; Floridia et al. 2008).

In HIV, drug dosing is currently administered in standard doses rather than weight based. Given the previously discussed sex differences, women are at increased risk of adverse effects including rashes, lipodystrophic changes, hepatotoxicity, and dyslipidemias (Bonfanti et al. 2003; Clark 2005; Currier et al. 2000; Floridia et al. 2008; Mazhude et al. 2002; Pacifici et al. 1996; Pernerstorfer-Schoen et al. 2001). Sex differences in the expression of cellular kinases leads to the variable effects of nucleoside reverse transcriptase inhibitors (NRTIs). These differences may lead to an increased frequency of lactic acidosis, an adverse effect more commonly encountered in obese women (Floridia et al. 2008; Moyle et al. 2002). Protease inhibitors (PI) including saquinavir and ritonavir have lower clearances and increased concentrations in women when compared to men (Floridia

et al. 2008; Pai et al. 2004). Women exposed to evirapine, a non-nucleoside reverse transcriptase inhibitor (NNRTI), or the other NNRTIs are at higher risk of adverse effects such as rash and hepatotoxicity when compared to men (Floridia et al. 2008; Sanne et al. 2005; van Leth et al. 2005).

Another unique situation for women affected with HIV is the management of their disease in the setting of pregnancy. Drugs that should be avoided include efavirenz due to the risk of birth defects, stavudine and didanosine due to lactic acidosis, as well as tenofovir due to effects on developing bone (Clumeck et al. 2008; Floridia et al. 2008).

Treatment may also increase the risk of premature delivery, with studies both in Europe and the United States finding a rate of premature delivery of 25% (Cotter et al. 2006; Floridia et al. 2008; Ravizza et al. 2007; Schulte et al. 2007; Townsend et al. 2007). Antiretrovirals also place the mother as well as the pregnancy at increased risk of commonly encountered complications such as fatty liver, diabetes, cholestasis, and preeclampsia (Floridia et al. 2008).

Pregnancy has also been shown to alter the pharmacokinetics of antiretrovirals. Both PI and NNRTI affect the CYP450 system. The use of ritonavir leads to decreased levels of nevirapine, indanavir, saquinavir, and nelfinavir likely the result of enhanced CYP3A4 activity in pregnancy (Floridia et al. 2008).

Chemotherapeutics

Many sex differences affect the use of chemotherapeutics. Fluorouracil (5-FU), initially used in the management of colorectal cancer, is now also used for cancers involving the head and neck, lung, and breast. In a study evaluating patients being treated for head and neck cancer, women were found to have a 10% median lower clearance than men (Milano et al. 1992). Another study of patients treated with 5-FU for colorectal cancer noted that women were more likely to suffer toxicity such as dehydration. Their findings corroborated previous trials in which women were found to have a higher incidence of neurological toxicity as well as nausea, vomiting, and alopecia (Oliver et al. 2013).

When female lung cancer patients were treated with combinations of cyclophosphamide, vincristine, cisplatin, doxorubicin, and etoposide, they had more severe leukotoxicity when compared to males. Noted differences may be due to the lower hepatic expression of P-glycoprotein, which leads to decreased clearance and increased plasma concentrations when compared to males (Davis 2005; Yamamoto et al. 2008).

Other agents used in the treatment of cancer include cisplatin, carboplatin, and docetaxel. Multiple clinical trials have found an increased incidence of side effects including nausea and vomiting in women (Harichand-Herdt and Ramalingam, 2009). When carboplatin and paclitaxel are used in the treatment of lung cancer, women suffer a greater incidence of both leukocytopenia and neutropenia (Yamamoto et al. 2008). Theories for the noted differences include the decreased ability of women to repair DNA damage caused by chemotheraputics within cancer cells because of mutations in the epithelial growth factor receptor (EGFR) (Harichand-Herdt and Ramalingam 2009).

Conclusion

Differences between men and women encompass many aspects of their physiology. Medicine is slowly starting to unravel the mysteries of how sex influences medication responses via changes in both pharmacokinetics and pharmacodynamics. Sex hormones may be responsible for influencing a majority of those changes. Modifications to clinical trial enrollment by the FDA have allowed further inclusion of women into drug trials, thus, describing some sex effects. Further studies and greater inclusion will aid in better delineating the role of sex on pharmaceutical effects.

Sex Differences Found in Women

- Increased fat stores and lower lean body mass, thus a single dosing approach leads to increased number of adverse events
- More side effects when exposed to placebo
- Increased gastric pH, decreased gastric enzymatic activity, decreased gastric transit time, and varying concentration of bile acids, all of which alter a drug's absorption
- Increased body fat composition leading to lower concentrations of lipid-soluble drugs, while increasing the risk of bioaccumulation
- Lower protein binding of pharmaceuticals leading to higher concentrations of active drug

---

- Lower rates of glucuronidation and hydrolyzation
- Increased activity of CYP3A4 and CYP2C19
- Decreased hepatic and renal clearance
- One-half to one-third less P-glycoprotein, increasing hepatic metabolism but leading to lower intestinal metabolism
- Higher risk of adverse effects
- Increased baseline QT_c, and increased risk of dysrhythmia in setting of QT-prolonging drugs
- Higher likelihood of using medication in an acute overdose
- Potential for alternative metabolism of intravenous lipid emulsion
- Increased risk of adverse events when being treated for HIV infection
- Higher likelihood of leukotoxicty and neurotoxicity when being treated for cancer

Case Conclusion

The presented patient demonstrated classic sex differences regarding her pharmaceutical use of zolpidem. She is a young female who was taking therapeutic dosing of a prescribed sleep medication at the currently recommended dosing. Given her impaired drug clearance due to her sex, she suffered ill consequences that resulted in her accident need for emergency evaluation and placed her at risk of legal prosecution as a result of driving under the influence of medications.

Gaps in Knowledge/Research Questions

There is a paucity of data on the subject of sex differences and medication efficacy and safety. Areas that need further research include the following:

Sex-specific effects of other drug transporters such as the sodium taurocholatecontransporting polypeptide (NTCP) and the organic cation transporter 2 (OCT2), which in animals have been shown to have sex-specific expression.

Human data on sex-specific differences in antidote effects, in particular newer agents such as intravenous lipid therapy and high-dose insulin euglycemia therapy.

References

Ammon, E., Schafer, C., Hofmann, U. & Klotz, U. 1996. Disposition and first-pass metabolism of ethanol in humans: Is it gastric or hepatic and does it depend on gender? *Clinical Pharmacology & Therapeutics*, **59**, 503–513.

Anderson, G.D. 2002. Sex differences in drug metabolism: Cytochrome P-450 and uridine diphosphate glucuronosyltransferase. *Journal of Gender-Specific Medicine*, **5**, 25–33.

Anderson, G.D. 2008. Gender differences in pharmacological response. *International Review of Neurobiology*, **83**, 1–10.

Athreya, B.H., Pletcher, J., Zulian, F., Weiner, D.B. & Williams, W.V. 1993. Subset-specific effects of sex hormones and pituitary gonadotropins on human lymphocyte proliferation in vitro. *Clinical Immunology and Immunopathology*, **66**, 201–211.

Baggio, G., Corsini, A., Floreani, A., Giannini, S. & Zagonel, V. 2013. Gender medicine: A task for the third millennium. *Clinical Chemistry and Laboratory Medicine*, **51**, 713–727.

Bano, S., Akhter, S. & Afridi, M.I. 2004. Gender based response to fluoxetine hydrochloride medication in endogenous depression. *Journal of the College of Physicians and Surgeons Pakistan*, **14**, 161–165.

Baraona, E., Abittan, C.S., Dohmen, K., Moretti, M., Pozzato, G., Chayes, Z.W., Schaefer, C. & Lieber, C.S. 2001. Gender differences in pharmacokinetics of alcohol. *Alcoholism: Clinical and Experimental Research*, **25**, 502–507.

Beierle, I., Meibohm, B. & Derendorf, H. 1999. Gender differences in pharmacokinetics and pharmacodynamics. *International Journal of Clinical Pharmacology and Therapeutics*, **37**, 529–547.

Benet, L.Z., Izumi, T., Zhang, Y., Silverman, J.A. & Wacher, V.J. 1999. Intestinal MDR transport proteins and P-450 enzymes as barriers to oral drug delivery. *Journal of Controlled Release*, **62**, 25–31.

Bonfanti, P., Gulisano, C., Ricci, E., Timillero, L., Valsecchi, L., Carradori, S., Pusterla, L., Fortuna, P., Miccolis, S., Magnani, C., Gabbuti, A., Parazzini, F., Martinelli, C., Faggion, I., Landonio, S., Quirino, T. & Vigevani, G. 2003. Risk factors for lipodystrophy in the CISAI cohort. *Biomedicine & Pharmacology*, **57**, 422–427.

Brosen, K. 1993. Isoenzyme specific drug oxidation: Genetic polymorphism and drug-drug interactions. *Nordic Journal of Psychiatry*, **47**, 21–26.

Centers for Disease Control. 2013. Vital signs: Overdoses of prescription opioid pain relievers and other drugs among women–United States, 1999–2010. *Morbidity and Mortality Weekly Report*, **62**, 537–542.

Chen, M.L., Lee, S.C., Ng, M.J., Schuirmann, D.J., Lesko, L.J. & Williams, R.L. 2000. Pharmacokinetic analysis of bioequivalence trials: Implications for sex-related issues in clinical pharmacology and biopharmaceutics. *Clinical Pharmacology & Therapeutics*, **68**, 510–521.

Clark, R. 2005. Sex differences in antiretroviral therapy-associated intolerance and adverse events. *Drug Safety*, **28**, 1075–1083.

Clumeck, N., Pozniak, A. & Raffi, F. 2008. European AIDS Clinical Society (EACS) guidelines for the clinical management and treatment of HIV-infected adults. *HIV Medicine*, **9**, 65–71.

Cohen, R.M., Nordahl, T.E., Semple, W.E. & Pickar, D. 1999. The brain metabolic patterns of clozapine- and fluphenazine-treated female patients with schizophrenia: Evidence of a sex effect. *Neuropsychopharmacology*, **21**, 632–640.

Compton, P., Charuvastra, V.C. & Ling, W. 2003. Effect of oral ketorolac and gender on human cold pressor pain tolerance. *Clinical and Experimental Pharmacology and Physiology*, **30**, 759–763.

Cotter, A.M., Garcia, A.G., Duthely, M.L., Luke, B. & O'sullivan, M.J. 2006. Is antiretroviral therapy during pregnancy associated with an increased risk of preterm delivery, low birth weight, or stillbirth? *Journal of Infectious Diseases*, **193**, 1195–1201.

Crosby, A.E., Han, B., Ortega, L.A., Parks, S.E. & Gfroerer, J. 2011a. Suicidal thoughts and behaviors among adults aged >/=18 years – United States, 2008–2009. *Morbidity and Mortality Weekly Report Surveillance Summary*, **60**, 1–22.

Crosby, A.E., Ortega, L. & Stevens, M.R. 2011b. Suicides – United States, 1999–2007. *Morbidity and Mortality Weekly Report Surveillance Summary*, **60** Suppl, 56–59.

Currier, J.S., Spino, C., Grimes, J., Wofsy, C.B., Katzenstein, D.A., Hughes, M.D., Hammer, S.M. & Cotton, D.J. 2000. Differences between women and men in adverse events and CD4+ responses to nucleoside analogue therapy for HIV infection. The Aids Clinical Trials Group 175 Team. *Journal of Acquired Immune Deficiency Syndrome*, **24**, 316–324.

Dafny, N. & Yang, P.B. 2006. The role of age, genotype, sex, and route of acute and chronic administration of methylphenidate: A review of its locomotor effects. *Brain Research Bulletin*, **68**, 393–405.

Dai, G., He, L., Chou, N. & Wan, Y.J. 2006. Acetaminophen metabolism does not contribute to gender difference in its hepatotoxicity in mouse. *Toxicological Sciences*, **92**, 33–41.

Davis, M. 2005. Gender differences in P-glycoprotein: Drug toxicity and response. *Journal of Clinical Oncology*, **23**, 6439–6440.

Dluzen, D.E., Tweed, C., Anderson, L.I. & Laping, N.J. 2003. Gender differences in methamphetamine-induced mRNA associated with neurodegeneration in the mouse nigrostriatal dopaminergic system. *Neuroendocrinology*, **77**, 232–238.

FDA. 2013a. FDA Drug Safety Communication: Risk of next-morning impairment and use of insomnia drugs; FDA requires lower recommended doses for certain drugs containing zolpidem (Ambien, Ambien CR, Edluar, and Zolpmist). Available at www.fda.gov/Drugs/DrugSafety/ucm334033.htm. Accessed January 15, 2014.

FDA. 2013b. FDA Drug Saftery Communication: FDA approves new label changes and dosing for zolpidem products and a recommendation to avoid driving the day after using Ambien CR. Available at www.fda.gov/Drugs/DrugSafety/ucm352085.htm. Accessed January 15, 2014.

Floridia, M., Giuliano, M., Palmisano, L. & Vella, S. 2008. Gender differences in the treatment of HIV infection. *Pharmacological Research*, **58**, 173–82.

Ford, J.M., Truman, C.A., Wilcock, G.K. & Roberts, C.J. 1993. Serum concentrations of tacrine hydrochloride predict its adverse effects in Alzheimer's disease. *Clinical Pharmacology & Therapeutics*, **53**, 691–695.

Franconi, F., Brunelleschi, S., Steardo, L. & Cuomo, V. 2007. Gender differences in drug responses. *Pharmacological Research*, **55**, 81–95.

Franconi, F. & Campesi, I. 2014. Pharmacogenomics, pharmacokinetics and pharmacodynamics: Interaction with biological differences between men and women. *British Journal of Pharmacology*, **171**, 580–594.

Franconi, F., Campesi, I., Occhioni, S., Antonini, P. & Murphy, M.F. 2012. Sex and gender in adverse drug events, addiction, and placebo. *Handbook of Experimental Pharmacology*, 107–126.

Frezza, M., DI Padova, C., Pozzato, G., Terpin, M., Baraona, E. & Lieber, C.S. 1990. High blood alcohol levels in women. The role of decreased gastric alcohol dehydrogenase activity and first-pass metabolism. *New England Journal of Medicine*, **322**, 95–99.

Grossman, M.I., Kirsner, J.B. & Gillespie, I.E. 1963. Basal and histalog-stimulated gastric secretion in control subjects and in patients with peptic ulcer or gastric cancer. *Gastroenterology*, **45**, 14–26.

Hagg, S., Spigset, O. & Dahlqvist, R. 2001. Influence of gender and oral contraceptives on CYP2D6 and CYP2C19 activity in healthy volunteers. *British Journal of Clinical Pharmacology*, **51**, 169–173.

Hamilton, J. & Yonkers, K. 1996. Sex differences in pharmacokinetics of psychotropic medication. Part I: Physiological basis for effects. In: H. U. Jensvold & J. Hamilton, eds. *Psychopharmacology and Women: Sex, Gender and Hormones*. Washington, DC: American Psychiatric Press.

Harichand-Herdt, S. & Ramalingam, S.S. 2009. Gender-associated differences in lung cancer: Clinical characteristics and treatment outcomes in women. *Seminars in Oncology*, **36**, 572–580.

Hartter, S., Wetzel, H., Hammes, E. & Hiemke, C. 1993. Inhibition of antidepressant demethylation and hydroxylation by fluvoxamine in depressed patients. *Psychopharmacology (Berlin)*, **110**, 302–308.

Henderson, J.P., Mellin, C. & Patel, F. 2005. Suicide – a statistical analysis by age, sex and method. *Journal of Clinical Forensic Medicine*, **12**, 305–309.

Hreiche, R., Morissette, P., Zakrzewski-Jakubiak, H. & Turgeon, J. 2009. Gender-related differences in drug-induced prolongation of cardiac repolarization in prepubertal guinea pigs. *Journal of Cardiovascular Pharmacology and Therapeutics*, **14**, 28–37.

James, A.F., Choisy, S.C. & Hancox, J.C. 2007. Recent advances in understanding sex differences in cardiac repolarization. *Progress in Biophysics and Molecular Biology*, **94**, 265–319.

Janse De Jonge, X.A., Boot, C.R., Thom, J.M., Ruell, P.A. & Thompson, M.W. 2001. The influence of menstrual cycle phase on skeletal muscle contractile characteristics in humans. *Journal of Physiology*, **530**, 161–166.

Jesmok, G.J., Woods, E.F., Ditzler, W.S. & Walsh, G. 1981. Fat emulsion catabolism in vitro and in vivo–sex related differences. *Journal of Parenteral and Enteral Nutrition*, **5**, 200–203.

Johnson, B.D., Zheng, W., Korach, K.S., Scheuer, T., Catterall, W.A. & Rubanyi, G.M. 1997. Increased expression of the cardiac L-type calcium channel in estrogen receptor-deficient mice. *Journal of General Physiology*, **110**, 135–140.

Kalow, W. & Tang, B.K. 1991. Use of caffeine metabolite ratios to explore CYP1A2 and xanthine oxidase activities. *Clinical Pharmacology & Therapeutics*, **50**, 508–519.

Kalra, B.S. 2007. Cytochrome P450 enzyme isoforms and their therapeutic implications: An update. *Indian Journal of Medical Sciences*, **61**, 102–116.

Kashuba, A.D., Bertino, J.S., Jr., Rocci, M.L., Jr., Kulawy, R.W., Beck, D.J. & Nafziger, A.N. 1998. Quantification of 3-month intraindividual variability and the influence of sex and menstrual cycle phase on CYP3A activity as measured by phenotyping with intravenous midazolam. *Clinical Pharmacology & Therapeutics*, **64**, 269–277.

Kawalek, J. 1979. The effect of bile acids in drug metabolism. *Nutrition and Cancer*, **1**, 13–18.

Kaye, C.M. & Nicholls, B. 2000. Clinical pharmacokinetics of ropinirole. *Clinical Pharmacokinetics*, **39**, 243–254.

Ketter, T.A., Flockhart, D.A., Post, R.M., Denicoff, K., Pazzaglia, P.J., Marangell, L.B., George, M.S. & Callahan, A.M. 1995. The emerging role of cytochrome P450 3A in psychopharmacology. *Journal of Clinical Psychopharmacology*, **15**, 387–398.

King, D.E., Herning, R.I., Gorelick, D.A. & Cadet, J.L. 2000. Gender differences in the EEG of abstinent cocaine abusers. *Neuropsychobiology*, **42**, 93–98.

Kornstein, S.G., Schatzberg, A.F., Thase, M.E., Yonkers, K.A., Mccullough, J.P., Keitner, G.I., Gelenberg, A.J., Davis, S.M., Harrison, W.M. & Keller, M.B. 2000. Gender differences in treatment response to sertraline versus imipramine in chronic depression. *American Journal of Psychiatry*, **157**, 1445–1452.

Kosten, T.R., Kosten, T.A., Mcdougle, C.J., Hameedi, F. A., Mccance, E.F., Rosen, M.I., Oliveto, A.H. & Price, L. H. 1996. Gender differences in response to intranasal cocaine administration to humans. *Biological Psychiatry*, **39**, 147–148.

Krecic-Shepard, M.E., Barnas, C.R., Slimko, J. & Schwartz, J.B. 2000a. Faster clearance of sustained release verapamil in men versus women: Continuing observations on sex-specific differences after oral administration of verapamil. *Clinical Pharmacology & Therapeutics*, **68**, 286–292.

Krecic-Shepard, M.E., Park, K., Barnas, C., Slimko, J., Kerwin, D.R. & Schwartz, J.B. 2000b. Race and sex influence clearance of nifedipine: Results of a population study. *Clinical Pharmacology & Therapeutics*, **68**, 130–142.

Kurokawa, J., Suzuki, T. & Furukawa, T. 2009. New aspects for the treatment of cardiac diseases based on the diversity of functional controls on cardiac muscles: Acute effects of female hormones on cardiac ion channels and cardiac repolarization. *Journal of Pharmacological Sciences*, **109**, 334–40.

Labbe, L., Sirois, C., Pilote, S., Arseneault, M., Robitaille, N.M., Turgeon, J. & Hamelin, B.A. 2000. Effect of gender, sex hormones, time variables and physiological urinary pH on apparent CYP2D6 activity as assessed by metabolic ratios of marker substrates. *Pharmacogenetics*, **10**, 425–438.

Lemmens, H.J., Burm, A.G., Hennis, P.J., Gladines, M. P. & Bovill, J.G. 1990. Influence of age on the pharmacokinetics of alfentanil. Gender dependence. *Clinical Pharmacokinetics*, **19**, 416–422.

Lown, K.S., Mayo, R.R., Leichtman, A.B., Hsiao, H.L., Turgeon, D.K., Schmiedlin-Ren, P., Brown, M.B., Guo, W., Rossi, S.J., Benet, L.Z. & Watkins, P.B. 1997. Role of intestinal P-glycoprotein (mdr1) in interpatient variation in the oral bioavailability of cyclosporine. *Clinical Pharmacology & Therapeutics*, **62**, 248–260.

Makkar, R.R., Fromm, B.S., Steinman, R.T., Meissner, M.D. & Lehmann, M.H. 1993. Female gender as a risk factor for torsades de pointes associated with cardiovascular drugs. *Journal of the American Medical Association*, **270**, 2590–2597.

Marazziti, D., Baroni, S., Picchetti, M., Piccinni, A., Carlini, M., Vatteroni, E., Falaschi, V., Lombardi, A. & Dell'osso, L. 2013. Pharmacokinetics and pharmacodynamics of psychotropic drugs: Effect of sex. *CNS Spectrums*, **18**, 118–127.

Masubuchi, Y., Nakayama, J. & Watanabe, Y. 2011. Sex difference in susceptibility to acetaminophen hepatotoxicity is reversed by buthionine sulfoximine. *Toxicology*, **287**, 54–60.

Mazhude, C., Jones, S., Murad, S., Taylor, C. & Easterbrook, P. 2002. Female sex but not ethnicity is a strong predictor of non-nucleoside reverse transcriptase inhibitor-induced rash. *AIDS*, **16**, 1566–1568.

Mccune, J.S., Lindley, C., Decker, J.L., Williamson, K. M., Meadowcroft, A.M., Graff, D., Sawyer, W.T., Blough, D.K. & Pieper, J.A. 2001. Lack of gender differences and large intrasubject variability in cytochrome P450 activity measured by phenotyping with dextromethorphan. *Journal of Clinical Pharmacology*, **41**, 723–731.

Mcgilveray, I.J. 2011. Bioequivalence studies of drugs prescribed mainly for women. *Journal of Population and Clinical Pharmacology*, **18**, e516–e522.

Mchugh, R.K., Devito, E.E., Dodd, D., Carroll, K.M., Potter, J.S., Greenfield, S.F., Connery, H.S. & Weiss, R. D. 2013. Gender differences in a clinical trial for prescription opioid dependence. *Journal of Substance Abuse Treatment*, **45**, 38–43.

Meibohm, B., Beierle, I. & Derendorf, H. 2002. How important are gender differences in pharmacokinetics? *Clinical Pharmacokinetics*, **41**, 329–342.

Milano, G., Etienne, M.C., Cassuto-Viguier, E., Thyss, A., Santini, J., Frenay, M., Renee, N., Schneider, M. & Demard, F. 1992. Influence of sex and age on fluorouracil clearance. *Journal of Clinical Oncology*, **10**, 1171–1175.

Miners, J.O., Attwood, J. & Birkett, D.J. 1983. Influence of sex and oral contraceptive steroids on paracetamol metabolism. *British Journal of Clinical Pharmacology*, **16**, 503–509.

Moller, C. & Netzer, R. 2006. Effects of estradiol on cardiac ion channel currents. *European Journal of Pharmacology*, **532**, 44–49.

Moyle, G.J., Datta, D., Mandalia, S., Morlese, J., Asboe, D. & Gazzard, B.G. 2002. Hyperlactataemia and lactic acidosis during antiretroviral therapy: Relevance, reproducibility and possible risk factors. *AIDS*, **16**, 1341–1349.

Munro, C.A., Mccaul, M.E., Wong, D.F., Oswald, L.M., Zhou, Y., Brasic, J., Kuwabara, H., Kumar, A., Alexander, M., Ye, W. & Wand, G.S. 2006. Sex differences in striatal dopamine release in healthy adults. *Biological Psychiatry*, **59**, 966–974.

Nakagawa, M., Ooie, T., Takahashi, N., Taniguchi, Y., Anan, F., Yonemochi, H. & Saikawa, T. 2006. Influence of menstrual cycle on QT interval dynamics. *Pacing and Clinical Electrophysiology*, **29**, 607–613.

Nemeroff, C.B., Devane, C.L. & Pollock, B.G. 1996. Newer antidepressants and the cytochrome P450 system. *American Journal of Psychiatry*, **153**, 311–320.

Nicolas, J.M., Espie, P. & Molimard, M. 2009. Gender and interindividual variability in pharmacokinetics. *Drug Metabolism Reviews*, **41**, 408–421.

Nicolson, T.J., Mellor, H.R. & Roberts, R.R. 2010. Gender differences in drug toxicity. *Trends in Pharmacological Sciences*, **31**, 108–114.

Oliver, J.S., Martin, M.Y., Richardson, L., Kim, Y. & Pisu, M. 2013. Gender differences in colon cancer treatment. *Journal of Womens Health (Larchmont)*, **22**, 344–351.

Pacifici, G.M., Evangelisti, L., Giuliani, L., Metelli, R.M. & Giordani, R. 1996. Zidovudine glucuronidation in human liver: interindividual variability. *International Journal of Clinical Pharmacology and Therapeutics*, **34**, 329–334.

Pai, M.P., Schriever, C.A., Diaz-Linares, M., Novak, R.M. & Rodvold, K.A. 2004. Sex-related differences in the pharmacokinetics of once-daily saquinavir soft-gelatin capsules boosted with low-dose ritonavir in patients infected with human immunodeficiency virus type 1. *Pharmacotherapy*, **24**, 592–599.

Parker, G., Parker, K., Austin, M.P., Mitchell, P. & Brotchie, H. 2003. Gender differences in response to differing antidepressant drug classes: Two negative studies. *Psychological Medicine*, **33**, 1473–1477.

Parsells Kelly, J., Cook, S.F., Kaufman, D.W., Anderson, T., Rosenberg, L. & Mitchell, A.A. 2008. Prevalence and characteristics of opioid use in the US adult population. *Pain*, **138**, 507–513.

Patel, H., Bell, D., Molokhia, M., Srishanmuganathan, J., Patel, M., Car, J. & Majeed, A. 2007. Trends in hospital admissions for adverse drug reactions in England: Analysis of national hospital episode statistics 1998–2005. *BMC Clinical Pharmacology*, **7**, 9.

Pernerstorfer-Schoen, H., Jilma, B., Perschler, A., Wichlas, S., Schindler, K., Schindl, A., Rieger, A., Wagner, O.F. & Quehenberger, P. 2001. Sex differences in HAART-associated dyslipidaemia. *AIDS*, **15**, 725–734.

Pirmohamed, M., James, S., Meakin, S., Green, C., Scott, A.K., Walley, T.J., Farrar, K., Park, B.K. & Breckenridge, A.M. 2004. Adverse drug reactions as cause of admission to hospital: Prospective analysis of 18 820 patients. *British Medical Journal*, **329**, 15–19.

Pollock, B.G. 1997. Gender differences in psychotropic drug metabolism. *Psychopharmacological Bulletin*, **33**, 235–241.

Pollock, B.G., Perel, J.M., Altieri, L.P., Kirshner, M., Fasiczka, A.L., Houck, P.R. & Reynolds, C.F. 1992. Debrisoquine hydroxylation phenotyping in geriatric psychopharmacology. *Psychopharmacological Bulletin*, **28**, 163–168.

Preskorn, S.H. 1997. Clinically relevant pharmacology of selective serotonin reuptake inhibitors. An overview with emphasis on pharmacokinetics and effects on oxidative drug metabolism. *Clinical Pharmacokinetics*, **32** Suppl 1, 1–21.

Pud, D., Yarnitsky, D., Sprecher, E., Rogowski, Z., Adler, R. & Eisenberg, E. 2006. Can personality traits and gender predict the response to morphine? An experimental cold pain study. *European Journal of Pain*, **10**, 103–112.

Ramchandani, V.A., Bosron, W.F. & Li, T.K. 2001. Research advances in ethanol metabolism. *Pathologie Biologie (Paris)*, **49**, 676–682.

Rao, S.S., Read, N.W., Brown, C., Bruce, C. & Holdsworth, C.D. 1987. Studies on the mechanism of bowel disturbance in ulcerative colitis. *Gastroenterology*, **93**, 934–940.

Ravizza, M., Martinelli, P., Bucceri, A., Fiore, S., Alberico, S., Tamburrini, E., Tibaldi, C., Guaraldi, G., Anzidei, G., Maccabruni, A., Crisalli, M.P. & Floridia, M. 2007. Treatment with protease inhibitors and coinfection with hepatitis C virus are independent predictors of preterm delivery in HIV-infected pregnant women. *Journal of Infectious Diseases*, **195**, 913–914; author reply 916–917.

Rickels, K. 1965. Some comments on non-drug factors in psychiatric drug therapy. *Psychosomatics*, **6**, 303–309.

Sanne, I., Mommeja-Marin, H., Hinkle, J., Bartlett, J.A., Lederman, M.M., Maartens, G., Wakeford, C., Shaw, A., Quinn, J., Gish, R.G. & Rousseau, F. 2005. Severe hepatotoxicity associated with nevirapine use in HIV-infected subjects. *Journal of Infectious Diseases*, **191**, 825–829.

Saxon, L., Hiltunen, A.J., Hjemdahl, P. & Borg, S. 2001. Gender-related differences in response to placebo in benzodiazepine withdrawal: A single-blind pilot study. *Psychopharmacology (Berlin)*, **153**, 231–237.

Schuetz, E.G., Furuya, K.N. & Schuetz, J.D. 1995. Interindividual variation in expression of P-glycoprotein in normal human liver and secondary hepatic neoplasms. *Journal of Pharmacological and Experimental Therapeutics*, **275**, 1011–1018.

Schulte, J., Dominguez, K., Sukalac, T., Bohannon, B. & Fowler, M.G. 2007. Declines in low birth weight and preterm birth among infants who were born to HIV-infected women during an era of increased use of maternal antiretroviral drugs: Pediatric Spectrum of HIV Disease, 1989–2004. *Pediatrics*, **119**, e900–e906.

Schwartz, J.B. 2003. The influence of sex on pharmacokinetics. *Clinical Pharmacokinetics*, **42**, 107–121.

Services, U.S.D.O.H.H. 2013. Selected prescription drug classes used in the past 30 days, by sex and age: United States, selected years 1988–1994 through 2007–2010. In PREVENTION, C.F.D.C.A. (ed.).

Spoletini, I., Vitale, C., Malorni, W. & Rosano, G.M. 2012. Sex differences in drug effects: Interaction with sex hormones in adult life. *Handbook of Experimental Pharmacology*, 91–105.

Tamminga, W.J., Wemer, J., Oosterhuis, B., Weiling, J., Wilffert, B., De Leij, L.F., De Zeeuw, R.A. & Jonkman, J.H. 1999. CYP2D6 and CYP2C19 activity in a large population of Dutch healthy volunteers: Indications for oral contraceptive-related gender differences. *European Journal of Pharmacology*, **55**, 177–184.

Tanaka, E. 1999. Gender-related differences in pharmacokinetics and their clinical significance. *Journal of Clinical Pharmacy and Therapeutics*, **24**, 339–346.

Townsend, C.L., Cortina-Borja, M., Peckham, C.S. & Tookey, P.A. 2007. Antiretroviral therapy and premature delivery in diagnosed HIV-infected women in the United Kingdom and Ireland. *AIDS*, **21**, 1019–1026.

Van Leth, F., Andrews, S., Grinsztejn, B., Wilkins, E., Lazanas, M.K., Lange, J.M. & Montaner, J. 2005. The effect of baseline CD4 cell count and HIV-1 viral load on the efficacy and safety of nevirapine or efavirenz-based first-line HAART. *AIDS*, **19**, 463–471.

Wadelius, M., Darj, E., Frenne, G. & Rane, A. 1997. Induction of CYP2D6 in pregnancy. *Clinical Pharmacology & Therapeutics*, **62**, 400–407.

Ward, D.S., Norton, J.R., Guivarc'h, P.H., Litman, R.S. & Bailey, P.L. 2002. Pharmacodynamics and pharmacokinetics of propofol in a medium-chain triglyceride emulsion. *Anesthesiology*, **97**, 1401–1408.

Wilcox, C.S., Cohn, J.B., Linden, R.D., Heiser, J.F., Lucas, P.B., Morgan, D.L. & Defrancisco, D. 1992. Predictors of placebo response: A retrospective analysis. *Psychopharmacological Bulletin*, **28**, 157–162.

Wilson, K. 1984. Sex-related differences in drug disposition in man. *Clinical Pharmacokinetics*, **9**, 189–202.

Yamamoto, H., Sekine, I., Yamada, K., Nokihara, H., Yamamoto, N., Kunitoh, H., Ohe, Y. & Tamura, T. 2008. Gender differences in treatment outcomes among patients with non–small cell lung cancer given a combination of carboplatin and paclitaxel. *Oncology*, **75**, 169–174.

Zhou, S., Yung Chan, S., Cher Goh, B., Chan, E., Duan, W., Huang, M. & Mcleod, H.L. 2005. Mechanism-based inhibition of cytochrome P450 3A4 by therapeutic drugs. *Clinical Pharmacokinetics*, **44**, 279–304.

Zyoud, S.H., Awang, R., Sulaiman, S.A. & Al-Jabi, S.W. 2010. A cross-sectional observation of the factors associated with deliberate self-poisoning with acetaminophen: Impact of gender differences and psychiatric intervention. *Human Psychopharmacology*, **25**, 500–508.

A Sex and Gender Based Perspective on Traumatic Injury

Jason Cohen, Stefan Merrill and Federico E. Vaca

Introduction

A 23-year-old woman, single mother of a young child, is driving home from a restaurant where she works as a server. As she rounds a curve, she sees several cars involved in a collision immediately in front of her. She tries to brake, but the road is icy and she skids, colliding with the other vehicles. The injured drivers and passengers are transported to the local hospital. She is diagnosed with a traumatic subarachnoid hemorrhage, an orbital wall fracture, multiple rib fractures, a pulmonary contusion, a splenic laceration, and a closed lower extremity fracture. She is resuscitated and admitted to the surgical intensive care unit. During her hospitalization, she undergoes several surgical procedures and is eventually transferred to a rehabilitation facility. How does gender impact her initial presentation and resuscitation? How can her biochemical and proteomic makeup change her body's response to stress and injury? What will the long-term impact of her trauma be on her quality of life?

Traumatic injury is a leading cause of death throughout the world and, currently, is the third leading cause of death for men and women younger than age 45 living in the industrialized world. Traumatic brain Injury (TBI) is the most common injury leading to death in trauma patients (Schoenberg et al. 2013). But only in the past decade have researchers investigated the effects of gender on outcomes from traumatic injury. The published work has demonstrated many conflicting results both in the preclinical/translational models and in direct clinical studies. Evidence has revealed an increasing incidence of severe traumatic injuries in women in the United States and throughout the world (Wohltman et al. 2001). Gender-based differences in risk-taking behavior and prevalence of participation in high-risk vocations/activities appear to be the major effectors of trauma type and the nature and extent of injury.

A review of the epidemiology of trauma reveals gender-based differences in the levels of severity and types of injury in every country where studies have been done. The burden of traumatic injury and post-traumatic morbidity varies by income and developmental status of the countries studied and accounts for some of the variability in mortality. However, even in countries designated "high income" by the World Health Organization where gender differences in morbidity and mortality from trauma would be expected to be minimized, a significant disparity remains (WHO – Global Health Observatory Data Repository 2013). Exposure to high-risk activities (machinery, firearms, motor vehicles) plays a large role in the causes and rates of trauma and trauma-related deaths. For example, more than 230 million motor vehicles are registered in the United States, and fewer than 5,000 in the Central African Republic (CAR). Motor vehicle crashes make a greater contribution to traumatic injury and death in the United States; however, because of limitations of resources including emergency and trauma care, the case fatality rate from trauma related to motor vehicle crashes is much greater in the CAR. This variability hinders attempts to quantify worldwide prevalence and carry out analysis of variance studies. Gender-related role behavior is magnified in working life, creating a downstream effect on work-related injuries, missed workdays, and inevitable financial implications. The majority (>60%) of missed workdays resulting from occupational injuries occurred in men – the median number of days missed was nine. Women who missed work as a result of occupational injuries tended to miss shorter periods of work – 7 days on median (CDC MMWR 2011a).

Within the United States itself, mechanisms of injury vary by sex. For example, the vast majority of firearms-related deaths occur in men (85% in 2013) (CDC VitalStats 2014; CDC WISQARS 2014). Examination of the data for emergency department visits for TBI in patients younger than age 19 demonstrates that head injuries in young men are most likely to result while playing football and head injuries in young women occur during playground activities (CDC MMWR 2011b). A report describing the impact of sex on adolescent trauma revealed that sex itself was not associated with differences in the number of injuries experienced by school-age patients once the investigators had controlled for risk-taking behavior, disciplinary issues, and the frequency of exercise (Alexander et al. 1995). These behavioral- and activity-based differences therefore account for significant disparities in the severity of overall injuries and the associated presentations further complicating the true impact of sex on outcomes in trauma patients.

Differences in the incidence and mechanisms of injury between the sexes affect Emergency Department care and treatment and also must be considered when planning public health interventions and injury prevention programs. However, the epidemiology of injury stratified by sex does not exclusively explain the differing outcomes between injured men and women. Multiple animal and human studies have demonstrated sex-based differences in immune-mediated reactions to trauma and, specifically, hemorrhagic shock (Angele and Faist 2000; Angele et al. 2000; Choudry et al. 2007). Following severe trauma, multiple inflammatory pathways are activated leading to increased production of cytokines and chemokines leading to the recruitment of immune-modulating cells to areas of injury as well as systemically (Lederer et al. 1999). This can lead to reduced host response to further infectious insult as well as direct end organ damage.

In males, this subsequent relative immuno-suppression (based on cytokine levels) following severe injury appears to be absent or greatly attenuated in females and castrated males. Animal models have suggested that these differences may be related to direct binding of sex hormones to receptors on immune system cells leading to down regulation (androgens) or stabilizing effects

(estrogen, progesterone, and estradiol) (Angele and Faist 2000; Angele et al. 2000). Alternatively, the cardiovascular and endothelial response to sex hormones may be responsible for these differences. Although the exact mechanisms remain unknown, some of the detrimental cytokine and inflammatory responses to trauma lower rates of multi-system organ dysfunction syndrome (MSODS) and sepsis following an initial traumatic insult. Many traumatic injuries are later complicated by infection and sepsis and contribute to further morbidity and mortality (Sauaia 1993). Thus, immunosuppression at the time of injury may be a major contributor to adverse outcomes. While most studies of older patients demonstrate a loss of the effect of gender on traumatic outcomes, a few investigations have reported conflicting results (e.g., Mostafa 2002). A German study showed *higher* mortality in older women than in their paired male counterparts, although this result may be explained by the increased incidence of head injury in the women and their overall older age (Schoenberg et al. 2013). While these sex steroid–mediated cytokine differences represent an appealing target for therapy, this has yet to be efficaciously translated into clinical practice.

Gender-Related Presentation of Disease/Injury

Anatomical differences between men and women may explain some of the effect of sex on the varying presentation of trauma patients. The shorter stature of women may result in an increase in lower body injuries following motor vehicle collisions (WHO – Gender and Road Traffic Injuries 2002). In a study on complications *after* trauma, women's shorter urethra may be responsible for the increase in urinary tract infections seen in women after traumatic injury when compared to men. Many variables affect the chance that one might sustain a traumatic injury, but some differences seen in outcomes are sex specific. Age and sex differences in microbiology and immunology also influence various outcomes and will be discussed in greater detail.

Investigators have shown the traumatically injured women are less likely to be as severely injured as men, more likely to have insurance,

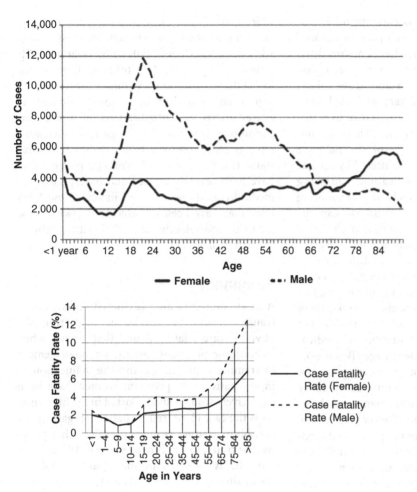

Figure 6.1 Trauma incidents and case fatality rate by age and gender

and less likely than men to present with self-inflicted injury. Men present at a higher frequency than women in all areas of traumatic injury until age 72, when the percentage of women treated for traumatic injury exceeds that of men, as recorded in the National Trauma Data Bank in 2013 (Figure 6.1) (American College of Surgeons, 2014).

Age Related

Trauma in the elderly is complicated by impaired hemostasis, adverse drug reactions and drug–drug interactions, and decreasing immune function. In reviews of the literature, it is clear that older adults had higher short- and long-term mortality rates than younger patients, higher in-hospital and post-hospital mortality for any given

ISS, and longer overall hospital stays (Jacoby et al. 2006). In elderly patients with abdominal trauma, the mortality rate is reported to range from two to three times greater than in younger people and more than a fourfold increase in thoracic trauma mortality (Sharma 2007; Wardle 1999). Sex is independently correlated with increased mortality in older adults (Jacoby et al. 2006).

In a systematic review by Jacoby et al., investigators cited multiple studies evaluating the relationship between sex and outcome for traumatically injured elders that consistently demonstrated that men had a higher risk of mortality than women (Jacoby et al. 2006). In these studies, women were more likely than men to be alive seven to eight years after injury. While differences in immunologic function by sex may contribute to this disparity in a manner similar to that seen in younger trauma patients, other reasons more specific to the elderly population need to be considered. Elders often have comorbidities with prescribed medications that may alter physiologic responses to trauma and acute injury, especially regarding pulmonary and cardiovascular reserves. Because of this, errors in triage decisions may occur when vital signs do not accurately reflect the severity of the patient's acute injury. Vital signs can be altered by cardiac and antihypertensive medications masking hypovolemia and early shock or exacerbating minor insults. Response to injury can be adversely affected by pharmacologic or physiologic alterations in hemodynamics and coagulation. Nevertheless, all of the difference in outcomes by sex in elderly trauma patients cannot necessarily be attributed to medications. In a study of nursing home patients in Israel, there was no difference in the number of different medication by sex, but the number of medications did increase with patient's age (Beloosesky et al. 2013). In a study in US nursing homes, elderly women were only slightly more likely than men to be taking more than nine drugs (OR 1.1, 95% CI, 1.00–1.20) (Dwyer et al. 2010). When only the most commonly prescribed medications were considered, there was no difference between the sexes. Patients taking more prescription medications have a greater risk of adverse drug reactions. Medications such as anticoagulants, antihypertensives, and sedatives can adversely affect an elderly patient's ability to cope with trauma. Nevertheless, no evidence shows a significant difference between sexes in the number or types of medications that elders take (Nguyen et al. 2006).

Variances in the prevalence of types of medical problems are another consideration that might contribute to differences between the sexes in injury presentation and outcomes in elderly patients. For example, osteoporosis is more common in elderly women and is associated with an increased risk of fractures from trauma. Elderly women are more likely than men to sustain rib fractures; however, the likelihood of mortality from these rib fractures was 2.35 (95% CI, 1.1 – 5.7) times higher in men. Likewise, the mortality and morbidity of hip fractures are widely reported with a large sex discrepancy among these patients.

More than 75% of those sustaining hip fractures are women, likely due to the effects of osteoporosis (Jordan and Cooper 2002). First-year mortality statistics range from 12% to 37%, likely related to anatomic location (Wolinsky et al. 1997). Significant mortality has been attributed to exacerbations or complications of preexisting conditions. Less than half of patients sustaining a hip fracture return to their baseline functional status (Keene et al. 1993). Younger patients who have been severely injured and have preexisting medical conditions also have increased mortality rates that have been reported to be twice those seen in equivalently injured healthy patients (Morris et al. 1990).

Pregnancy

A discussion regarding sex-based differences in trauma would be remiss in neglecting the obvious care-related issues that arrive when treating the pregnant patient. The management of trauma in pregnancy and the delineation of injury patterns in pregnant women have been extensively studied and reported in the literature. As is the case in all trauma patients regardless of sex, blunt trauma is more prevalent that penetrating trauma in pregnant women. Women are more likely to suffer intimate partner violence (IPV) during pregnancy. Therefore, emergency health care providers must have a higher index of suspicion for IPV and should systematically screen all pregnant patients presenting for the evaluation of an injury or vague illness. Such interventions have been demonstrated to decrease the effects of IPV and to improve pregnancy-related outcomes (Kiely et al. 2010).

In the United States, trauma is the leading cause of death in pregnant women (Fildes et al. 1992). Surprisingly though, some studies have reported that pregnant women have a lower mortality rate than nonpregnant women presenting with similar injury severity and injury severity scores (John et al. 2011). This can be understood by the fact that traumatic injury proportionally causes the most deaths during pregnancy.

Procedures commonly performed on trauma patients in the emergency department require special consideration in the traumatically injured pregnant woman (Figure 6.2). While an in-depth

Estimation of fetal age by physical exam or ultrasound	Uterine fundus at umbilicus equals about 22 weeks gestation
Determine Rh status if bleeding	Consider Rhogam in Rh negative mother
Understand implications of gravid uterus on procedures and anatomy	Changes in FAST scan and landmarks to be used in procedures like tube thoracostomy
Do not limit diagnostic and resuscitative efforts in the setting of pregnancy	Utilize CT and x-ray per usual protocol to diagnose traumatic injury in pregnant patients

Figure 6.2 Keys to resuscitation of the traumatically injured pregnant woman

discussion is beyond the scope of this chapter, it is crucial to recognize that anatomy and physiology change throughout gestation, and the emergency health care provider must keep these changes in mind when evaluating the patient or planning a procedure. For example, when placing a chest tube in women in the third trimester of pregnancy, the tube must be inserted one intercostal space above the usual site of insertion between the fourth and fifth ribs to avoid injuring the diaphragm that is elevated because of the size and position of the gravid uterus. Pregnancy-related alterations in evaluation and treatment must be studied and practiced by the emergency health care provider prior to confronting a crashing pregnant trauma patient so that habits of muscle memory and routine do not interfere with the rendering of effective care in critical situations.

Beyond routine trauma care, the emergency health care provider should be prepared to perform the following additional critical interventions for the pregnant trauma patient: establishment of fetal age (changes in physical exam), maintaining patient in a left lateral decubitus position (to decrease effect of uterus on inferior vena cava), determination of Rh status (administration of rhogam as indicated to prevent subsequent fetal hydrops), carrying out all appropriate imaging for the type and severity of injuries in the same manner and as thoroughly as would be done in the non-pregnant trauma patient (care of fetus is predicated on care of mother), and screening for intimate partner violence (Zelop 2013).

Immunology/Hormones

Some of the most interesting and important research on sex differences in trauma patients has focused on the effects of hormones. Several studies have reported menstruating women who

suffer a traumatic injury or sepsis have increased survival rates. The immune function of women who are immediately preovulatory remains fully active after severe trauma, in contradistinction to young men and oophorectimized or postmenopausal women, whose immune function is impaired after significant trauma (Choudhry et al. 2007). One explanation of this phenomenon is that estradiol enhances cell-mediated and humoral immunity while androgens suppress the immune system. In animal models, castration has been shown to improve survival after trauma. Premenopausal women are less likely to develop many of the life-threatening complications of trauma, such as adult respiratory distress syndrome (ARDS), pneumonia, sepsis, pulmonary emboli, or acute renal failure. However, women who develop these complications have a greater case fatality rate than men. Women with any of these complications have an odds ratio of death of 1.2 compared to men. If they avoid these complications, they are 26% less likely to die from similar traumatic injuries than men (Haider et al. 2009).

Sex hormones may be important therapeutic options in trauma. However, interpreting their significance in certain populations can be complicated by exogenous hormone intake and clinical human studies have not demonstrated efficacy (Angele et al. 2012).

LGBT Patients

The emergency health care provider must be aware of the more common hormone regimens used by transsexual patients and the implications of those regimens on the morbidity and mortality related to trauma. Male patients transitioning to female use combinations of antiandrogens, GnRH agonists, and estrogens, which, theoretically, could improve their survival from traumatic injury if the data demonstrating the relationship of mortality from traumatic injury to hormonal changes associated with the menstrual cycle can be extrapolated to exogenous hormone ingestion (Gooren and Tangpricha 2013). However, hormones supplements for gender transition are not always taken as prescribed by physicians, or not always purchased in pharmacies. They can be acquired online from vendors whose sources are unregulated and may lack quality control and testing. Providers should be aware of potential complications of exogenous hormone ingestion, such as increased rate of venous thromboembolic events and accelerated cardiovascular disease. Females transitioning to male use androgen therapies such as testosterone. Sex hormones in these cases are, of course, not being taken by the patient to improve outcomes in trauma and sepsis but may have a significant pejorative effect on outcomes.

Traumatic Brain Injury

The rates of TBI related to ED visits increased in 2010 for both men and women (Figure 6.3) (Centers for Disease Control 2011b). A recent study showed that women who had sustained a TBI during the luteal phase of their menstrual cycle, when progesterone levels were high, had lower quality of life health-rating scores than women who sustained a TBI when progesterone levels were low and estrogen was high (Wunderle et al. 2013). When examined in a murine model,

all female mice suffering from TBI survived the initial injury in the acute period, as compared to 72% of the male mice. Female mice had less impairment in cerebral blood flow and better recovery than male mice. The improved survival in the females was posited to be the result of the ability of the females to maintain a higher and more consistent mean arterial blood pressure and therefore more consistent cerebral perfusion pressure in the face of elevated estrogen levels. The investigators suggest that estrogen may be neuroprotective, with beneficial effects on the cerebral microvasculature, inducing the production of endothelial nitric oxide synthase, which has an important antioxidant effect limiting oxidant-mediated damage through a direct antioxidant effect (Roof and Hall 2000).

Multiple other models have demonstrated improved outcomes when the brain injury was treated with adjunctive progesterone. Animal models of injury have found beneficial effects on both anatomic and functional outcomes along with decreases in associated biomarkers of injury and inflammation. Progesterone has been found to cross the blood-brain barrier and decrease levels of cerebral edema and associated expression of pro-apoptotic genes (Stein 2011). This has been followed by three small human clinical trials that, while positive, have yet to demonstrate sufficient strength of evidence to recommend progesterone therapy for traumatic brain injured patients (Ma et al. 2012). Several large, prospective clinical

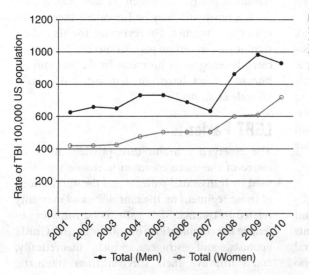

Figure 6.3 Rates of traumatic brain injury by sex – United States, 2001–2010
Source: Center for Disease Control: 2014. Available at www.cdc.gov/traumaticbraininjury. Accessed July 1, 2014.

trials are currently being conducted in several countries that, it is hoped, will provide clear direction as to progesterone's utility and efficacy in preventing the severe morbidity associated with TBI (ProTECT III and SyNAPSe).

Provider and Team Differences

Beyond understanding the role that sex plays in the trauma patient, it is important to consider the implications of gender differences among health care providers and in the resuscitation team. Significant research has been done investigating the qualities of skilled and effective trauma teams, including team composition and communication styles, but no studies have been done evaluating the differences between male and female trauma team leaders. Historically, men have held more leadership roles; therefore, "maleness" and masculine characteristics including competitiveness, aggression, and dominance have become associated with leadership. These characteristics may not truly be the most effective for trauma team leadership. In fact, women's leadership characteristics such as the ability to cooperate and engender collaboration in others, manifesting and encouraging empathy, and providing emotional support to the patient and the team may be equally important or more useful in successfully coordinating a team approach to trauma management. It may be that there are greater differences between leaders of the same sex reflecting their personalities and social and emotional backgrounds than identifiable gender-based leadership characteristics (Moran 1992). Leadership qualities are generally situationally dependent. Leaders who succeed are those whose skills fit the situation or who rise to the occasion. It is not difficult to imagine that providers who choose to work in the specialties of trauma surgery or emergency medicine might have intrinsic personality-based leadership characteristics that are not gender specific. Beyond leadership, gender seems to affect other aspects of doctor–patient interactions. For example, a study revealed that nurses (the majority of whom are women) provide less analgesia to men than to women. Conversely, physicians of both sexes are more likely to undertreat female patients in pain (Chen et al. 2008; Nevin 1996).

A study published in 2012 in the United States demonstrated a surprising bias in the triaging of injured patients to designated trauma receiving centers in countries where such centers exist. The investigators found that pre-hospital providers were more likely to transport injured men than injured women to trauma centers (41% vs. 31%, p<0.0001). This bias was maintained even after the researchers controlled for age, comorbidities, injury severity score, and bodily region injured. This bias was also seen when the investigators reported on physician decisions to transfer patients to trauma centers from non-trauma designated emergency medicine facilities (36% vs. 24% p<0.0001) (Gomez et al. 2012). The impact of this discrepancy has not been individually teased out but can be assumed to be dramatic given the demonstrated mortality benefit of 30% when direct pre-hospital transfer to a trauma center is achieved (Haas et al. 2012).

Long-Term Sequelae

Advances in medical care have increased survival after traumatic injury, especially after severe multi-system trauma and TBI. These patients often require ongoing community support to facilitate their return to functional daily activities and life. Given the differences in the prevalence of significant trauma and degree of severity of injuries between the sexes and the many complex sociocultural, economic, and political differences associated with gender, there is a profound social and economic difference in the long-term effects of temporary and permanent disability. Women are less likely to hold jobs with adequate health or disability insurance and may be unable to pay for assistance with child care if they are injured. Furthermore, men, in many cultures, are the sole provider of income for the household. Thus, the impact of severe injury on men and women will be different with varied and significant acute manifestations and long-term repercussions. No published articles examine the differences by gender in the long-term outcome, both socioeconomically and medically, following severe traumatic injury. The studies that are available primarily examine differences in outcome after TBI. Some other papers focus on the psychological sequelae of trauma in the form of post-traumatic stress disorder (PTSD).

One study on the long-term consequences of mild TBI revealed that women tended to have an increased incidence of persistent symptoms including dizziness, fatigue, headache, anxiety, and depression (Farrace and Alves 2000). Conversely, long-term executive function and cognitive flexibility are more likely to be preserved in women than in men when patients are assessed one year following TBI (Colantonio et al. 2010). Some studies have demonstrated improved community integration for women after TBI. However, a differential persistence of symptoms was seen between men and women for up to 10 years post injury (Doninger et al. 2003; Schopp et al. 2001; Bay et al. 2009).

PTSD is now widely recognized as a significant problem following any kind of traumatic injury but especially TBI and injuries requiring treatment in an intensive care unit. Although women have a lower incidence of traumatic injuries than men, they develop PTSD at up to twice the rate that men do. This increased rate is found even after controlling for injury/trauma type and severity (Breslau et al. 1998; Ditlevsen and Elkit 2010). Interestingly, the increased rate of PTSD seen in women seems to reverse with age; men older than age 50 have an increased prevalence of PTSD (Creamer and Parslow 2008). It may be that gender-based differences in the rates of PTSD reflect men's tendencies to underreport symptoms and women's tendencies to over report symptoms of PTSD (Ditlevsen and Elkit 2010).

Conclusion

Our patient survived her motor vehicle collision and was in the hospital for four weeks; she was then discharged to inpatient rehabilitation for two weeks. She had persistent memory loss and was frequently dizzy. She was able to climb a flight of stairs but had to rest at the top. She reported persistent pain in her injured leg and could not bear weight on it for more than 10 to 15 minutes. She reported frequent anxiety and experienced vivid recollections of having uncomfortable things done to her in the intensive care unit. She was unable to sleep for more than an hour at a time. She was unable to return to work because of her symptoms and her physical condition and needed to move in with her extended family as she could not afford additional care for her daughter.

There is still much to be learned about gender differences in the treatment of trauma. Unfortunately, many of the biochemical

mechanisms that appeared to explain gender differences in preclinical studies have not translated into the clinical realm, especially the preclinical models of inflammation. Greater attention and more research in developing a broader understanding of these underlying pathways are needed. Defining the differences in trauma response between genders is crucial to developing an understanding of these mechanisms and identifying potential treatments. Acknowledging and focusing on these differences will also help clinicians devise more effective public health and injury prevention strategies.

References

Alexander C.S., Somerfield M.R., Ensminger M.E., Kim Y.J., Johnson KE. 1995. Gender differences in injuries among rural youth. *Injury Prevention*, **1**, 15–20.

Alspach J.G. 2012. Is there gender bias in critical care? *Critical Care Nursing*, **32**(6), 8–14.

American College of Surgeons, Committee on Trauma. 2014. National Trauma Database Annual Report 2013. Available at www.facs.org/quality-programs/trauma/ntdb/docpub. Accessed July 30, 2014.

Angele M.K., Schwacha M.G., Ayala A., & Chaudry I.H. (2000). Effect of gender and sex hormones on immune responses following shock. *Shock*, **14**(2), 81–90.

Angele M.K., Pratschke S., & Chaudry I.H. 2012. Does gender influence outcomes in critically ill patients? *Critical Care*, **16**(3), 129–130.

Angele M.K. & Faist E. 2000. Gender-specific immune response following shock: Clinical and experimental data. *European Journal of Trauma*, **26**(6), 267–277.

Bay E., Sikorskii A., & Saint-Arnault D. 2009. Sex differences in depressive symptoms and their correlates after mild-to-moderate traumatic brain injury. *Journal of Neuroscience Nursing*, **41**(6), 298–309.

Breslau N., Kessler R.C., Chilcoat H.D., Schultz L.R., Davis G.C., & Andreski P. 1998. Trauma and posttraumatic stress disorder in the community: The 1996 Detroit Area Survey of Trauma. *Archives of General Psychiatry*, **55**(7), 626–632.

Beloosesky Y., Nenaydenko O., Gross Nevo R.F., Adunsky A., & Weiss A. 2013. Rates, variability, and associated factors of polypharmacy in nursing home patients. *Clinical Interventions in Aging*, **8**, 1585–1590.

Centers for Disease Control and Prevention – Morbidity and Mortality Weekly Report. 2011a. Nonfatal Occupational Injuries and Illnesses Among Older Workers – United States, 2009. Available at www.cdc.gov/mmwr/preview/mmwrhtml/mm6016a3.htm?s_cid=mm6016a3_w#tab. Accessed January 9, 2014.

Centers for Disease Control and Prevention – Morbidity and Mortality Weekly Report. 2011b. Nonfatal Traumatic Brain Injuries Related to Sports and Recreation Activities Among Persons Aged ≤19 Years – United States, 2001–2009. Available at www.cdc.gov/mmwr/preview/mmwrhtml/mm6039a1.htm?s_cid=mm6039a1_w#tab3. Accessed January 5, 2014.

Centers for Disease Control and Prevention – National Center for Health Statistics. VitalStats. Available at www.cdc.gov/nchs/vitalstats.htm. Accessed January 9, 2014.

Centers for Disease Control and Prevention – National Center for Injury Prevention and Control. Web-based Injury Statistics Query and Reporting System (WISQARS) [online]. Accessed January 9, 2014.

Chen E.H., Shofer F.S., Dean A.J., Hollander J.E., Baxt W.G., Robey J.L., Sease K.L., Mills A.M. 2008. Gender disparity in analgesic treatment of emergency department patients with acute abdominal pain. *Academic Emergency Medicine*, 15(5), 414–418.

Choudhry M.A., Bland K.I., & Chaudry I.H. 2007. Trauma and immune response–effect of gender differences. *Injury*, 38(12), 1382–1391.

Colantonio A., Harris J.E., Ratcliff G., Chase S., Ellis K. 2010. Gender differences in self reported long term outcomes following moderate to severe traumatic brain injury. *BMC Neurology*, 10(102).

Creamer M. & Parslow R. 2008. Trauma exposure and posttraumatic stress disorder in the elderly: A community prevalence study. *American Journal of Geriatric Psychiatry*, 16(10), 853–856.

Ditlevsen D. and Elkit A. 2010. The combined effect of gender and age on post traumatic stress disorder: Do men and women show differences in the lifespan distribution of the disorder? *Annals of General Psychiatry*, 9(32).

Doninger N.A., Heinemann A.W., Bode R.K., Sokol K., & Corrigan J.D. 2003. Predicting community integration following traumatic brain injury with health and cognitive status measures. *Rehabilitation Psychology*, 48(6).

Dwyer L.L., Han B., Woodwell D.A., & Rechtsteiner E.A. 2010. Polypharmacy in nursing home residents in the United States: Results of the 2004 National Nursing Home Survey. *The American Journal of Geriatric Pharmacotherapy*, 8(1), 63–72.

Fildes J., Reed L., Jones N., Martin M., & Barrett J. 1992. Trauma: The leading cause of maternal death. *Journal of Trauma*, 32(5), 643–645.

Gomez D., Haas B., de Mestral C., Sharma S., Hsiao M., Zagorski B., Rubenfeld G., Ray J., & Nathens A.B. 2012. Gender-associated differences in access to trauma center care: A population-based analysis. *Surgery*, 152(2):179–185.

Gooren L.J. and Tangpricha V. 2013. Treatment of Transsexualism. UptoDate. Available at www.uptodate.com. Accessed July 1, 2014.

Haas B., Stukel T.A., Gomez D., Zagorski B., De Mestral C., Sharma S.V., Rubenfeld G.D., & Nathens A.B. 2012. The mortality benefit of direct trauma center transport in a regional trauma system: A population-based analysis. *Journal of Trauma and Acute Care Surgery*, 72(6), 1510–1515.

Haider A.H., Crompton J.G., Oyetunji T., Stevens K.A., Efron D.T., Kieninger A.N., Chang D.C., Cornwell E.E., 3rd, & Haut E.R. 2009. Females have fewer complications and lower mortality following trauma than similarly injured males: A risk adjusted analysis of adults in the National Trauma Data Bank. *Surgery*, 146(2), 308–315.

Jacoby S.F., Ackerson T.H., & Richmond T.S. 2006. Outcome from serious injury in older adults. *Journal of Nursing Scholarship*, 38(2), 133–140.

John P.R., Shiozawa A., Haut E.R., Efron D.T., Haider A., & Cornwell E.E., 3rd et al. 2011. An assessment of the impact of pregnancy on trauma mortality. *Surgery*, 149(1), 94–8.

Jordan K.M. and Cooper C. 2002. Epidemiology of osteoporosis. *Best Practice and Research: Clinical Rheumatology*, 16(5), 795–806.

Keene G.S., Parker M.J., & Pryor G.A. 1993. Mortality and morbidity after hip fractures. *British Medical Journal*, 307(6914):1248–1250.

Kiely M., El-Mohandes A., El-Khorazaty M., & Gantz M. 2010. An integrated intervention to reduce intimate partner violence in pregnancy: A randomized trial. *Obstetrics & Gynecology*, 115(2), 273–283.

Lederer, J.A., Rodrick, M.L., & Mannick, J.A. 1999. The effects of injury on the adaptive immune response. *Shock*, 11(3), 153–159.

Moran B. 1992. Gender Differences in Leadership. Library Trends. 40. The Board of Trustees, University of Illinois; pp. 475–491.

Morris J.A., Jr., MacKenzie E.J., Damiano A.M., & Bass S.M. 1990. Mortality in trauma patients: The interaction between host factors and severity. *Journal of Trauma*, 30(12), 1476–1482.

Mostafa G., Huynh T., Sing R.F., Miles W.S., Norton H.J., & Thomason M.H. 2002. Gender-related outcomes in trauma. *Journal of Trauma*, 53(3), 430–435.

Nevin K. 1996. Influence of sex on pain assessment and management. *Annals of Emergency Medicine*, 27(4), 424–426.

Nguyen J.K., Fouts M.M., Kotabe S.E., & Lo E. 2006. Polypharmacy as a risk factor for adverse drug reactions in geriatric nursing home residents. *The American Journal of Geriatric Pharmacotherapy*, 4(1), 36–41.

Roof R.L. & Hall E.D. 2000. Gender differences in acute CNS trauma and stroke: Neuroprotective effects of estrogen and progesterone. *Journal of Neurotrauma*, **17**(5), 367–388.

Sauaia A., Moore F.A., Moore E.E., Haenel J.B., & Read R.A. 1993. Pneumonia: Cause or symptom of postinjury multiple organ failure? *American Journal of Surgery*, **166**(6), 606–610.

Schoenberg C., Kauther M.D., Hussmann B., Keitel J., Schmitz D., & Lendemans S. 2013. Gender-specific differences in severely injured patients between 2002 and 2011: Data analysis with matched-pair analysis. *Critical Care*, **17**(6), R277.

Schopp L., Shigaki C., Johnstone B., & Kirlpatrick H. 2001. Gender differences in cognitive and emotional adjustment to traumatic brain injury. *Journal of Clinical Psychology in Medical Settings*, **8**, 181.

Sharma O.P., Oswanski M.F., Sharma V., Stringfellow K., & Raj S.S. 2007. An appraisal of trauma in the elderly. *The American Surgeon*, **73**(4), 354–358.

Stein D.G. 2011. Is progesterone a worthy candidate as a novel therapy for traumatic brain injury? *Dialogues in Clinical Neuroscience*, **13**(3), 352–359.

Wardle T.D. 1999. Co-morbid factors in trauma patients. *British Medical Bulletin*, **55**(4), 744–756.

Wolinsky F.D., Fitzgerald J.F., & Stump T.E. 1997. The effect of hip fracture on mortality, hospitalization, and functional status: A prospective study. *American Journal of Public Health*, **87**(3), 398.

World Health Organization. n.d. Gender and Health: Gender and Road Traffic Injuries. Available at www.who.int/gender/documents/road_traffic/a85576/en/index.html. Accessed January 12, 2014.

World Health Organization. 2013. Global Health Observatory Data Repository. Available at http://apps.who.int/gho/data/node.main.886?lang=en. Accessed January 4, 2014.

Wunderle K., Hoeger K.M., Wasserman E., & Bazarian J.J. 2014. Menstrual phase as predictor of outcome after mild traumatic brain injury in women. *Journal of Head Trauma Rehabilitation*. **29**(5), E1–8.

Zelop, C.M. 2013. Cardiopulmonary arrest in pregnancy. UpToDate. Available at www.uptodate.com. Accessed July 9, 2014.

7

Sex and Gender Differences in the Presentation and Treatment of Cerebrovascular Emergencies

Tracy Madsen and Karen Furie

Opening Case

EL is a 63-year-old woman with a history of migraine, hypertension, and hyperlipidemia who presented to the Emergency Department with a persistent, severe, right-sided headache and right-sided weakness that had lasted 30 minutes before resolving. EL had frequently experienced right-sided "migraines," although she had never experienced numbness or weakness with her migraines in the past. On exam, EL was neurologically intact and denied any symptoms other than her headache. As her weakness had completely resolved and her headache seemed similar to prior episodes, EL was treated symptomatically and discharged home with primary care follow-up.

Introduction

Cerebrovascular emergencies are among the most life-threatening and time-sensitive conditions that emergency medicine (EM) physicians are expected to diagnose and treat in the acute care setting; it is essential that physicians are aware of the sex and gender differences in the presentation, diagnosis, and treatment of these emergent conditions. In the United States, there are 795,000 new strokes each year, and stroke is the leading cause of disability and the fifth-leading cause of death.[1] Headaches, which may be the primary presenting symptom of subarachnoid hemorrhage (SAH) and intracerebral hemorrhage (ICH), account for 3 million Emergency Department (ED) visits in the United States;[2] there are many sex and gender differences in the epidemiology, pathophysiology, and course of these conditions. Seizure, a complication of cerebrovascular disease, also shows sex and gender differences relevant to ED providers. The frequency with which ED providers treat patients with neurovascular

emergencies as well as the high morbidity and mortality of these illnesses make it essential that EM physicians understand how sex and gender affect disease risk, presentation, management, and outcomes. In this chapter, the term "sex" will be used to discuss differences between men and women that are due to biologic or physiologic processes; "gender" will be used to discuss differences between men and women that may be influenced by social and cultural roles and expectations.

Discussion

Ischemic Stroke

Disease Risk and Prevention

Compared to men, women have a higher lifetime risk of stroke (both ischemic and hemorrhagic) but a lower age-specific incidence of stroke because women have longer life expectancies and are approximately five years older at the time of their initial stroke.[3] EM physicians routinely perform risk assessment during the diagnosis and disposition of suspected stroke patients; multiple sex differences in stroke risk factor prevalence should be considered. Women are more likely to have hypertension and atrial fibrillation as risk factors for stroke; men are more likely to have large artery atherosclerosis, diabetes, and myocardial infarctions.[4–7] ED providers should also be aware that both diabetes and metabolic syndrome increase the risk of stroke more dramatically in women than in men.[3,8] In addition, there are known sex differences in the utility of antithrombotic medications for primary stroke prevention: Aspirin is effective at preventing stroke in women but not in men; consequently, it is imperative that women receive antiplatelet therapy for primary prevention of stroke.

Older women have a greater prevalence of atrial fibrillation than older men; therefore, they have more cardio-embolic strokes when compared to men.[6,9–11] It is particularly concerning that in spite of the increased incidence of cardio-embolic strokes in women, women with stroke and atrial fibrillation are less likely to be started on anticoagulant therapy.[7,12–15] Multiple studies have also shown that women are less likely to be discharged on aspirin after suffering a stroke.[13–15] EM providers should be especially vigilant in identifying atrial fibrillation in ED stroke patients and appropriately initiating anticoagulation therapy.

Stroke risk factors specific to women include pregnancy and its complications, hormonal contraception, and hormone replacement therapy (HRT). Stroke causes approximately 12% of deaths during pregnancy, and the greatest risks occur during the third trimester and the peripuerperal period.[16] Complications of pregnancy lead to a dramatically increased stroke risk during the pregnancy itself; however, the risks can persist for up to 30 years after delivery.[17] Conditions associated with increased risk of stroke include preeclampsia, eclampsia, hypertension of pregnancy, and gestational diabetes. For example, women with a history of preeclampsia or eclampsia have almost twice the odds of stroke in the 10 years following their pregnancy.[17] Women using exogenous hormones, primarily estrogen, are also at increased risk for primary stroke. Two randomized controlled trials studying estrogen for primary stroke prevention, the Women's Health Initiative (WIH) Study and the Women's Estrogen Stroke Trial (WEST), found estrogen to be of no benefit for stroke prevention; women on estrogen in the WIH study were actually at increased risk of stroke.[18]

Migraine with aura is another important risk factor for stroke in women. Migraine headaches are three times more common in women than in men, and among all patients with migraine, the risk of stroke is more pronounced in women.[19] Migraine will be discussed in more depth in the "Migraines/Headache" section of the chapter.

Sex Differences in the Biology and Physiology of Stroke

The etiology of sex differences in stroke is multifactorial, but estrogen is thought to play a major role in the brain's response to injury. During acute ischemia, in preclinical models, estrogen acts as a neuroprotectant through its actions on neurons, glial cells, and endothelial cells. In animal and cell models, estrogen down regulates inflammation, decreases disruption of the blood-brain barrier, reduces cell death, and causes vasodilation of cerebral vessels; however, these mechanisms have not been confirmed in humans.[20] Estrogen's effects on inflammation and apoptosis are altered in the setting of specific genetic polymorphisms as well, making the pathophysiology even more complex.[20–23] Despite preclinical knowledge that estrogen acts as a neuroprotectant, there has not yet been research investigating estrogen as a potential beneficial treatment in the acute setting for humans with ischemic stroke. Other preclinical data have revealed additional genetic differences between male and female cells that contribute to different responses to injury and ischemia, even in the absence of sex hormones.[20,24] In preclinical models of cerebral ischemia without the influence of sex hormones, novel treatments designed to decrease inflammation seem to have more effect in male cells, suggesting additional mechanisms for sex differences in the brain's response to injury.[20,24,25] For example, in animal models, kappa opioid receptor agonists thought to decrease nitric oxide production in acute ischemic stroke reduce brain infarct volume in males but not in females, even in the absence of endogenous sex hormones.[24] Future research should (a) investigate estrogen as a possible ED treatment for acute ischemic stroke and (b) consider that current and future ED therapies for ischemic stroke may have sex-specific benefits and responses.

ED Presentation/Clinical Manifestations

As has been described in acute coronary syndromes, women are more likely to have nontraditional symptoms of stroke including pain, change in level of consciousness, and non-neurologic symptoms.[26,27] Women are also more likely to have stroke mimics.[28–30] There are no known consistent gender differences, however, in the frequency of traditional symptoms including hemiparesis and unilateral sensory changes. In one study that surveyed patients admitted with acute stroke, women were 42% more likely to report at least one nontraditional symptom.[27] ED physicians should be aware of the frequency of atypical symptoms in stroke to minimize potential diagnostic and treatment delays.

Since both intravenous (IV) as well as intraarterial (IA) therapies for ischemic stroke are time sensitive, delay to ED presentation is a critical issue for both men and women. Some studies have shown gender differences in the time between symptom onset and ED arrival, but other data conflict, likely because of methodological differences across studies.[31–36] Living alone and having an unwitnessed onset of symptoms are associated with longer pre-hospital delays and may be contributors to gender disparities in treatment; these factors affect women more often than men because of women's longer life expectancies.[4,37] Future ED-based research should investigate methods to decrease pre-hospital delays for those living alone or with unwitnessed stroke.

Diagnosis

A non-contrast CT scan is the initial imaging modality of choice for patients presenting with stroke symptoms. Studies of gender disparities in stroke care show that women are less likely to receive rapid brain imaging, which is defined by the American Heart Association and American Stroke Association as non-contrast CT within 25 minutes of arrival.[38,39] In a large study of patients in a national stroke registry, women were 15% less likely to have initial brain imaging completed within 25 minutes in unadjusted analysis and 7% less likely to have rapid brain imaging in adjusted analysis.[38] Studies have also found that women wait longer for physician evaluation, but these findings have not been replicated consistently.[32,40]

In addition, women are less likely to have echocardiography and carotid ultrasound performed during their stroke evaluation. These are both important tools in the evaluation of stroke etiology but in the past have been less directly relevant to ED providers as compared to neurologists. Relevance to ED providers will increase, however, as ED physicians assume care for patients in TIA observation units.[3]

Acute Management

In addition to being aware of gender disparities in diagnostic imaging, ED providers should be aware of gender disparities in the use of standard ED stroke treatments. In multiple observational studies, women were less likely to receive IV tissue plasminogen activator (tPA) for acute ischemic stroke.[7,31,33,41–43] In one meta-analysis of 18 studies, women were between 19% and 30% less likely to receive IV tPA.[42] In some populations, gender disparities in the use of IV tPA are attenuated after adjusting for variables including age, National Institutes of Health Stroke Scale (NIHSS), and other eligibility criteria, but these factors do not completely explain the treatment differences.[42] Other contributing factors to the discrepancy in the use of tPA may include delays to ED arrival, delays to CT scan, and women's presentation with nontraditional symptoms; however, the literature suggests that these factors do not completely explain the disparities. Future researchers should investigate the current status of gender disparities in the use of IV tPA. Recent data from national stroke registries have shown increasing rates of tPA use over time, but it is unknown whether gender disparities remain or whether the use of organized stroke care has reduced these disparities.[44,45]

In addition, there may be gender disparities in the use of intra-arterial therapies in the acute treatment of stroke.[45] This area of research is not as well developed as research on IV tPA, but one large study of patients from a national US database revealed that women were 36% less likely than men to receive cerebral angiography.[45] This study was limited by a lack of data on the specific intra-arterial procedures performed. Further investigation is necessary to evaluate the presence of disparities in specific intra-arterial therapies including intra-arterial tPA and mechanical thrombectomy.

Treatment Response

Disparities in the use of IV tPA have been especially notable in light of data suggesting that IV tPA is more beneficial to women than men. A 2006 pooled analysis of patients from tPA clinical trials showed that women treated with tPA were 10% more likely to be able to carry out their usual daily activities at 90 days when compared to those receiving placebo, while no such treatment response was found in men.[46] Other small studies are supportive of this finding, including one small retrospective study that found that women receiving tPA were more likely to have vessel recanalization on post-stroke imaging.[47] There has been speculation that women's improved response to treatment with tPA may be related to variations in fibrinolysis, but the differences in response to tPA and the factors causing those differences need to be confirmed. If there are in fact genetic, hormonal, or other biologic differences between women and men that impact the effectiveness of tPA, it is imperative that these be identified so ED therapies can be used with greater specificity and efficacy.

Clinical Outcomes

Gender differences in mortality from stroke vary across age categories, but because of women's longer life expectancies, the total number of stroke deaths is higher for women than for men. There are no consistent gender differences in case fatality from stroke after adjusting for factors such as age and stroke severity.[3]

Data on functional outcomes in ischemic stroke are clearer: Women consistently fare more poorly than men. Specifically, women are more likely to be disabled three months after stroke and have limitations in activities of daily living (ADLs) and lower health-related quality of life scores one year after a stroke when compared to men.[4,6,12,48,49] Women are also less likely to return home after stroke and more likely to be discharged to chronic care facilities.[5,12] Studies of gender differences in functional outcomes after stroke typically include both treated and untreated patients and do not consistently adjust for use of tPA. Some of the factors that may contribute to worse functional outcomes for women may include older age and more comorbidities at the time of the stroke, although these do not completely explain the difference. In the future, investigations of ED diagnostic tools such as prognostic biomarkers or clinical decision rules may help ED providers identify both women and men at risk for poor outcomes.

Hemorrhagic Stroke

Disease Risk/Prevention

Spontaneous intracerebral hemorrhages (ICH) represent only a small portion of strokes overall; approximately 10% to 15% of new strokes are spontaneous hemorrhagic strokes,[50] and the incidence of ICH has been estimated to be 246 per 100,000 person-years.[51] In one study of 266 patients in China, ICH was twice as common in men as compared to women.[52] In a meta-analysis across multiple countries, however, there were no differences in the incidence of ICH between men and women.[51] Risk factors for ICH include hypertension, diabetes, and use of caffeine, tobacco, and alcohol. These factors may increase risk differentially in men versus women. For example, both hypertension and excessive alcohol use increased the risk of ICH in men more significantly than in women in a group of 18- to 49-year-olds.[53]

Another potential risk factor for ICH that differs by gender is the use of stimulant substances, including ephedrine, a weight-loss supplement used twice as frequently by women.[54] Multiple case series suggest that ephedrine use is associated with ICH, but one large retrospective study of more than 700 ICH patients did not confirm this finding. Its results did, however, suggest an increased ICH risk with higher doses of ephedrine.[55] The dose-dependent association between ephedrine and ICH needs to be confirmed in a larger sample of ephedrine users. Similarly, cocaine use is associated with spontaneous ICH, but its use is more common in men. In a small study of patients with ICH, however, there were no gender differences in the proportion of patients who had used cocaine prior to their ICH.[56]

Finally, preclinical data suggest that certain genetic mutations that increase patients' risks for poor outcomes after ICH may have sex-specific effects. For example, polymorphisms in apolipoprotein E (APOE), a gene that influences brain injury and inflammation in ICH, have sex-specific effects on the outcomes of ICH in rodents.[57]

Management/Treatment Response

Few studies have focused on differences in responses to specific treatments for ICH by gender, including blood pressure control and surgical intervention. Despite this lack of data, inferences based on surrogate measures demonstrate that women are more likely to have limitations in care after having an ICH. For example, in one study, women with ICH were more than three times more likely to have do not resuscitate

(DNR) orders initiated within 24 hours of diagnosis as compared to men, even after adjusting for factors such as age and volume of hemorrhage.[58] In the same study, women were more likely to be admitted to the floor for comfort care and were less likely to be admitted to the intensive care unit.

Blood pressure management is a mainstay of therapy for ICH. It is unknown whether there are gender differences in the treatment of blood pressure in the setting of acute ICH, but some data suggest a difference between women and men in the response to lowering blood pressure. In one study of more than 100 patients, a more rapid decrease in blood pressure in the first 24 hours after ICH was more strongly associated with increased mortality in men as compared to women.[59]

Outcomes

ICH is a condition with high morbidity and mortality; in-hospital mortality rates can reach 25%, and 30-day mortality rates are often as high as 50%.[50,52] No consistent evidence shows whether there are true gender differences in outcomes after ICH. In studies that include patients with sub- or supratentorial hemorrhages, women are more likely to have cerebellar hemorrhages, death within seven days, and worse functional outcomes.[58,60,61] In another study that included only patients with supratentorial bleeds, men and women had the same mortality rates.[62] Some data even suggest lower mortality in women.[63] Diversity in the populations, as well as other confounding factors, may help explain the conflicting findings in the relationship between sex and ICH outcomes. One study of these outcomes revealed a significant interaction between sex and age, with women older than age 70 having a higher risk of poorer outcomes.[64] There are large knowledge gaps in the area of gender and ICH, and future research relevant to the acute care of ICH patients should focus on differences in risk factors, presentation, management, and prognosis.

Subarachnoid Hemorrhage (SAH)

Disease Risk/Prevention

The prevalence of both unruptured intracranial aneurysms (UIA) and subarachnoid hemorrhage (SAH) are higher in women than men; women older than age 50 are two to three times more likely to have SAH when compared to men.[65–67] Furthermore, ruptured intracranial aneurysm is the most common etiology of SAH, and after the sixth decade of life, women are twice as likely to have an UIA.[65] The reason for the increased prevalence of both SAH and UIA in women is unclear. One hypothesis is that estrogen protects against the development of aneurysms by increasing vessel collagen deposition and strength, and postmenopausal women lose this protective effect.[67] This is supported by data showing that HRT reduces SAH risk.[67–69] Conversely, the use of combined oral contraceptives increases the risk of SAH, but this is not true across all studies.[68,70] The risk of SAH has not been found to be elevated during pregnancy.[68]

SAH has many risk factors in addition to sex, including hypertension, advanced age, non-white race, family history of SAH, autosomal dominant polycystic kidney disease, smoking, and alcohol use. The risk of SAH is greater for women who smoke than for men who smoke.[69,71] In one study, cigarette smoking increased the risk of SAH by a factor of nine in women but only by three in men.[69] ED providers must be aware of these risk factors when evaluating patients with symptoms suggestive of SAH and should include the risk of SAH in their counseling message to smokers.

Natural History

The risk factors for rupture of an UIA include aneurysm size, patient age, and smoking. Between 20% and 50% of cerebral aneurysms will rupture; the annual risk of rupture of UIA ranges from 0.05% per year to 1.5% per year.[72,73] No published data address the influence of sex on the natural history of unruptured aneurysms. An increased prevalence of aneurysms in women is likely the major contributor to the increased incidence of SAH.[67] Of those with SAH, women are more likely to have multiple aneurysms and internal carotid aneurysms, but the size of the ruptured aneurysm does not differ by sex.[67]

Clinical Manifestations/ED Presentation

Symptoms of SAH include thunderclap headache, exertional onset, emesis, syncope, meningismus, and photophobia.[72] It is unknown whether there are gender differences in the presenting symptoms of SAH, although data suggest that the frequencies of coma and decreased Glasgow Coma Scale (GCS) are similar in men and women.[67,74] One small study showed no difference in rates of sentinel headaches between men and women with SAH.[75] Overall, women with headaches are more likely to use the ED, but it is not known if this is true in patients with UIA or SAH. In addition to having an increased incidence of SAH, women have higher rates of migraine and chronic headache, making the diagnosis of SAH potentially more difficult. In studies of SAH misdiagnosis, though, where the most common incorrect diagnoses were migraine and tension headache, women were not more likely to be misdiagnosed.[76]

Diagnosis

The diagnostic standard for identifying SAH is a non-contrast CT scan followed by a lumbar puncture and neurosurgical consultation.[72] It is not known whether there are gender differences in the use of either CT or spinal tap as diagnostic approaches in patients with suspected SAH. Small datasets suggest no gender differences in sentinel headaches, but this should be confirmed with future research, given the risk of missed SAH diagnosis if CT and lumbar puncture are not performed.[75,76] Additional recommended imaging for those with suspected SAH includes CT angiography and/or MR angiography. There are no sex-specific recommendations in use of imaging, and it is unknown whether gender differences exist in the use of these imaging modalities. This is an important direction for future research, as there are known differences in prevalence of SAH between men and women.[65]

Acute Management

Management of ruptured aneurysms includes admission to an intensive care unit, prevention of vasospasm, and definitive treatment for the aneurysm with either surgical or endovascular therapy.[72] Men are less likely than women to receive early definitive therapy for SAH, and those with delayed surgical and/or endovascular treatments are more likely to have disability following SAH.[67,77] The reason for the delayed therapy in men remains unclear, although the higher rates of both internal carotid aneurysms and

multiple aneurysms in women may contribute to the delay.[67,77]

Clinical Outcomes

Research has not demonstrated clear differences in mortality from SAH by sex, although the data remain conflicting.[67,78] Age is a predictor of mortality, and women with SAH are typically older; this should be taken into account by ED providers. Women, however, report a lower quality of life following SAH as defined by difficulty performing daily activities, depression, and anxiety, even after adjusting for SAH severity.[79,80] This may be because more women live alone, a finding in other stroke types, but the etiologies of these results have not been confirmed in studies of SAH.

Migraines/Headache

Disease Risk/Prevention

Women have a higher risk of most primary headache syndromes including migraine and tension headache.[81-84] Specifically, migraine is two to three times more common in women than in men, affecting 12% to 25% women versus 5% to 9% of men.[81-84] Women are also at higher risk for various types of secondary headache syndromes including temporal arteritis, cerebral venous thrombosis, idiopathic intracranial hypertension, trigeminal neuralgia, and temporal mandibular disorders.[85-87]

ED providers must also be aware that chronic headache syndromes increase the risks for other medical, somatic, and psychiatric conditions that include stroke, cardiovascular disease, fibromyalgia, depression, and anxiety.[83] Of note, migraine with aura has a stronger association with cardiovascular comorbidities including stroke, myocardial infarction, and death from cardiovascular disease as compared to migraine without aura.[19,88] There are also sex differences in the comorbidities associated with migraine. One study found men with migraine were more likely to have comorbid medical conditions including hypertension and diabetes, while women with migraine were more likely to have fibromyalgia, depression, and anxiety.[89] Another study, however, found that women with migraine with aura were more than twice as likely to have had an ischemic stroke, but no association was found between stroke and migraine in men.[88] The exact pathophysiology of the association between migraine and ischemic events may be related to endothelial dysfunction that occurs with chronic migraine, but this needs association will require further confirmation.[90] Finally, ED providers must be aware of constellations of stroke risk factors that occur in women: Women who have migraine, smoke cigarettes, and use oral contraception are 10 times more likely to have an ischemic stroke compared to those without migraine who do not use cigarettes or hormonal contraception.[91]

Natural History

Approximately 5% of patients with episodic or intermittent migraine will develop chronic or daily migraine, which leads to more frequent ED visits and more lost days of work and school.[92] The rate of progression to daily headache seems to be similar in women and men.[92]

Other aspects of the natural history of migraine, however, differ between women and men because of fluctuating female sex hormones. Both elevated estrogen and hormonal fluctuations in estrogen trigger migraine.[83] Menstruation is often a time when migraines are more frequent, more severe, and longer lasting; this increased frequency is seen more commonly in migraines without aura.[83,93] Some women even suffer from "menstrual migraine," headache present only during menstruation. In women who suffer from migraine without aura, migraines become less frequent during pregnancy and menopause, when sex hormone levels are more stable.[94] In pregnant women presenting to the ED who have increased headache frequency or a new type of headache, alternate diagnoses including preeclampsia should be considered.

Clinical Manifestations/ED Presentation

Among migraine patients, the frequency of presentation to the ED differs by gender; women migraineurs visit the ED almost five times more frequently than men.[2] Overall, some estimate that women account for 80% of US health care costs for migraine.[2] Clinical aspects of migraine also differ by gender. Women report migraines that are more frequent and last longer and are more

severe when compared to men's reports.[83] Women more commonly report a visual scotoma preceding the migraine, as well as more nausea, photophobia, and phonophobia.[83,95] Migraines that mimic stroke are of special interest to ED providers. Hemiplegic migraines are about three times more common in women than men, but elucidating sex differences in other associated headache symptoms that may mimic stroke will require further research.[96]

Diagnosis

Migraine is primarily a clinical diagnosis. The ED evaluation of acute headache, however, often includes diagnostic testing to exclude other etiologies of headache including SAH and cerebral venous thrombosis. ED providers should consider the sex differences in prevalence of these alternative diagnoses when making a diagnosis of migraine.

Acute Management/Treatment Response

Men are three times less likely to seek treatment for headaches, 54% less likely to receive prescription medications for headache, and 37% less likely to use preventative medications for migraine.[97] Reasons for these disparities are unclear but may be related to gender differences in response to pain or a greater frequency of undiagnosed migraines in men. There are clear gender differences in recommended headache treatments during pregnancy and during menstrually triggered headaches. Some of the medications used to treat acute migraine have possible teratogenic effects that must be considered before they are prescribed to pregnant patients with migraine. Acetaminophen and metoclopramide are first-line options for pregnant patients, although sumatriptan has also been used.[98] Optimal treatment of menstrual migraine differs from that of typical migraine; if severe menstrual migraine is suspected, referral to a specialist and treatment with oral hormones to induce amenorrhea should be considered.[99]

Gender differences exist in the response to some medications used for acute headache in the ED, but more research is needed. For example, in one study women were more likely to have recurrent migraines following treatment with triptans for acute headache; nevertheless, this pattern of ostensible recurrence may have been a result of longer-lasting, more severe migraines in women.[100] Both animal and human studies have shown that women experience less analgesia and more side effects from opiates including morphine. Narcotics for primary headache syndromes, however, should be avoided in both men and women.[101,102]

Clinical Outcomes

Functional outcomes differ by gender with women reporting more lost productivity and disability from their headaches. As reported by the World Health Organization, migraine is the 12th most common cause of disability in women but the 19th most common when the data for men and women were combined.[83] On average, women with migraine miss 8.3 days of work per year compared to 3.8 days for men, and work-related disability as a result of migraine is worse for menstrual migraines than non-menstrual migraines.[103,104]

Seizure/Status Epilepticus

Many aspects of seizure disorders manifest sex and gender differences relevant to ED providers. Overall, the prevalence of seizure is higher in men than in women, probably because of higher prevalence of trauma, substance use, stroke, and central nervous system infection in men.[105] Idiopathic generalized seizure disorder, a subtype of seizure with a purely genetic cause, however, is more common in women.[105] In addition, psychogenic non-epileptic seizures, or pseudo-seizures, are more common in women than men and require different treatment strategies than true epileptic events.[106]

Hormones affect seizure frequency as many women experience exacerbation of their epilepsy during menstruation. Catamenial epilepsy is defined as a twofold increase in seizure frequency during menstruation or around the time of ovulation and is thought to occur in up to one-third of women with epilepsy.[107] In addition to the typical seizure triggers such as sleep deprivation and alcohol use, hormonal fluctuation should be considered by ED providers treating women with seizures.

Status epilepticus, a sustained period of seizure activity and common ED emergency, requires urgent treatment. Status epilepticus is more common in men, as is mortality from it.[105] The increased mortality probably results from the greater frequency of seizure triggers in men, including trauma, but it may also be related to the effects of sex hormones on the seizure threshold.[105] Management of status epilepticus is similar in men and women, but ED physicians should consider how sex and gender might affect treatment response. Many antiepileptic medications (AEDs) are weight based, and there is a clear association between sex and weight. Inaccurate dosing may lead to continued seizure activity and/or oversedation with a need for acute airway protection. In addition, emergency providers must consider potential teratogenic effects of common AEDs.[108] Finally, ED providers must counsel their women patients with epilepsy who are taking AEDs that these medications decrease the effectiveness of oral contraceptives as they stimulate the metabolism of both estrogen and progesterone. Drug interactions between AEDs and contraceptives can also lead to lower plasma concentrations of AEDs if they are taken concomitantly and thus to more seizures.[109]

The differential diagnosis of seizure and status epilepticus in pregnant women must include eclampsia. Women with a history of epilepsy are also more likely to have complications of pregnancy including eclampsia, placental abruption, and preterm labor.[110,111] These women are more likely to have an increase in seizure frequency during pregnancy.[112] Seizures from eclampsia must be considered in all pregnant women from week 20 of gestation up to 4 weeks postpartum, even in those without hypertension or other classic signs of preeclampsia such as headache and visual changes.[113,114] Patients with suspected eclampsia should be managed with blood pressure control, magnesium, and AEDs.

Future research should investigate potential sex differences in the effectiveness of antiepileptic medications, particularly those used to manage status epilepticus. Further research also needs to focus on the possibility that AED dosing may need to be adjusted during times of hormonal fluctuation such as menopause.

Conclusion

Cerebrovascular emergencies have high prevalence, high morbidity, and high mortality. There are important sex and gender differences in many aspects of these conditions including disease risks, presentation, management, and outcomes. Many of these differences may stem from biologic and pathophysiologic differences between men and women, although sociocultural gender roles also contribute. ED providers must be aware of these differences and incorporate them into their care for both men and women presenting to the ED with cerebrovascular emergencies.

Case Conclusion

Four days later, EL experienced a recurrence of her right-sided weakness that did not resolve so she re-presented to the Emergency Department. She continued to have a headache as well. On this visit, EL had a stroke scale of 4 and was evaluated for acute stroke with a CT scan. The scan showed evidence of a subacute left-sided stroke. She was out of the time window for IV tPA but was given antiplatelet therapy and admitted to the hospital. During the hospitalization, EL was diagnosed with cardio-embolic stroke and paroxysmal atrial fibrillation. Despite some mild improvements, she continued to have left-sided deficits and was discharged to acute rehabilitation.

This case reinforces the concepts that migraine is a risk factor for stroke and that gender differences include nontraditional presenting symptoms of stroke in women. Consequently, this patient had a delayed hospital presentation and was out of the window for thrombolysis. ED providers face many challenges when considering sex and gender differences in the diagnosis and treatment of acute neurologic emergencies.

Gaps in Knowledge/Research Questions

Despite all the known sex and gender differences in cerebrovascular emergencies, there are many unanswered questions. See Table 6.1 for examples of recommended future research directions. It is essential that future research questions on gender differences in cerebrovascular emergencies be translated to clinical knowledge so that clinicians may optimize the care of their patients.

Table 6.1 Future Research Directions

Topic	Research Direction
Stroke	• Identify biologic mechanisms behind sex differences in stroke with the ultimate goal of translating this knowledge into more effective and specific stroke treatments for both women and men. • Identify factors contributing to gender disparities in treatment of acute stroke. • Investigate how increasing use of stroke networks may help eliminate any existing gender disparities in stroke care.
SAH	• Investigate potential gender differences in the ED evaluation of suspected SAH, specifically in the use of diagnostic procedures including CT and lumbar puncture. • Evaluate ED-based interventions to reduce SAH risk factors such as smoking.
Migraine/Headache	• Investigate gender differences in responses to commonly prescribed medications for migraine in the ED and apply this knowledge to optimize therapy for migraine. • Investigate factors that lead to recurrent ED visits for headache with the objective of translating this knowledge into strategies to reduce the need for frequent visits for migraine. • Investigate gender differences in migraine as a stroke mimic and use this information to better guide clinicians in treatment of patients with symptoms of acute stroke.
Other	• Investigate potential sex differences in the effectiveness of antiepileptic medications across the life cycle with special attention to times of hormonal fluctuation such as menopause.

References

1. Centers for Disease Control and Prevention, Stroke Facts. n.d. Available at www.cdc.gov/nchs/fastats/stroke.htm. Accessed January 22, 2014.

2. Lucado J, Paez, K, Elixhauser, A. Headaches in U.S. hospitals and Emergency Departments, 2008. *Healthcare Cost and Utilization Project: Statistical Brief* 2011; **111**:1–12.

3. Reeves MJ, Bushnell CD, Howard G et al. Sex differences in stroke: Epidemiology, clinical presentation, medical care, and outcomes. *The Lancet Neurology* 2008; **7**(10):915–926.

4. Di Carlo A, Lamassa M, Baldereschi M et al. Sex differences in the clinical presentation, resource use, and 3-month outcome of acute stroke in Europe: Data from a multicenter multinational hospital-based registry. *Stroke: A Journal of Cerebral Circulation* 2003; **34**(5):1114–1119.

5. Niewada M, Kobayashi A, Sandercock PA, Kaminski B, Czlonkowska A. Influence of gender on baseline features and clinical outcomes among 17,370 patients with confirmed ischaemic stroke in the international stroke trial. *Neuroepidemiology* 2005; **24**(3):123–128.

6. Roquer J, Campello AR, Gomis M. Sex differences in first-ever acute stroke. *Stroke: A Journal of Cerebral Circulation* 2003; **34**(7):1581–1585.

7. Reeves MJ, Fonarow GC, Zhao X, Smith EE, Schwamm LH. Quality of care in women with ischemic stroke in the GWTG program. *Stroke: A Journal of Cerebral Circulation* 2009; **40**(4):1127–1133.

8. Galassi A, Reynolds K, He J. Metabolic syndrome and risk of cardiovascular disease: A meta-analysis. *The American Journal of Medicine* 2006; **119**(10):812–819.

9. Arboix A, Oliveres M, Garcia-Eroles L, Maragall C, Massons J, Targa C. Acute cerebrovascular disease in women. *European Neurology* 2001; **45**(4):199–205.

10. Gray LJ, Sprigg N, Bath PM et al. Sex differences in quality of life in stroke survivors: Data from the Tinzaparin in Acute Ischaemic Stroke Trial (TAIST). *Stroke: A Journal of Cerebral Circulation* 2007; **38**(11):2960–2964.

11. Kolominsky-Rabas PL, Weber M, Gefeller O, Neundoerfer B, Heuschmann PU. Epidemiology of ischemic stroke subtypes according to TOAST criteria: Incidence, recurrence, and long-term survival in ischemic stroke subtypes: A population-based study. *Stroke: A Journal of Cerebral Circulation* 2001; **32**(12):2735–2740.

12. Glader EL, Stegmayr B, Norrving B et al. Sex differences in management and outcome after stroke: A Swedish national perspective. *Stroke: A Journal of Cerebral Circulation* 2003; **34**(8):1970–1975.

13. Holroyd-Leduc JM, Kapral MK, Austin PC, Tu JV. Sex differences and similarities in the management and outcome of stroke patients. *Stroke: A Journal of Cerebral Circulation* 2000; **31**(8):1833–1837.

14. McInnes C, McAlpine C, Walters M. Effect of gender on stroke management in Glasgow. *Age and Ageing* 2008; **37**(2):220–222.

15. Simpson CR, Wilson C, Hannaford PC, Williams D. Evidence for age and sex differences in the secondary prevention of stroke in Scottish primary care. *Stroke: A Journal of Cerebral Circulation* 2005; **36**(8):1771–1775.

16. Del Zotto E, Giossi A, Volonghi I, Costa P, Padovani A, Pezzini A. Ischemic stroke during pregnancy and puerperium. *Stroke Research and Treatment* 2011; 606–780.

17. Bushnell C, McCullough LD, Awad IA et al. Guidelines for the prevention of stroke in women: A statement for healthcare professionals from the American Heart Association/American Stroke Association. *Stroke: A Journal of Cerebral Circulation* 2014; **45**(5):1545–1588.

18. Rossouw JE, Anderson GL, Prentice RL et al. Risks and benefits of estrogen plus progestin in healthy postmenopausal women: Principal results from the Women's Health Initiative randomized controlled trial. *JAMA: The Journal of the American Medical Association* 2002; **288**(3):321–333.

19. Kurth T, Gaziano JM, Cook NR, Logroscino G, Diener HC, Buring JE. Migraine and risk of cardiovascular disease in women. *JAMA: The Journal of the American Medical Association* 2006; **296**(3):283–291.

20. Bushnell CD, Hurn P, Colton C et al. Advancing the study of stroke in women: Summary and recommendations for future research from an NINDS-Sponsored Multidisciplinary Working Group. *Stroke: A Journal of Cerebral Circulation* 2006; **37**(9):2387–2399.

21. Hurn PD, Brass LM. Estrogen and stroke: A balanced analysis. *Stroke: A Journal of Cerebral Circulation* 2003; **34**(2):338–341.

22. Wise PM, Dubal DB, Rau SW, Brown CM, Suzuki S. Are estrogens protective or risk factors in brain injury and neurodegeneration? Reevaluation after the Women's Health Initiative. *Endocrine Reviews* 2005; **26**(3):308–312.

23. Yang SH, Liu R, Perez EJ, Wang X, Simpkins JW. Estrogens as protectants of the neurovascular unit against ischemic stroke. *Current Drug Targets.*

CNS and Neurological Disorders 2005; 4(2):169–177.

24. Chen CH, Toung TJ, Hurn PD, Koehler RC, Bhardwaj A. Ischemic neuroprotection with selective kappa-opioid receptor agonist is gender specific. *Stroke: A Journal of Cerebral Circulation* 2005; 36(7):1557–1561.

25. Li H, Pin S, Zeng Z, Wang MM, Andreasson KA, McCullough LD. Sex differences in cell death. *Annals of Neurology* 2005; 58(2):317–321.

26. Labiche LA, Chan W, Saldin KR, Morgenstern LB. Sex and acute stroke presentation. *Annals of Emergency Medicine* 2002; 40(5):453–460.

27. Lisabeth LD, Brown DL, Hughes R, Majersik JJ, Morgenstern LB. Acute stroke symptoms: Comparing women and men. *Stroke: A Journal of Cerebral Circulation* 2009; 40(6):2031–2036.

28. Martinez-Ramirez S, Vidal A, Querol L et al. Frequency and outcome of patients wrongly treated with intravenous thrombolysis. *Cerebrovascular Diseases* 2008; 25 (Suppl 2):27.

29. Tsivgoulis G, Alexandrov AV, Chang J et al. Safety and outcomes of intravenous thrombolysis in stroke mimics: A 6-year, single-care center study and a pooled analysis of reported series. *Stroke: A Journal of Cerebral Circulation* 2011; 42(6):1771–1774.

30. Zinkstok SM, Engelter ST, Gensicke H et al. Safety of thrombolysis in stroke mimics: Results from a multicenter cohort study. *Stroke: A Journal of Cerebral Circulation* 2013; 44(4):1080–1084.

31. Foerch C, Misselwitz B, Humpich M, Steinmetz H, Neumann-Haefelin T, Sitzer M. Sex disparity in the access of elderly patients to acute stroke care. *Stroke: A Journal of Cerebral Circulation* 2007; 38(7):2123–2126.

32. Menon SC, Pandey DK, Morgenstern LB. Critical factors determining access to acute stroke care. *Neurology* 1998; 51(2):427–432.

33. de Ridder I, Dirks M, Niessen L, Dippel D, Investigators P. Unequal access to treatment with intravenous alteplase for women with acute ischemic stroke. *Stroke: A Journal of Cerebral Circulation* 2013; 44(9):2610–2612.

34. Azzimondi G, Bassein L, Fiorani L et al. Variables associated with hospital arrival time after stroke: Effect of delay on the clinical efficiency of early treatment. *Stroke: A Journal of Cerebral Circulation* 1997; 28(3):537–542.

35. Lacy CR, Suh DC, Bueno M, Kostis JB. Delay in presentation and evaluation for acute stroke: Stroke Time Registry for Outcomes Knowledge and Epidemiology (S.T.R.O.K.E.). *Stroke: A Journal of Cerebral Circulation* 2001; 32(1):63–69.

36. Morris DL, Rosamond W, Madden K, Schultz C, Hamilton S. Prehospital and emergency department delays after acute stroke: The Genentech Stroke Presentation Survey. *Stroke: A Journal of Cerebral Circulation* 2000; 31(11):2585–2590.

37. Tanaka Y, Nakajima M, Hirano T, Uchino M. Factors influencing pre-hospital delay after ischemic stroke and transient ischemic attack. *Internal Medicine* 2009; 48(19):1739–1744.

38. Kelly AG, Hellkamp AS, Olson D, Smith EE, Schwamm LH. Predictors of rapid brain imaging in acute stroke: Analysis of the Get With the Guidelines – Stroke program. *Stroke: A Journal of Cerebral Circulation* 2012; 43(5):1279–1284.

39. Centers for Disease Control and Prevention. Prehospital and hospital delays after stroke onset – United States, 2005–2006. *MMWR. Morbidity and Mortality Weekly Report* 2007; 56(19):474–478.

40. Sun Y, Teow KL, Heng BH, Ooi CK, Tay SY. Real-time prediction of waiting time in the emergency department, using quantile regression. *Annals of Emergency Medicine* 2012; 60(3):299–308.

41. Fonarow GC, Smith EE, Saver JL et al. Timeliness of tissue-type plasminogen activator therapy in acute ischemic stroke: Patient characteristics, hospital factors, and outcomes associated with door-to-needle times within 60 minutes. *Circulation* 2011; 123(7):750–758.

42. Reeves M, Bhatt A, Jajou P, Brown M, Lisabeth L. Sex differences in the use of intravenous rt-PA thrombolysis treatment for acute ischemic stroke: A meta-analysis. *Stroke: A Journal of Cerebral Circulation* 2009; 40(5):1743–1749.

43. Reid JM, Dai D, Gubitz GJ, Kapral MK, Christian C, Phillips SJ. Gender differences in stroke examined in a 10-year cohort of patients admitted to a Canadian teaching hospital. *Stroke: A Journal of Cerebral Circulation* 2008; 39(4):1090–1095.

44. Schwamm LH, Ali SF, Reeves MJ et al. Temporal trends in patient characteristics and treatment with intravenous thrombolysis among acute ischemic stroke patients at Get With The Guidelines – Stroke hospitals. *Circulation. Cardiovascular Quality and Outcomes* 2013; 6(5):543–549.

45. Towfighi A, Markovic D, Ovbiagele B. Sex differences in revascularization interventions after acute ischemic stroke. *Journal of Stroke and Cerebrovascular Diseases: The Official Journal of the National Stroke Association.* 2013.

46. Kent DM, Price LL, Ringleb P, Hill MD, Selker HP. Sex-based differences in response to recombinant tissue plasminogen activator in acute ischemic stroke – A pooled analysis of randomized clinical

trials. *Stroke: A Journal of Cerebral Circulation* 2005; **36**(1):62–65.

47. Savitz SI, Schlaug G, Caplan L, Selim M. Arterial occlusive lesions recanalize more frequently in women than in men after intravenous tissue plasminogen activator administration for acute stroke. *Stroke: A Journal of Cerebral Circulation* 2005; **36**(7):1447–1451.

48. Gall SL, Tran PL, Martin K, Blizzard L, Srikanth V. Sex differences in long-term outcomes after stroke: Functional outcomes, handicap, and quality of life. *Stroke: A Journal of Cerebral Circulation* 2012; **43**(7):1982–1987.

49. Gargano JW, Reeves MJ. Sex differences in stroke recovery and stroke-specific quality of life: Results from a statewide stroke registry. *Stroke: A Journal of Cerebral Circulation* 2007; **38**(9):2541–2548.

50. Broderick J, Connolly S, Feldmann E et al. Guidelines for the management of spontaneous intracerebral hemorrhage in adults: 2007 update: A guideline from the American Heart Association/American Stroke Association Stroke Council, High Blood Pressure Research Council, and the Quality of Care and Outcomes in Research Interdisciplinary Working Group. *Circulation* 2007; **116**(16):e391–413.

51. Van Asch CJ, Luitse MJ, Rinkel GJ, van der Tweel I, Algra A, Klijn CJ. Incidence, case fatality, and functional outcome of intracerebral haemorrhage over time, according to age, sex, and ethnic origin: A systematic review and meta-analysis. *The Lancet Neurology* 2010; **9**(2):167–176.

52. Hu YZ, Wang JW, Luo BY. Epidemiological and clinical characteristics of 266 cases of intracerebral hemorrhage in Hangzhou, China. *Journal of Zhejiang University. Science. B.* 2013; **14**(6):496–504.

53. Feldmann E, Broderick JP, Kernan WN et al. Major risk factors for intracerebral hemorrhage in the young are modifiable. *Stroke: A Journal of Cerebral Circulation* 2005; **36**(9):1881–1885.

54. Blanck HM, Serdula MK, Gillespie C et al. Use of nonprescription dietary supplements for weight loss is common among Americans. *Journal of the American Dietetic Association* 2007; **107**(3):441–447.

55. Morgenstern LB, Viscoli CM, Kernan WN et al. Use of ephedra-containing products and risk for hemorrhagic stroke. *Neurology* 2003; **60**(1):132–135.

56. Martin-Schild S, Albright KC, Hallevi H et al. Intracerebral hemorrhage in cocaine users. *Stroke: A Journal of Cerebral Circulation* 2010; **41**(4):680–684.

57. Lei B, Mace B, Bellows ST et al. Interaction between sex and apolipoprotein e genetic background in a murine model of intracerebral

hemorrhage. *Translational Stroke Research* 2012; **3**(1):94–101.

58. Nakagawa K, Vento MA, Seto TB et al. Sex differences in the use of early do-not-resuscitate orders after intracerebral hemorrhage. *Stroke: A Journal of Cerebral Circulation* 2013; **44**(11):3229–3231.

59. Qureshi AI, Bliwise DL, Bliwise NG, Akbar MS, Uzen G, Frankel MR. Rate of 24-hour blood pressure decline and mortality after spontaneous intracerebral hemorrhage: A retrospective analysis with a random effects regression model. *Critical Care Medicine* 1999; **27**(3):480–485.

60. Ganti L, Jain A, Yerragondu N et al. Female gender remains an independent risk factor for poor outcome after acute nontraumatic intracerebral hemorrhage. *Neurology Research International* 2013; http://dx.doi.org/10.1155/2013/219097.

61. Cadilhac DA, Dewey HM, Vos T, Carter R, Thrift AG. The health loss from ischemic stroke and intracerebral hemorrhage: Evidence from the North East Melbourne Stroke Incidence Study (NEMESIS). *Health and Quality of Life Outcomes* 2010; **8**:49.

62. Falcone GJ, Biffi A, Brouwers HB et al. Predictors of hematoma volume in deep and lobar supratentorial intracerebral hemorrhage. *JAMA Neurology* 2013; **70**(8):988–994.

63. Zia E, Engstrom G, Svensson PJ, Norrving B, Pessah-Rasmussen H. Three-year survival and stroke recurrence rates in patients with primary intracerebral hemorrhage. *Stroke: A Journal of Cerebral Circulation* 2009; **40**(11):3567–3573.

64. Umeano O, Phillips-Bute B, Hailey CE et al. Gender and age interact to affect early outcome after intracerebral hemorrhage. *PloS One* 2013; **8**(11). DOI:10.1371/journal.pone.0081664

65. de Rooij NK, Linn FH, van der Plas JA, Algra A, Rinkel GJ. Incidence of subarachnoid haemorrhage: A systematic review with emphasis on region, age, gender and time trends. *Journal of Neurology, Neurosurgery, and Psychiatry* 2007; **78**(12):1365–1372.

66. Vlak MH, Algra A, Brandenburg R, Rinkel GJ. Prevalence of unruptured intracranial aneurysms, with emphasis on sex, age, comorbidity, country, and time period: A systematic review and meta-analysis. *The Lancet Neurology* 2011; **10**(7):626–636.

67. Kongable GL, Lanzino G, Germanson TP et al. Gender-related differences in aneurysmal subarachnoid hemorrhage. *Journal of Neurosurgery* 1996; **84**(1):43–48.

68. Algra AM, Klijn CJ, Helmerhorst FM, Algra A, Rinkel GJ. Female risk factors for subarachnoid hemorrhage: A systematic review. *Neurology* 2012; **79**(12):1230–1236.

69. Lindekleiv H, Sandvei MS, Njolstad I et al. Sex differences in risk factors for aneurysmal subarachnoid hemorrhage: A cohort study. *Neurology* 2011; **76**(7):637–643.

70. Feigin VL, Rinkel GJ, Lawes CM et al. Risk factors for subarachnoid hemorrhage: An updated systematic review of epidemiological studies. *Stroke: A Journal of Cerebral Circulation* 2005; **36**(12):2773–2780.

71. Okamoto K, Horisawa R, Ohno Y. The relationships of gender, cigarette smoking, and hypertension with the risk of aneurysmal subarachnoid hemorrhage: A case-control study in Nagoya, Japan. *Annals of Epidemiology* 2005; **15**(10):744–748.

72. Brisman JL, Song JK, Newell DW. Cerebral aneurysms. *The New England Journal of Medicine* 2006; **355**(9):928–939.

73. Juvela S, Porras M, Poussa K. Natural history of unruptured intracranial aneurysms: Probability and risk factors for aneurysm rupture. *Neurosurgical Focus* 2000; **8**(5):Preview 1.

74. Eden SV, Meurer WJ, Sanchez BN et al. Gender and ethnic differences in subarachnoid hemorrhage. *Neurology* 2008; **71**(10):731–735.

75. Pereira JL, de Albuquerque LA, Dellaretti M et al. Importance of recognizing sentinel headache. *Surgical Neurology International* 2012; **3**:162.

76. Kowalski RG, Claassen J, Kreiter KT et al. Initial misdiagnosis and outcome after subarachnoid hemorrhage. *JAMA: The Journal of the American Medical Association* 2004; **291**(7):866–869.

77. Siddiq F, Chaudhry SA, Tummala RP, Suri MF, Qureshi AI. Factors and outcomes associated with early and delayed aneurysm treatment in subarachnoid hemorrhage patients in the United States. *Neurosurgery* 2012; **71**(3):670–677; discussion 677–678.

78. Johnston SC, Selvin S, Gress DR. The burden, trends, and demographics of mortality from subarachnoid hemorrhage. *Neurology* 1998; **50**(5):1413–1418.

79. Katati MJ, Santiago-Ramajo S, Perez-Garcia M et al. Description of quality of life and its predictors in patients with aneurysmal subarachnoid hemorrhage. *Cerebrovascular Diseases* 2007; **24**(1):66–73.

80. Passier PE, Visser-Meily JM, van Zandvoort MJ, Rinkel GJ, Lindeman E, Post MW. Predictors of long-term health-related quality of life in patients with aneurysmal subarachnoid hemorrhage. *NeuroRehabilitation* 2012; **30**(2):137–145.

81. Leonardi M, Steiner TJ, Scher AT, Lipton RB. The global burden of migraine: Measuring disability in headache disorders with WHO's Classification of Functioning, Disability and Health (ICF). *The Journal of Headache and Pain* 2005; **6**(6):429–440.

82. Lipton RB, Scher AI, Kolodner K, Liberman J, Steiner TJ, Stewart WF. Migraine in the United States: Epidemiology and patterns of health care use. *Neurology* 2002; **58**(6):885–894.

83. Macgregor EA, Rosenberg JD, Kurth T. Sex-related differences in epidemiological and clinic-based headache studies. *Headache* 2011; **51**(6):843–859.

84. Stovner L, Hagen K, Jensen R et al. The global burden of headache: A documentation of headache prevalence and disability worldwide. *Cephalalgia: An International Journal of Headache* 2007; **27**(3):193–210.

85. Bruce BB, Kedar S, Van Stavern GP et al. Idiopathic intracranial hypertension in men. *Neurology* 2009; **72**(4):304–309.

86. Coutinho JM, Ferro JM, Canhao P et al. Cerebral venous and sinus thrombosis in women. *Stroke: A Journal of Cerebral Circulation* 2009; **40**(7):2356–2361.

87. Dieleman JP, Kerklaan J, Huygen FJ, Bouma PA, Sturkenboom MC. Incidence rates and treatment of neuropathic pain conditions in the general population. *Pain* 2008; **137**(3):681–688.

88. Le H, Tfelt-Hansen P, Russell MB, Skythe A, Kyvik KO, Olesen J. Co-morbidity of migraine with somatic disease in a large population-based study. *Cephalalgia: An International Journal of Headache* 2011; **31**(1):43–64.

89. Tietjen GE, Herial NA, Hardgrove J, Utley C, White L. Migraine comorbidity constellations. *Headache* 2007; **47**(6):857–865.

90. Tietjen EG. Migraine and ischaemic heart disease and stroke: Potential mechanisms and treatment implications. *Cephalalgia: An International Journal of Headache* 2007; **27**(8):981–987.

91. MacClellan LR, Giles W, Cole J et al. Probable migraine with visual aura and risk of ischemic stroke: The stroke prevention in young women study. *Stroke: A Journal of Cerebral Circulation* 2007; **38**(9):2438–2445.

92. Munakata J, Hazard E, Serrano D et al. Economic burden of transformed migraine: Results from the American Migraine Prevalence and Prevention (AMPP) Study. *Headache* 2009; **49**(4):498–508.

93. Granella F, Sances G, Pucci E, Nappi RE, Ghiotto N, Napp G. Migraine with aura and

reproductive life events: A case control study. *Cephalalgia: An International Journal of Headache* 2000; **20**(8):701–707.

94. Aegidius K, Zwart JA, Hagen K, Stovner L. The effect of pregnancy and parity on headache prevalence: The Head-HUNT study. *Headache* 2009; **49**(6):851–859.

95. Boardman HF, Thomas E, Croft PR, Millson DS. Epidemiology of headache in an English district. *Cephalalgia: An International Journal of Headache* 2003; **23**(2):129–137.

96. Lykke Thomsen L, Kirchmann Eriksen M, Faerch Romer S et al. An epidemiological survey of hemiplegic migraine. *Cephalalgia: An International Journal of Headache* 2002; **22**(5):361–375.

97. Diamond S, Bigal ME, Silberstein S, Loder E, Reed M, Lipton RB. Patterns of diagnosis and acute and preventive treatment for migraine in the United States: Results from the American Migraine Prevalence and Prevention study. *Headache* 2007; **47**(3):355–363.

98. O'Quinn S, Davis RL, Gutterman DL, Pait GD, Fox AW. Prospective large-scale study of the tolerability of subcutaneous sumatriptan injection for acute treatment of migraine. *Cephalalgia: An International Journal of Headache* 1999;**19**(4):223–231; discussion 200.

99. Sulak P, Willis S, Kuehl T, Coffee A, Clark J. Headaches and oral contraceptives: Impact of eliminating the standard 7-day placebo interval. *Headache* 2007; **47**(1):27–37.

100. Visser WH, Jaspers NM, de Vriend RH, Ferrari MD. Risk factors for headache recurrence after sumatriptan: A study in 366 migraine patients. *Cephalalgia: An International Journal of Headache* 1996; **16**(4):264–269.

101. Cepeda MS, Carr DB. Women experience more pain and require more morphine than men to achieve a similar degree of analgesia. *Anesthesia and Analgesia* 2003; **97**(5):1464–1468.

102. Fillingim RB, Ness TJ, Glover TL et al. Morphine responses and experimental pain: Sex differences in side effects and cardiovascular responses but not analgesia. *The Journal of Pain: Official Journal of the American Pain Society* 2005; **6**(2):116–124.

103. Granella F, Sances G, Allais G et al. Characteristics of menstrual and nonmenstrual attacks in women with menstrually related migraine referred to headache centres. *Cephalalgia: An International Journal of Headache* 2004; **24**(9):707–716.

104. Lipton RB, Stewart WF, Diamond S, Diamond ML, Reed M. Prevalence and burden of migraine in the United States: Data from the American Migraine Study II. *Headache* 2001; **41**(7):646–657.

105. McHugh JC, Delanty N. Epidemiology and classification of epilepsy: Gender comparisons. *International Review of Neurobiology* 2008; **83**:11–26.

106. Bora IH, Taskapilioglu O, Seferoglu M et al. Sociodemographics, clinical features, and psychiatric comorbidities of patients with psychogenic nonepileptic seizures: Experience at a specialized epilepsy center in Turkey. *Seizure: The Journal of the British Epilepsy Association* 2011; **20**(6):458–461.

107. Herzog AG, Klein P, Ransil BJ. Three patterns of catamenial epilepsy. *Epilepsia* 1997; **38**(10):1082–1088.

108. Tomson T, Battino D. Teratogenic effects of antiepileptic medications. *Neurologic Clinics* 2009; **27**(4):993–1002.

109. O'Brien MD, Guillebaud J. Contraception for women with epilepsy. *Epilepsia* 2006; **47**(9):1419–1422.

110. Yerby MS. Epilepsy and pregnancy. New issues for an old disorder. *Neurologic Clinics* 1993; **11**(4):777–786.

111. Veiby G, Daltveit AK, Engelsen BA, Gilhus NE. Pregnancy, delivery, and outcome for the child in maternal epilepsy. *Epilepsia* 2009; **50**(9):2130–2139.

112. Pennell PB. Antiepileptic drug pharmacokinetics during pregnancy and lactation. *Neurology* 2003; **61**(6 Suppl 2):S35–42.

113. Kaplan PW. The neurologic consequences of eclampsia. *The Neurologist* 2001; **7**(6):357–363.

114. Lubarsky SL, Barton JR, Friedman SA, Nasreddine S, Ramadan MK, Sibai BM. Late postpartum eclampsia revisited. *Obstetrics and Gynecology* 1994; **83**(4):502–505.

Chapter

8

From Title IX to the Q angle: Sex and Gender in Acute Care Orthopedics and Sports Medicine

Neha Raukar and Kimberly Templeton

An Introduction to Sex and Gender in Acute Care Orthopedics and Sports Medicine

This chapter focuses on the effect of sex and gender on the epidemiology, pathophysiology, diagnosis, and treatment of acute orthopedic and sports-related injuries. Topics include the athletic energy imbalance; ligamentous and joint pathology, especially ACL tears and shoulder instability; musculoskeletal pain syndromes; osteoporosis and fragility fractures; and concussion. Acute management and counseling strategies are highlighted as well as future directions and research questions.

Exercise is considered to be an important part of a balanced lifestyle, and women who play sports are healthier, get better grades, are less likely to experience depression and to use alcohol, cigarettes, and drugs than their sedentary counterparts (Penedo 2005). In addition, women who begin playing sports during high school or college are more likely to remain physically active as adults. Women's participation in athletic activities has increased significantly in the past few decades, and there has been a concomitant increase in the incidence of women presenting for medical treatment for a wide variety of acute, subacute, and chronic musculoskeletal complaints. As the importance of women's health has grown among health care providers and consumers alike, sex and gender differences in musculoskeletal injury patterns between men and women have attracted increasing research support and clinical endorsement.

Although women have historically always participated in certain circumscribed and "appropriate" athletic events, opportunities and choices for women interested in athletics had been limited. The women's movement, beginning with suffrage in the early twentieth century, empowered women to challenge traditional sex roles, including women's roles in sports; at the same time, the increasing number of women's colleges provided women with access to more types of physical activity and competitive sporting events in a milieu devoid of men. In spite of these changes, women's participation in organized, competitive sports remained limited. For example, track events for women were not routinely part of the Olympics until 1960; the first women's Olympic marathon was held in 1984. Until 1972, collegiate women were banned from participating in so-called dangerous or challenging athletic events, such as the marathon, because officials of the Amateur Athletic Union (AAU) believed that competing in physically stressful activities would be harmful to reproductive function in the woman (Macy, 1996). These restrictions changed with the passage of Title IX of the Educational Amendment of 1972, which mandated that equal money and opportunities be made available to both sexes at publicly funded institutions. Since then, there has been more than a tenfold increase in women's participation in both high school and collegiate athletics. In 1972, 3.7% of high school athletes were women. In 1971–1972, fewer than 30,000 women participated in college sports. In 2010–2011, that number exceeded 190,000 – about six times the pre–Title IX rate (Irick, 2011).

Male and female athletes have different injury patterns because of anatomic, hormonal, neuromuscular, and sport-specific differences. While many studies have focused on individual joint injuries, a more comprehensive review of all joints and the injuries associated with each joint, categorized and analyzed by gender, will someday provide a more thorough guide for injury prevention in all sports. Currently, research has clearly demonstrated that knee injuries, especially those of the anterior cruciate ligament (ACL) (Griffin, 2000) and the patellofemoral joint (Fulkerson, 2000), have consistently demonstrated sex specificity. Epidemiologic research on other joints including the ankle, elbow, and shoulder has revealed suggestive trends in sex based injury specificity. The following section emphasizes knee injuries while pointing out germane material on other joint injuries.

Sports-Related Injuries by Anatomic Region

Case

A 17-year-old basketball player presents with a painful, swollen right knee. She is unable to bear weight on the right leg because of pain in her knee, which she cannot flex or extend. She sustained this injury twisting her knee while landing a jump during a game.

Clinical Questions

- *How would you approach this patient?*
- *Is there a physical exam maneuver that will help identify the injury?*
- *What are the sex-specific elements in diagnosis and management that you should consider?*

Knee – Anterior Cruciate Ligament

The anatomy, physiology, and biomechanical differences of the knee and, in particular, the anterior cruciate ligament (ACL) between men and women have been extensively researched. The anterior cruciate ligament provides sagittal and rotational stability to the knee. Women are two to eight times more likely to sustain a tear of the ACL than men (Renstrom et al., 2008). More than 38,000 ACL injuries occur in women every year; in spite of extensive research and attempts at prevention by athletic trainers and sports medicine physicians, there has been no significant decrease in the number of injuries. ACL tears can have significant short- and long-term impact on athletes, interfering with their participation in sports and precipitating the early onset of osteoarthritis. While men are more likely to sustain an ACL injury from contact-related trauma, as is

commonly seen in football players wearing cleats who have been tackled, women are significantly more likely to sustain ACL tears from non-contact injury. Non-contact injuries typically arise when the athlete attempts to cut/pivot, to decelerate rapidly, or to attempt to land a jump. These activities frequently result in what researcher Mary Lloyd Ireland (Buschbacher et al. 2008) has termed the "point of no return": loss of control of the hip/pelvis while the hip is internally rotated, the knee is in valgus, the tibia is externally rotated, and the foot is pronated and externally rotated relative to the ankle. This anomalous and unstable position puts abnormal strain on the ACL, immediately after initial foot contact. Women's sports most highly associated with an ACL injury are basketball, soccer, alpine skiing, and lacrosse, although every sport that involves running, turning, or jumping puts women athletes at risk.

The relative impacts of anatomy, sex hormone levels, and neuromuscular control on the risk of ACL injury have been the subject of considerable investigation. Lower extremity alignment differs between the sexes in multiple planes; however, the impact of this difference on risk of ACL injury remains controversial. The most common alignment issues that seem to be significant are that women have greater hip adduction, knee valgus, and foot pronation than men, and these anatomical differences increase strain on the ACL. Other differences in lower extremity anatomy between men and women that have been studied to determine their relative impact on ACL injury risk include differences in femoral condyle width, tibial slope, lateral compartment alignment, and size of the femoral "notch" with particular attention to the relationship between the notch and ACL size. These anatomic factors may increase the inherent instability of women's knee joints when landing or pivoting and place additional stress directly on the ACL; nevertheless, most studies note significant overlap for both men and women between athletes with some or all of these anatomical risk factors and the actual likelihood of sustaining an ACL injury. None of these factors has been proven to be a significant prognostic indicator of an athlete's potential for ACL injury. Of course, anatomy is a static factor and cannot be altered. Thus identifying risk factors in any given athlete may trigger the initiation of an effective prevention program that allows the athlete to continue to play while decreasing the potential for ACL injury (Liable 2013).

Women's connective tissue tends to be more lax than men's because of differences in sex hormone concentrations. Temporal variations in sex hormone levels in individual women also seem to increase the risk of ACL injury. Estrogen and relaxin receptors have been identified on synoviocytes. Estrogen decreases collagen production; thus, rising estrogen serum concentrations increase laxity and impair the athletes' ability to repair microtrauma to the ACL. Relaxin increases soft tissue laxity. Joint laxity appears to be greatest during the pre-ovulatory (follicular and ovulatory) phase of the menstrual cycle, and a variety of studies (Wojtys et al. 2002; Hewett et al. 2007) have suggested that the risk of ACL injuries increases during this phase while varying throughout the menstrual cycle. Unfortunately, most of the studies connecting the relationship of the risk of ACL injury with the menstrual cycle were retrospective. More recent prospective studies examining the relationship between measured sex hormone levels and ACL injury have not supported a risk of ACL injury that waxes and wanes with the athlete's menstrual cycle (Bell et al. 2014); however, this continues to be investigated. Thus women athletes should not modify their sports activities during the menstrual cycle, and no evidence supports the use of exogenous hormone therapy to regulate the menstrual cycle to decrease risk of ACL injury.

Some researchers have suggested that inherent sex differences in neuromuscular control can explain women's increased risk of ACL injury (e.g., Shultz et al. 2015); however, sex-based variability in approaches to conditioning and training may contribute. While there is undoubtedly some impact on risk of ACL injury from anatomic factors and hormonal fluctuations, these factors are much less amenable than neuromuscular control to direct intervention and prevention. Some research strongly correlates lower extremity landing positions with ACL injury risk (e.g., Homan et al. 2013, Hewett et al. 1999, Hewett et al. 2005). When an athlete lands with her hips and knees extended, there is anterior translation of the tibia on the femur and increased valgus stress on the knee, both of which contribute to additional strain on the ACL. Both hamstring activation and stiffness provide resistance to anterior tibial translation and valgus stress of the knee, leading to reduced strain on the ACL. Prior to menarche, girls land their jumps with the same body kinesthetics as boys; afterward, for reasons that have not yet been elucidated, women tend to land jumps with their hips in internal rotation, their feet flat, and their hips and knees fully extended. This anatomical landing position, when combined with static hip adduction and valgus stress of the knee, places considerable additional strain on the ACL.

Women's post-menarchal landing pattern also reflects sex differences in neuromuscular activation. Women exhibit hamstring strength that is less than quadriceps strength and have a longer activation time to reach peak hamstring force; men's quadriceps and hamstring strength and activation time are equivalent. In addition, under conditions of muscle fatigue, women's hamstring activation becomes even slower, and the peak hamstring torque is decreased; men's peak torque and activation remain unchanged (Iguchi et al. 2014). Athletes who consistently land in positions that represent the extremes of normal ranges have the greatest risk of ACL injury. Researchers have not determined the point at which abnormal motion is significant enough to increase the risk of ACL injury, and why some athletes sustain ACL injuries while others with similar landing kinematics do not.

Patients who have sustained an ACL tear present with pain and acute hemarthrosis. Their knees swell immediately after the injury. They may or may not be able to bear weight. The pain, guarding, and swelling all interfere with a comprehensive physical examination of the knee, especially the Lachman or anterior drawer test, which is helpful in uncovering asymmetric ACL laxity. Patients with a history and physical findings that are consistent with an ACL tear should be immediately referred for further evaluation and management. Evaluation involves obtaining an MRI (Figure 8.1) to confirm the diagnosis and to assess for additional joint injury, particularly meniscal tears. The patient should be counseled to ice the knee, limit weight bearing, and initiate range of motion exercises to prevent arthro-fibrosis.

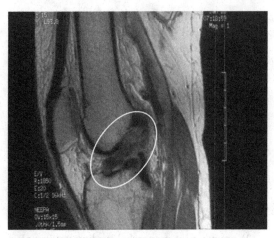

Figure 8.1 Sagittal T1 weighted MRI image demonstrating an ACL tear (Raukar)

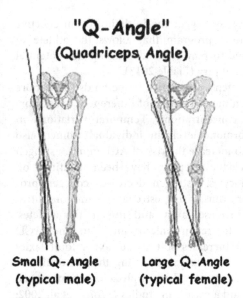

Figure 8.2 The Q Angle (Becker)

Although the ACL can be reconstructed after injury, stabilizing the knee and decreasing "giving way" episodes, reconstruction does not protect patients from developing secondary osteoarthritis (OA) as a direct result of articular cartilage injury sustained at the time of ACL damage. Women, in particular, are at greater risk than men for developing OA of the knee after ACL injury and may develop OA at an earlier age, often 10 years after the initial injury. ACL injury and the subsequent development of osteoarthritis can be life altering; therefore, prevention of ACL injury is crucial. Effective prevention programs incorporate strengthening of the muscles and ligaments that support the knee and protect the ACL and posterior cruciate ligament (PCL) and stretching exercises, balance training, plyometrics, and an emphasis on learning and practicing appropriate and safe landing positions (i.e., landing with both hips and knees flexed, on the balls of the feet, the so-called light as a feather landing).

Other Knee Injuries

The anatomic lower extremity alignment in women that predisposes them to ACL injuries (i.e., internal rotation of the hip and valgus stress of the knee with external rotation of the tibia) also creates excessive force on the patellofemoral joint, increasing women's risk of patellofemoral subluxation (Arom et al. 2013). The Q angle is the angle formed by a line drawn from the anterior superior iliac spine to the center of the patella and a line drawn from central patella to the tibial tubercle, measured and subtracted from 180 degrees (Figure 8.2). Women have an increased Q angle (17 degrees vs. 14 degrees in men) placing them at greater risk for patellofemoral subluxation (Waterman et al. 2012) because of the direct effect of this angle on the force vector of the quadriceps. There is some controversy about the relative impact of the Q angle, which is measured statically when the athlete is at rest and may not accurately reflect active alignments and stresses on the knee during sports. While the static and active alignment of women's lower extremities as well as their relatively more lax connective tissue seem to be responsible for their increased risk of patellofemoral subluxation and anterior knee pain syndromes, the incidences of patellar dislocation and knee dislocation do not differ by sex (Iguchi 2014). These injuries always result from a significant impact, rather than the repetitive trauma that leads to anterior knee pain or patella subluxation. Furthermore, knee dislocation leads to vascular compromise and peroneal nerve injury more frequently in men (Natushara 2014), most likely reflecting the increased shearing forces associated with the dislocating trauma that is the usual cause of this injury (Peskun et al. 2012).

Clinical Pearls

Women are more prone to sustain ACL injuries, with a female:male ration of 7:1.

The acute care provider must maintain a high level of suspicion for ACL injury when a female athlete presents with an acutely swollen knee after landing a jump or performing a rapid change of direction while running ("a cutting maneuver"). This risk is higher if she has sustained a prior ACL injury.

Delays in diagnosis, stabilization, and treatment may result in significant knee stiffness and loss of Range of Motion, which must be addressed prior to surgical reconstruction.

Women suspected of having an ACL tear should ice their knee, limit weightbearing, and urgently follow up with their orthopedic surgeon.

Ankle/Foot

Sports-related injuries of the foot and ankle are often multifactorial. Differences between men and women in the neuromuscular control of landing mechanisms also affect the loading stresses of the foot and ankle. This variable loading mechanism is believed to underlie the increased risk of fifth metatarsal fractures and Achilles tendon ruptures in men. Overall, men sustain more ankle sprains than women; nevertheless, in specific sports, such as basketball, women are four times more likely than men to sustain type 1, but not type 2 or 3 ankle sprains, syndesmotic injuries, or ankle fractures (Lynch, 2002). Surprisingly, although kinesthetics vary across sports, men demonstrate no sport-specific increase in the risk of ankle injury. Sex hormones do not seem to play a role in women's propensity for ankle sprains. While rising estradiol levels increase women's ankle joint laxity, there is no established correlation between phase of the menstrual cycle and risk of injury.

One of the most common pathologies of the foot is hallux valgus, a painful syndrome caused by the lateral deviation of the great toe (Hecht and Lin 2014; Perera 2011). Women are twice as likely as men to have hallux valgus. The pathogenesis is complex but seems to be related to wearing shoes with a small toe box (Nguyen et al. 2010). The incidence of hallux valgus deformity has been reported in as many as 48% of women who wear "fashion" shoes, as compared to 16% to 33% of shoe-wearing men and 2% of the unshod. Interestingly, even in barefoot populations, hallux valgus deformity is more common in women than in men (Shine 1965; McLennan 1966).

Upper Extremity

Almost no data compare male and female athletes' upper extremity injury rates. The sex differences in ACL injury rate patterns have not been demonstrated for upper extremity injuries. Upper extremity injury rates by sex appear to reflect the kinesthetics and motor tasks associated with particular sports and their attendant risks. For example, sports involving a repetitive overhead throwing motion such as softball and baseball consistently demonstrate a high incidence of shoulder or elbow injury (Bigliani 1997; Kvitne et al. 1995). While a single traumatic event in any sport may cause injury, repetitive overuse more commonly leads to failure and damage of one or more of the musculoskeletal structures of the upper extremity.

Case

A 17-year-old woman who is right-hand dominant presents to the ED with an obvious right shoulder deformity. She was pitching a softball game and suddenly felt her shoulder "lock." Since then, she has been holding her arm close to her side, adducted, with her shoulder externally rotated.

Clinical Questions

- *How should you approach the work up in this patient?*
- *What are the sex-specific elements in diagnosis and management that you should consider?*

Shoulder

Fewer sex-specific differences have been reported for the shoulder than for the knee. The shoulder is the most commonly dislocated joint; the estimated incidence rate for shoulder dislocation is 23.9 per 100,000 (Zachilli 2010). When describing shoulder dislocations, health care providers generally use the location of the humeral head (e.g., anterior vs. posterior). Other classification systems are more useful for identifying the mechanism of instability. Using these descriptors, shoulder dislocations can be described in three ways:

- Traumatic or atraumatic
- Voluntary or involuntary
- Unidirectional or multidirectional

Traumatic dislocations are more common in men (71.8%) and demonstrate unidirectional instability; atraumatic dislocations are more common in women with multidirectional instability patterns (Zachilli 2010). Sports that put repetitive strain on the shoulder joint such as softball, swimming, volleyball, and gymnastics are associated with the greatest rates of shoulder dislocation among women athletes.

In the United States, the prevalence of shoulder instability (including dislocation and subluxation) in athletes has been documented for both men and women. The overall incidence rate is 23.9 per 100,000 person-years with male incidence at 34.90 per 100,000 person-years, and occurs 2.64 times more frequently in men than women (Zacchilli 2010).

The shoulder is a complex ball and socket joint: The humeral head sits on a shallow glenoid that is deepened by a collagenous labrum and capsule and supported by surrounding soft tissues. Dynamic stabilizers of the glenohumeral joint include the rotator cuff muscles, the scapulo-thoracic muscles, and the long head of the biceps tendon. Static stabilizers include the bony anatomy, the fibro-cartilaginous labrum, and the glenohumeral joint capsule. Shoulder instability variances between the sexes can be attributed to static restraints (collagen elasticity due to the action of hormones), dynamic restraints (altered stabilizer muscle firing patterns), and differences in proprioception. Multidirectional instability is characterized by symptomatic global laxity of the glenohumeral joint and is believed to be more prevalent in women. Female athletes are thought to have greater glenohumeral instability than their male counterparts (Borsa et al. 2000) because their shoulders demonstrate more anterior glenohumeral joint laxity, less anterior joint stiffness, and more joint hypermobility (Cameron 2010). It is important to note that pre-injury measurements of shoulder laxity may not reflect true dynamic instability or a predisposition to dislocation.

Women have decreased proprioceptive responsiveness in their shoulder joints, which causes a slowing of the reactive contraction of the supporting muscles, increasing the risk of

structural damage to the shoulder in response to stress (Blasier et al. 1994; Blasier 1992). When compared to nonathletic subjects, both male and female athletes participating in overhead throwing sports displayed greater joint stiffness; these studies suggest that conditioning and training decrease joint laxity. Shoulder joint laxity is also asymmetric; anterior and posterior laxity differs and this variance is found in men and women (Comstock 2013; McFarland et al. 1996). This directional asymmetry is nonspecific and demonstrates no consistent pattern: It is not known whether this asymmetry plays a role in injury risk for either sex.

Labral tears, particularly tears of the superior aspect of the labrum that involve the biceps anchor, are common in athletes who throw overhand. Burkhart and Morgan proposed that the superior labrum tears from anterior to posterior, so-called SLAP lesions, are caused by a "peel-back" mechanism in these athletes, resulting from the increased strain at the biceps anchor during the late cocking phase of the throw when the shoulder is at maximum external rotation (Burkhart & Morgan 1998). Kuhn et al. showed an increased incidence of SLAP lesions in male baseball pitchers, supporting the peel-back theory (Kuhn et al. 2005). Shoulder injuries are prevented primarily by engaging in specific stretching and strengthening exercises of the rotator cuff and proper warm-up routines prior to strenuous shoulder activity. The risk for labral tears seems to be sports specific: No available data indicate sex-specific differences.

The majority of rotator cuff injuries suffered by overhead throwing athletes involve articular-sided partial-thickness tears of the rotator cuff, which are caused by acute tensile overload, repetitive microtrauma, or both (White et al. 2014; Burkhart et al. 2003). This pattern of injury is commonly found postero-superiorly, at the junction of the infraspinatus (IS) and supraspinatus (SS) tendon insertions (Jobe 1995; Walch et al. 1992; Minachi 2002). As women get older, the risk of rotator cuff injuries involving the IS and SS tendons increases. The most common etiologies of rotation cuff–related pain or injury for both men and women are subacromial impingement syndromes or repetitive microtrauma. This form of rotator cuff injury, which is strongly correlated with aging, is much more common in women, especially those in the 55- to 59-year-old group (Jobe 1995).

Elbow

Most elbow injuries in athletes are due to repetitive overuse from overhead activities, throwing, or elbow weight-bearing sports such as gymnastics. Depending on the specific nature of the athlete's sport, these injuries occur in predictable anatomic locations. For example, for both sexes, an increased incidence of injuries has been reported in the capitellum as a result of repetitive trauma in upper extremity weight-bearing activities (Baker et al. 2010). During the late cocking and acceleration phases of the throwing motion, tremendous valgus stress is placed on the elbow joint. The resulting distractive forces along the medial aspect of the elbow create tensile stress for structures such as the ulnar collateral ligament (UCL), common flexor tendon, and ulnar nerve. The radio-capitellar joint is subjected to compressive forces, and the postero-medial joint, particularly the humeral-olecranon articulation, experiences shear forces. These biomechanics often lead to a constellation of elbow injuries in the throwing athlete that are often referred to as the "valgus overload syndrome" (Cain et al. 2003; Chen et al. 2001). Injuries include UCL sprains or tears, common flexor tendon inflammation or tear, ulnar neuritis, and osteoarthritic changes of the ulnohumeral joint (Anderson et al. 2010).

Most women have shorter upper extremities than men, an increased valgus-carrying angle, decreased upper extremity strength, and increased ligamentous laxity in the elbow (Ireland and Ott 2004). However, because of the excessive stress placed on the elbow during the overhand pitching motion of baseball as opposed to softball, which is pitched underhand, severe elbow injuries, such as UCL tears, remain more common in male athletes. Elbow dislocations are the result of trauma and are not the result of ligamentous laxity or structural anatomic differences in the elbow between the sexes. Trauma is more common in men; therefore, elbow dislocations are more common in men. Men tend to have stronger and larger upper extremity musculature; therefore, elbow dislocations in women can result from less forceful injuries such as falling on an outstretched hand. The incidence rate ratio of elbow dislocations males:females is 1.02 (5.26 per 100,000 for males and 5.16 per 100,000 for females) (Stoneback et al. 2012).

Hand and Wrist

Contact injuries in sports such as ice or field hockey or lacrosse can result in fractures of the hand or wrist. Overuse injuries to the wrist are common in gymnastics, golf, weightlifting, racquet sports, and bicycling. In gymnastics, the upper extremity becomes a weight-bearing limb; studies have found the incidence of wrist pain in gymnasts to be as high as 73% (Diffiori 1996). The differential diagnosis in chronic wrist pain in any athlete includes triangular fibrocartilage tears, ulnar impaction syndrome, dorsal wrist ganglion, dorsal wrist capsulitis, and carpal instability. Other possible sources of wrist pain are hamate fracture, carpal tunnel syndrome, tendinitis, and ulnar nerve compression. This constellation of injuries appears to be sports specific; no consistent data demonstrate sex-based differences in incidence or prevalence of these hand and wrist injuries.

Musculoskeletal Pain Syndromes

Pain is a common presenting complaint for patients seeking treatment in an Emergency Department; one study found that 40.6% of patients who presented to the ED with a musculoskeletal complaint had a non-acute, low-severity problem (Naturshara 2014). In 2004, 13.8% of the 110 million ED visits were directly attributable to a primary musculoskeletal disorder; more than one-third of these visits were categorized as either semi-urgent or nonurgent (McCraig 2006), including visits for "chronic pain." Back pain is one of the most common chief complaints of patients presenting to the ED (Pitts, 2006), and a majority of those patients are women. Patients with chronic neck or low back pain who have no inciting trauma, no systemic symptoms, and no significant changes in neurologic findings do not require acute evaluation or intervention. Neither plain films nor CT scans nor MRIs are of demonstrated benefit in the ED or acute care setting.

Chronic regional pain syndrome (CRPS), also known as reflex sympathetic dystrophy, is a known occasional sequela of orthopedic trauma, including fractures and crush injuries.

Surprisingly, it can also be seen after minimal injuries and after minor procedures, including needlesticks. Patients with CPS often present with pain out of proportion to the inciting injury, such as patients with limb ischemia from peripheral vascular disease. They can present at any time after their event. Unfortunately, the cause of the pain has not been elucidated and treatment is challenging. CRPS is much more common in women, with a prevalence ratio of 4:1 females: males (Field 2013).

Contractures are a permanent tightening of soft tissue caused by fibrosis, specifically, fibrosis of ligaments, tendons, and muscles. Histologically, contractures are characterized by inflammation, myofibroblast proliferation, and dense scar formation. Examples of contractures include Dupuytren's (contractures of the palmar fascia), Ledderhose (contractures of the plantar fascia), and adhesive capsulitis (contractures of the glenohumeral joint capsule). Classically associated with alcoholism, these conditions can also be the result of diabetes, trauma, and chronic phenytoin use. Men are primarily affected by Dupuytren's and Ledderhose's contractures, while women have a higher incidence of adhesive capsulitis. Dupuytren's contracture is reported to be up to nine times more common in men than in women.

Case

A 17-year-old woman has been training for the past six months to make the varsity high school track team. She has been running six to seven miles per day, six days a week, and biking on the seventh day. She has not changed her diet and eats as much as she did before she started training, but her parents report she is strict about limiting her fat intake. She states she is "the most athletic that she has ever been." She presents with a four-week history of progressive right leg pain that initially started at the end of one of her runs but now occurs as soon as she starts to run. She even feels the pain when she walks up and down stairs; the pain is impinging on her lifestyle. Physical exam reveals bony point tenderness along the mid-shaft of her tibia on the right. There is no warmth or erythema suggestive of cellulitis or infection. The patient states she is not sexually active; however, her last menses was three months prior to this presentation. A urine pregnancy test was negative.

Clinical Questions

- How would you approach the work up in this patient?
- What do you do if radiographs are negative?
- What are the sex- and gender-specific elements in diagnosis and management that you should consider?
- Are there specific referrals that should be made, and to whom?

Athlete Energy Imbalance

Athletic energy imbalance (AEI), which was formerly known as the female athlete triad, was first described by Drinkwater in 1984 and defined by the American College of Sports Medicine in 1993. The definition has evolved and is currently defined as low energy availability, menstrual disturbance, and low bone mineral density (Nazem and Ackerman 2012). Menstrual irregularity can include hypothalamic primary or secondary amenorrhea, luteal phase deficiency, or oligomenorrhea; disordered eating may include anorexia or bulimia or, most frequently, an inadequate number of calories consumed relative to the athlete's expenditure. The most common self-imposed dietary restriction is limiting consumption of fat. These athletes will also have inadequate bone mass that can span a spectrum from osteopenia to osteoporosis. Since each of the three AEI entities is a continuum of deficiency and pathology, the triad of AEI can be seen in both competitive and recreational athletes. While insufficient caloric consumption with a negative effect on bone health is most common in women, it can also be seen in men.

AEI can produce morbidity and even mortality in relatively young women (Torrsveit 2005). The long-term effects are often not appreciated or diagnosed until they become irreversible. There is a severe deficiency in health care practitioners' knowledge, understanding, recognition, and diagnosis of AEI. In one study, an unacceptably large proportion of physicians were unable to name all three components (Troy et al. 2006). In addition, health care workers, coaches, and team physicians may consider athletes with AEI to be "healthy," as their diet may not appear abnormal and their physical appearance may conform to societal norms for an athletic woman who is "cut" or "toned." Often these athletes are not appropriately screened for components of the triad. However, health care providers, trainers, and coaches must assess caloric intake in relationship to known training expenditure. Athletes are frequently unwilling to address this condition, even after having sustained an injury, because their low body weight may make them successful in their sport. This condition is most often seen in a population of athletes who engage in a high level of competition from a young age, particularly in sports where leanness or a slender appearance affects performance, such as gymnastics, ice skating, cycling, and track.

It was once believed that the three components of this condition were separate entities with some interrelationship: The energy deficiency resulting from disordered eating could be associated with the development of menstrual disturbances; these hormonal disturbances might contribute to bone loss. It is now believed that each component of the triad is deeply interrelated with the other components: Relative low caloric intake results in both menstrual dysfunction and bone loss. The bone loss seen with AEI represents a low bone turnover state, in contrast to the accelerated bone resorption seen with estrogen deficiency. Markers of bone formation normalize in the face of increased caloric intake or decreased caloric expenditure before menses resume.

The reproductive and skeletal deficits are the result of a relative lack of energy from disordered eating in the face of increased energy expenditure. Energy availability is the difference between dietary energy intake and energy expenditure. In animal studies, reducing caloric intake by more than 30% consistently caused infertility and skeletal demineralization (Merry and Holehan 1979). The resting metabolism of the young adult is 30 kcal·kg^{-1} FFM·d^{-1}. Usually, when energy requirements are not met, hunger is triggered; however, in the athlete practicing dietary restriction, the energy deficit produced by exercise does not necessarily trigger hunger or that athlete does not respond to that hunger. When the energy available to young female athletes is reduced by more than 33% from 45 to less than 30 kcal·kg^{-1} FFM·d^{-1}, a cascade is triggered with attendant effects on sports performance and bone demineralization (Loucks and Heath 1994). Acute care

practitioners must be aware of AEI to identify these patients, mostly female athletes, when they present for an injury or other complaint. If possible, these patients should be counseled on appropriate caloric intake, apprised of the athletic and health implications of AEI, asked to keep a food log, and encouraged to share this food log with their sports nutritionist or family physician.

Menstrual irregularity is the second part of the triad and is theorized to arise from decreased production of GnRH by the hypothalamus (hypothalamic amenorrhea). The effects of primary or secondary amenorrhea, oligomenorrhea, and luteal phase deficiency on the hormonal profile are different. The end result, though, is reproductive dysfunction with an altered cholesterol profile.

The third arm of this condition, low bone mass, typically manifests as a stress fracture (or fatigue fracture). Stress fractures occur in athletes whose long bones are subjected to the cumulative effects of repeated microtrauma, without time for bone healing; healing is particularly impaired in athletes whose bone metabolism has slowed. Both bone microtrauma and slowed bone metabolism are seen in patients with athlete energy imbalance. For those athletes with normal bone mineralization, stress fractures are seen when the athletes rapidly change their training regimen or increase their intensity of activity; stress fractures are also seen in female military cadets (Cosman et al. 2013). Female athletes who present to the ED should be specifically asked about their menses, caloric intake, and exercise regimen; if there is evidence of amenorrhea, they should be referred to a gynecologist.

The young menstruating female should gain 2% to 4% of bone mass annually; unfortunately, the amenorrheic female loses 2% of her bone mineral density (BMD) per year. Even if a normal menstrual cycle is achieved after a period of menstrual irregularity, BMD rarely fully recovers (Rose 2001). Most women achieve 95% of their peak bone mass by age 18; unless other health conditions intervene, bone mass remains relatively stable from age 30 until menopause. Those who do not achieve optimal peak bone mass are more likely to sustain fragility fractures at an earlier age. Thus, BMD gained during adolescence is essential for adult skeletal health (Skolnick 1993).

Bone mineral density is measured against a standard that has been developed by sampling normal, healthy women of similar age.

In 1993, an international consensus conference sponsored by what is now known as the International Osteoporosis Foundation and the American National Osteoporosis Foundation (Anonymous 1993) defined osteoporosis as: "A systemic skeletal disease characterized by low bone mass and micro-architectural deterioration of bone tissue with a consequent increase in bone fragility and susceptibility to fracture." This definition has persisted. In 1994, this definition was operationalized by the World Health Organization (WHO, 1994). Osteoporosis was defined as a BMD more than 2.5 standard deviations below the mean value of young health women while osteopenia was defined as 1.0 standard deviation below this norm. Patients with osteopenia and osteoporosis have an increase in the rate of fractures that doubles with each standard deviation in their BMD below normal (Treasure and Serpell 2001).

The true prevalence of athlete energy imbalance is unknown. Two studies compared female athletes in particular classes of sports to an age-matched population of elite female athletes in "thin build" sports. Thirty-one percent of the elite female athletes in these sports had eating disorders, as compared to 5.5% of the control population (Byrne and McLean 2002). Twenty-five percent of female elite athletes in endurance sports, aesthetic sports, and weight-class sports had clinical eating disorders as compared to 9% of a control population of women. The percentage of eating disorders was even more pronounced in collegiate gymnasts with whom the prevalence of eating disorders can be as great as 62% (Rosen and Hough 1988). Menarche is often delayed in female athletes. Secondary amenorrhea has a prevalence of 2% to 5% in the general population but has a reported prevalence of up to 65% in long-distance runners (Dusik 2001). Female athletes who participated in "lean sports" had a higher rate of menstrual dysfunction (24.8%) than those that participated in so-called non-lean sports (13.1%).

In general, exercise increases bone mineral density. AEI reverses this positive effect of exercise because of relatively inadequate caloric intake

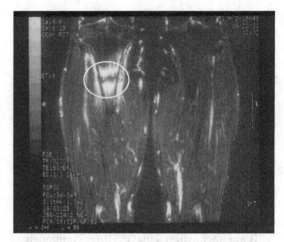

Figure 8.3 Area of increased metabolic activity and fracture line is highlighted (Raukar)

and nutritional deficiencies. Repetitive, subthreshold stress on bones that are abnormally weak because of demineralization and that are not allowed adequate healing and remodeling time increases fracture risk. Stress fractures account for 20% of all injuries in sports medicine clinics (Fredericson et al. 2006) (Figure 8.3).

Stress fractures in athletes are seen most frequently in the tibia, femoral neck, metatarsals, and pubic rami and are four to ten times more common in women than in men. Fatigue or stress fractures are typically seen in women with low bone mass who have recently changed (usually increased) their training regimen. Women, especially runners, who sustain stress fractures of their tibia have been found to have lower extremity muscles that fatigue more quickly than those without fractures. Muscle fatigue results in additional stress being placed on the bone. The hip adduction and hindfoot eversion, seen more commonly in female runners, increase the risk of fatigue fractures, especially of the tibia.

The female athlete who presents to the ED with a stress fracture should be referred to an orthopedist, not only for management of her stress fracture but also for an investigation of her overall bone health.

Patients with a history and physical examination findings consistent with stress fractures should be evaluated with plain radiographs. However, these radiographs may be misleading, as no gross fracture may be noted; in more advanced phases of stress fracture, periosteal reaction will eventually be seen. If there is significant concern, and plain radiographs are unremarkable, the bone can be further evaluated with magnetic resonance imaging to demonstrate the fracture.

The athlete presents with injury, pain, disability, and decreased performance. Stress fractures in female athletes are generally an indicator of athlete energy imbalance. The clinician should initiate a frank discussion with the patient in the acute care setting at the time of injury, as this interaction may provide a teachable moment. These patients should immediately limit their weight bearing and follow-up with an orthopedist as soon as possible. The urgency of follow-up is especially important for athletes with suspected stress fractures of the femoral neck which, if not treated properly, can progress to become displaced fractures requiring extensive surgical intervention with concomitant severe pain, disability, and loss of function. Identification and treatment of patients with athlete energy imbalance require a high index of suspicion, an awareness of the presentation and diagnostic approach, appropriate acute management of the fracture, and focused referral to initiate a multidisciplinary intervention addressing the underlying root causes and setting the athlete on a course to improve his or her bone health. These athletes are at high risk for developing fragility fractures at an early age. Early diagnosis, treatment, and referral are imperative to assure their long-term bone health and physical well-being.

> **Clinical Pearls**
>
> *Women are more prone to stress (fatigue) fractures*
>
> *All women with stress fractures should be asked about their menses, dietary restrictions, and exercise/training regimen*
>
> *Stress fractures are not always apparent on plain radiographs. If an athlete presents for acute care having increased her training regimen and subsequently developed bony point tenderness, even if radiographs are negative, she should be treated as a stress fracture and should not return to training or play until further evaluation. Evaluation should be urgent for suspected stress fractures of the femoral neck, which usually require prophylactic surgical stabilization.*

> *If a stress fracture is suspected or diagnosed in the ED, the patient will require follow up with their primary care provider, an orthopedist, and a gynecologist if the athlete is female. Patients should limit weight bearing until orthopedic evaluation.*
>
> *The patient should be encourage to keep a food log and this should be shared with a nutritionist or their primary care provider.*

Case

A 75-year-old male presents with right hip pain after a fall from standing. He was reaching up to get his coffee cup, lost his balance, and fell. He has a history of vertebral compression fractures but does not complain of any new back pain at this time.

Clinical Questions

- *How would you approach the work up in this patient?*
- *What specifically do you have to consider in a man with an osteoporotic fracture?*
- *What are the gender-specific elements in management and disposition that you should consider?*
- *Are there specific referrals that should be made and to whom?*
- *For those patients who are discharged with an osteoporotic fracture, can interventions be started in the ED that will decrease their future fracture risk?*

Low-Impact Fractures

Osteoporosis is defined as a generalized metabolic bone disease characterized by both decreased bone density and poor bone quality (NIH Consensus Statement 2000). Osteoporosis leads to an increase in the frequency of fractures of the hip, humerus, spine, and wrist. Osteoporosis is a global public health problem affecting more than 200 million people worldwide. In the United States, osteoporosis is considered a major health threat for almost 44 million Americans, almost 55% of the population older than age 50 – 10 million with osteoporosis and another 34 million with osteopenia or low bone mass. Once considered a disease only of women, research has demonstrated that men are also at significant risk of developing osteoporosis. Men currently represent approximately 20% to 40% of patients with osteoporosis (Roger et al. 2011). Men with osteoporosis tend to be older than osteoporotic women and are more likely to develop osteoporosis as a result of another health condition or disease; thus, these men have bleak survival outcomes.

Bone is dynamic: It is in a constant state of resorption and regeneration. Peak bone mass has accumulated in most people by the age of 30. After 30, bone resorption occurs at a faster rate than bone formation. The bony micro-architecture deteriorates, changing the protein structure and content of bone, reducing the overall bone mineral density (BMD) and bone strength resulting in an increased risk of low-impact fractures. Osteoporosis is caused by (a) inadequate peak bone mass formation during adolescence, (b) excessive bone resorption after menopause or as a result of a chronic health condition and the treatment for that condition (e.g., COPD treated with chronic prednisone), or (c) a combination of the two. Low-impact fractures are most common in the spine, hip, proximal humerus, and distal radius. Low-impact fractures of these bones are indicators of clinical osteoporosis. Acute care providers must recognize the acute injuries that signify a presentation of osteoporosis and must be prepared to intervene in these patients as they have a markedly elevated risk for future fractures.

Nearly 2 million osteoporosis-related fractures occur each year in the United States. According to the National Osteoporosis Foundation, by the year 2025 more than 3 million Americans will suffer osteoporosis-related fractures. In the United States, the rates of hip and wrist fragility fractures are equal with an annual incidence of 300,000 each. The lifetime risk for an osteoporotic fracture of any bone requiring clinical attention is equal to the risk of cardiovascular disease, at about 40% (Kanis 2002). In women, the risk of hip fracture is more than the collective risk of uterine, ovarian, and breast cancer; in men, the incidence of an osteoporotic fracture is equal to the risk of sustaining a myocardial infarction and exceeds the risk of lung and prostate carcinoma combined (Binkley 2009). Osteoporotic fractures cost $19 billion annually. Between 1995 and 2009,

the rate of hospitalization for osteoporosis-related injury and illness increased by 55%; 67% of these patients presented to EDs. Ninety percent were at least 65 years old, and 89% were women, who sustained these injuries at a rate six times greater than men (Russo 2009). In 2006 in the United States, hospitalization for injuries sustained as a result of osteoporosis exceeded $2.4 billion. Hip fractures were the most expensive osteoporotic injury and required the longest hospital stay. Although the majority of osteoporotic fractures occur in women, men have higher rates of fracture-related mortality. Outcomes after osteoporotic hip fractures requiring surgical repair are worse for men (Abrahamsen et al. 2009).

In patients with osteoporosis, fractures of the femoral neck, proximal humerus, and distal radius occur as the result of falls from standing. Even minimal trauma such as sneezing, rolling over in bed, bending over to perform activities of daily living, or falling out of a chair cause osteoporotic vertebral compression fractures. About 700,000 vertebral fractures are diagnosed annually in the United States. It is important to remember that most of these are incidental findings seen on X-rays obtained for other reasons. Elders in the United States are staying more active as they age and are sustaining more significant trauma. The acute care practitioner must remember that low bone mass can lead to more significant fractures than might have been anticipated from the mechanism of injury. Conversely, elders, especially women, with fractures from minimal trauma are likely to have osteoporosis.

Osteoporosis is diagnosed by measuring bone mineral density using dual-energy X-ray absorpitometry (DEXA) or quantitative CT (qCT) of the spine, hip, and/or forearm. The World Health Organization (WHO) defines osteoporosis as a bone mineral density that is 2.5 standard deviations or more below the mean peak bone mass, which is the bone mass of an average, young, healthy adult. Reference ranges for DEXA scans are sex based. The National Osteoporosis Foundation recommends BMD testing for all women age 65 and older and all men age 70 and older. Patients with significant risk factors should have their first DEXA scan at age 50. Risk factors (summarized in Table 8.1) include low body weight, history of prior fracture, family history

Table 8.1 Risk Factors for Osteoporosis

Modifiable	Non-modifiable
Low intake of calcium or vitamin D	Older age
Reduced intake of fruit and vegetables	Female gender
Increased intake of caffeine, sodium, or animal protein	Small frame/low body weight
Sedentary lifestyle	Menopause
Smoking/alcohol use	Family history
Medication use*	History of broken bones or height loss
*Medications Glucocorticoids >5 mg for >3 months Certain chemotherapy agents Lithium Phenytoin Proton pump inhibitors Selective seratonin reuptake inhibitors	Chronic health conditions or their treatment

of osteoporosis, smoking, excessive alcohol intake, and long-term use of certain medications, such as corticosteroids. However, a clinical diagnosis can be made in individuals who sustain a low-trauma or fragility fracture, such as a fall from standing height.

Osteoporosis itself is rarely lethal; nevertheless, the fractures that result from osteoporosis are a significant source of morbidity and mortality. Fragility fractures of the hip and spine are associated with an increase in the patient's baseline mortality rate of 10% to 20%. An osteoporotic hip fracture has a one-year mortality of 17% to 25% in women and 31% in men. Men have larger and stronger bones; therefore, it takes longer for their bone mass to decrease to the osteoporotic fracture threshold. Consequently, osteoporotic fractures occur later in life in men, when they have more comorbidities and thus higher mortality. At 6 months, only 15% of patients sustaining a fragility fracture of the hip regain their pre-fracture level of function (Marottoli et al. 1992). Even seemingly less significant fractures, such as those of the distal radius, are important as they impose functional limitations on the patient and serve as harbingers of more disabling fractures, such as those of the hip or spine.

Fractures as a result of minimal trauma in elders are a clear sign of clinical osteoporosis; intervention is essential to prevent future fractures with their attendant morbidity and mortality. Unfortunately, only a small percentage of patients who sustain fragility fractures are evaluated or treated for their low bone mass: Nearly 80% of patients with clinical osteoporosis, that is, those who present with an osteoporotic fracture, are never identified or treated (Nguyen et al. 2004). All fragility fractures warrant intervention and initiation of measures to prevent future fractures. Even after hip fractures, a recent study reported that patients were not being screened or treated for their osteoporosis. Only 19% received DEXA scans and appropriate treatment; interestingly, women were nearly three times more likely than men to receive proper treatment (Antonelli et al. 2014). Evaluation of bone health should occur at the time of a patient's initial presentation with a fragility fracture. The clinician should obtain baseline laboratories, with measurement of serum 25-OH vitamin D levels. There is some evidence that serum albumin and creatinine should also be measured (Liang-Yu et al. 2012; Jørgensen 2007). Additional testing, including DEXA scan or quantitative CT, should be obtained once the patient has recuperated from the acute injury. In cases of fragility fractures that result from falls, other health conditions that caused or contributed to the fall must be addressed and the patient's home and social situation must be assessed to prevent future falls and fractures. Although both sexes and all races are at risk for low bone mass and related fractures, white men and minorities of both sexes are even less likely than white women to have their bone health evaluated and treated (Kiebzak et al. 2002; Shekelle et al. 2007; Miller et al. 2005).

Initial plain radiographs of symptomatic areas in patients with minor trauma, low bone mass, and poor bone quality may not demonstrate the fracture, especially when the hip is involved. If the history and physical examination are consistent with fracture, and the plain X-rays are negative, the clinician must order further evaluation of the bone. Limited MRI of the region can help in identifying a fracture and can also reveal other conditions that might be causing pain. Technetium bone scanning can be utilized, if MRI is not readily available. The efficacy of computerized tomography for diagnosing occult fractures in patients with osteoporosis has not been substantiated in the literature (Cabarrus et al. 2008).

Treatment

Patients presenting with fragility fractures of the spine, humeral neck, or distal radius should be stabilized in the acute care setting and referred to an orthopedist for definitive treatment of their fracture and work-up and treatment for low bone mass. Healing is often delayed in patients with poor bone mass. Fractures of the femoral neck require urgent surgical treatment. In the past, surgery had often been delayed while the patient's other health problems were assessed and treated. However, there is evidence that treating these fractures surgically within 48 hours leads to a decreased complication rate, decreased length of stay, and decreased short- and long-term morbidity and mortality, as well as more rapid improvements in mobility (AAOS, 2014). Surprisingly, patients with comorbidities seem to benefit the most from early surgical intervention. Ultrasound-guided regional anesthesia administered in the ED for patients with hip fractures decreased the requirements for opioid narcotics with their attendant side effects in elders, decreased preoperative pain scores overall, and decreased postoperative delirium (Beaudoin et al. 2013).

Osteoporosis can be successfully treated and its rate of progression slowed or reversed, even in very elderly patients. Treatment of osteoporosis requires a combination of non-pharmacological and pharmacological approaches (Table 8.2), but, in spite of the complexity of the regime, intervention has been shown to be cost effective. Fracture risk can be reduced by 77% for vertebral fractures and 40% for hip fractures. Patients often have difficulty adhering to treatment regimes, even when the cost of medication is low often because osteoporosis is asymptomatic (like hypertension) until the patient sustains a fracture.

Behavioral issues that increase the risk of osteoporosis, such as smoking, alcohol intake, lack of exercise, and dietary deficiency should be addressed. Patients who take calcium

Table 8.2 Treatment Options for Osteoporosis

Non-pharmacological	Pharmacological
Calcium	
Vitamin D	Anabolic agents (parathyroid hormone)
Exercise	Antiresorptive agents (selective estrogen receptor modulators, calcitonin, bisphosphonates)

supplementation as a sole intervention seem to have a decreased risk of fractures, particularly vertebral fractures. Supplementation with calcium and vitamin D increases bone mass and improves elders' muscle strength, function, and balance (Gielen et al. 2011). Vitamin D and calcium supplementation, regular exercise, and pharmacologic treatment with bisphosphonates or other anti-resorptive agents can increase bone mass; at the very least, this regimen slows the progression of osteoporosis and lowers the risk for future fractures.

Clinical Pearls

Osteoporotic fractures are those that occur with a low energy mechanism and result in fractures of the wrist, spine, humerus, and hip.

Since osteoporosis begins at an earlier age in women than men, the prevalence of fragility fractures is greater in women.

Men who sustain fragility fractures, especially of the hip, have a higher mortality rate than women.

Most patients with fragility fractures are never evaluated for osteoporosis and are never started on treatment, even though treatment has been shown to reduce future fracture risk.

Emergency Medicine providers should refer all patients who present with fragility fractures to an orthopedist and should consider starting treatment with Calcium and Vitamin D, especially for those patients discharged from the ED.

There are few indications that justify delaying surgical treatment for patients presenting with fragility fractures of the proximal femur.

Case

A 16-year-old female presents to the ED with a head injury: She ran into the goalpost during a soccer game. She states she did not lose consciousness but is nauseated and complains of a headache. She states that she has a history of migraines. Her father wants to know when she can return to play; her mother wants to know whether this injury might put her at risk for other "problems." (This type of question can often be a subtext for psychological or educational problems). On examination, she has a GCS of 15, with a normal neurologic exam and some mild balance issues, especially with tandem gait. Her neurologic exam did not deteriorate after a three-hour observation period.

Clinical Questions

- How would you approach the work-up of this patient?
- Should you obtain a CT of the head?
- What are the sex- and gender-specific elements in diagnosis and management that you should consider?
- Should you taking a different approach when counseling a female athlete with a head injury than when counseling a man?

Concussion

The word "concussion" is derived from the Latin *concutere*, which means "to shake violently." Muhammad ibn Zakarīya Rāzi, a Persian physician practicing in the tenth-century CE, was the first person to use the term "cerebral concussion" and was the first to distinguish concussion from other types of head injury.

This definition has evolved, and there are now more than 75 definitions and grading systems for concussion. The most accepted definition was presented at the first International Conference on Concussion in Sport in Vienna in 2001 (Figure 8.4).

The Centers for Disease Control and Prevention (CDC) estimate that of the more than 2.4 million traumatic brain injuries (TBI) that occurred in 2009 (Coronado et al. 2012), at least 75% were classified as concussions or other mild TBIs. The impact of concussion on the acute

Concussion is defined as a complex pathophysiological process affecting the brain that is induced by traumatic biomechanical forces. Several common features that incorporate clinical, pathological, and biomechanical injury concepts in defining the nature of a concussive head injury state that a concussion:

- may be caused either by a direct blow to the head, face, neck, or elsewhere on the body with an impulsive force transmitted to the head.
- typically results in the rapid onset of short-lived impairment of neurological function that resolves spontaneously.
- may result in neuropathological changes, but the acute clinical symptoms largely reflect a functional disturbance rather than structural injury.
- results in a graded set of clinical syndromes that may or may not involve loss of consciousness. Resolution of the clinical and cognitive symptoms typically follows a sequential course.
- is typically associated with grossly normal structural neuroimaging studies.

Figure 8.4 Definition of concussion (Aubry et al. 2002)

care health care provider's practice is significant. Between 2001 and 2010, there was a 75% increase in the number of ED visits by children for the diagnosis and management of sports- and other trauma-related concussions (CDC).

The increase in the incidence of the concussion diagnosis is the result of better recognition and increased reporting. Several factors have sparked a growing awareness of and concern about sports-related concussions by parents, coaches, players, and health care providers. These factors include legislation mandating education of coaches, athletes, and parents; public head injury prevention campaigns such as the CDC's Head's Up campaign; broad media attention given to professional athletes who have suffered and died as a result of head injuries; and focus on legal settlements involving professional organizations.

The rate of sports-related concussion is dependent on the sex of the athlete, the sport being played, the level of play, the nature of "practices," and the physical environment in which the games are played. Football players sustain the most reported concussions overall; the most concussions in female athletes are seen in soccer players (Table X). When studying the influence of sex on the risk of concussion by examining sports for men and women that have comparable rules and equivalent protective equipment, such as hockey and soccer, the evidence suggests that women have a higher risk for concussion than men at both the high school and collegiate levels (Table X).

Biomechanical factors may contribute to women's increased risk of concussions. It has been postulated that the forces that generate the rotational acceleration of the brain that leads to concussion can be mitigated and absorbed by the muscles of the neck. Women athletes have a smaller neck muscle mass and less neck muscle strength than men. Comstock reported that athletes with smaller and weaker necks had an increased rate of concussions, and that for each pound of increase in neck strength, the probability of concussion decreased by 5% (Comstock 2013). Greater isometric neck strength and more rapid anticipatory activation were independently associated with decreased linear and rotational acceleration of the head in all planes of motion (Eckner et al. 2014). Since neck muscle mass and strength are potentially modifiable risk factors for concussion, some believe that neck strengthening may limit the transmitted forces and rotational acceleration that underlies all concussion injuries.

Wilcox studied male and female hockey players wearing helmets that were instrumented with accelerometers. He found that the threshold acceleration at which men and women sustained concussions seemed to be different. Instrumented helmets directly record linear acceleration and indirectly allow calculation of rotational acceleration. Female athletes in his study sustained concussions at lower linear and rotational accelerational forces than their male counterparts (Wilcox 2013).

Other factors may explain the relatively greater propensity for female athletes to report concussions. Traditionally, our culture has permitted women to be more honest and verbal than men about physical symptoms of injury. Furthermore, there is considerable social, parental, coaching, and societal pressure on male athletes to return to competition and hide symptoms (Dick 2009). These pressures are not as trenchant or directive for female athletes.

The symptoms of a concussion are classically divided into four categories: somatic, cognitive, emotional, and sleep related (Aubry, 2002). While headache is the most common complaint in concussed athletes, there are many other symptoms. The number and magnitude of these symptoms are directly related to the increased metabolic needs of injured neural white matter in the context of injury and altered cerebral blood flow. This metabolic mismatch instigates the constellation of concussion symptoms that brings the athlete to medical attention (Giza et al. 2001). It is not known whether sex plays a role in this metabolic mismatch.

In general, high school and collegiate female athletes with concussions have more reported symptoms than men; their symptoms are more likely to affect their activities of daily living and last for a longer period of time. Concussed female athletes are more likely to report headaches, dizziness, fatigue, and difficulty with concentration than men and present with twice the level of cognitive impairment when post-injury testing is compared to their pre-injury baseline (Covassin et al. 2012).

The metabolic mismatch instigated by brain injury from concussion results in the patient's signs and symptoms; therefore, the medical community has promulgated a regimen of physical and cognitive rest to support recovery (Giza et al. 2001). The mainstay of concussion treatment is focused on mitigating post-concussive symptoms through a period of inactivity, followed by planned, graduated return to social, scholastic, and athletic activity (Aubry et al. 2002). In addition, clinicians should prescribe mild pharmacologic intervention with agents to control nausea, dizziness, and pain.

Women are more likely to manifest post-concussion syndrome (PCS) (King 2014) at one and three months after injury in both traumatic and sports-related concussions (SRC) in series of patients presenting to the ED. Adult women are approximately three times more likely than men to report post-concussion symptoms three months after SRC. One study found that the phase of the menstrual cycle at time of injury seemed to influence the quality of life at one month post injury; specifically, if the female athlete was injured when serum progesterone concentration was high, that is, during the luteal phase of her menstrual cycle, she had significantly lower injury scores at one month post injury than women injured during the follicular phase of their cycle and also than women taking oral contraceptives (Wunderle et al. 2013).

Computerized neuropsychological testing (NPT) for patients with TBI and SRC is now widely available and easy to administer. It is often administered preseason to obtain a baseline for athletes participating in sports with an increased risk of head injury. NPT provides objective testing and scores on cognitive function in domains such as memory, reaction time, and impulsivity. Testing is repeated when the athlete is concussed, allowing comparison with the athlete's own baseline scores and national age- and sex-specific norms, helping clinicians make appropriate assessments about diagnosis, treatment, recovery, and decisions about return to school and athletic play.

Sports medicine practitioners' growing understanding of known sex differences in NPT performance at baseline and the specific changes seen after concussion can then be used to create guidelines focusing on tracking recovery from SRC in injured athletes and identifying specific nuances in the deficits of each concussed athlete to provide tailored treatment interventions. For example, at baseline, pre-concussion, women report more concussion-like symptoms, collegiate women perform better on verbal memory tests, and men score higher on visual memory tasks. After concussion, female athletes have significantly prolonged reaction times, have even worse scores on visual memory tasks, and are twice as likely to demonstrate cognitive impairment than men.- (Broshek et al. 2005). Research has not revealed the short- and long-term significance of these differences. The most effective and efficacious treatment regimens for concussion have not yet been proven in large clinical trials, nor has the literature reported on sex-specific approaches or even more complex individualized regimes that reflect symptoms, NPT performance, and other factors that have not yet been defined. Clearly, a "one size fits all" approach, which is the current standard, will prove to be inappropriate and ineffective in evaluating and treating this important and debilitating problem.

Clinical Pearls

Women are more prone to sustain concussions, either because of a lower biomechanical threshold, decreased neck muscle mass and strength, or a gender-related reporting bias.

Concussions result in a different constellation of symptoms in women than men.

Women take longer to recover from concussions than men.

Directions for Further Research

Researchers must clarify the pathophysiologic processes that are the basis of sex differences in the cause of musculoskeletal injury, including ligamentous laxity, differences in proprioception, and strength. The differences in survival from osteoporotic fractures needs to be explored and the role of the acute care provider in mitigating those risks needs to be investigated. Concussion affects both athletes and trauma patients, and there are distinct differences in presentation, response to treatment, and long-term recovery between men and women. Current approaches to diagnosis and treatment of musculoskeletal disease are often based on studies that preferentially include mostly men. Strides have been made in orthopedics, especially in joint replacement, to account for differences in the female anatomy. Current approaches to diagnosis and treatment of musculoskeletal conditions are often based on studies that preferentially include one sex, for example osteoporosis in women and concussion in men. Strides have been made to account for sex-based differences, but more needs to be done.

References

AAOS 2014 www.aaos.org/Research/guidelines/HipFx Guideline.pdf.

Abrahamsen B, van Staa T, Ariely R, Olson M, Cooper C. Excess mortality following hip fracture: A systematic epidemiological review. *Osteoporosis International* 2009; **20**(10):1633–1650.

Anderson MW, Alfort BA. Overhead throwing injuries of the shoulder and elbow. *Radiologic Clinics of North America* 2010; **48**:1137–1154.

Anonymous. Consensus development conference: diagnosis, pro-phylaxis and treatment of osteoporosis. *American Journal of Medicine* 1993; **94**:646–650.

Antonelli M, Einstadter D, Magrey M. Screening and treatment of osteoporosis after hip fracture: comparison of sex and race. *Journal of Clinical Densitometry: The Official Journal of the International Society for Clinical Densitometry* 2014; **17**(4):479–483.

Arom GA, Yeranosian MG, Petrigliano FA, Terrell RD, McAllister DR. The changing demographics of knee dislocation: A retrospective database review. *Clinical Orthopaedics and Related Research* 2013; **472**(9):2609–2614.

Aubry M, Cantu R, Dvorak J, Graf-Baumann T, Johnston K, Kelly J, Lovell M, McCrory P, Meeuwise W, Schamasch P. Concussion in Sport Group: Summary and Agreement Statement of the First International Conference on Concussion in Sport, Vienna. *British Journal of Sports Medicine* 2002; **36**(1):6–10.

Baker CL 3rd, Romeo AA, Baker CL Jr. Osteochondritis dissecans of the capitellum. *American Journal of Sports Medicine* 2010; **38**(9):1917–1928.

Beaudoin FL, haran JP, Liebmann O. A comparison of ultrasound-guided three-in-one femoral nerve block versus parenteral opioids alone in analgesia in Emergency Department patients with hip fractures: A randomized controlled trial. *Academic Emergency Medicine* 2013; **20**(6):584–591.

Bell DR, Blackburn JT, Hackney AC, Marshall SW, Beutler A, Padua DA. Jump-landing biomechanics and knee-laxity change across the menstrual cycle in women with anterior cruciate ligament reconstruction. *Journal of Athletic Training* 2014; **49**(2):154–162.

Bigliani LU, Codd TP, Connor PM et al. Shoulder motion and laxity in the professional baseball player. *American Journal of Sports Medicine* 1997; **25**:609–613.

Binkley N. A perspective on male osteoporosis. *Best Practice and Research: Clinical Rheumatology* 2009; **23**:755–768.

Blasier RB, Carpenter JE, Huston LJ. Shoulder proprioception. Effect of joint laxity, joint position. *Orthopedic Reviews* 1994; 234–250.

Blasier RB, Goldberg RE, Tothman ED. Anterior shoulder stability: Contributions of rotator cuff forces and capsular ligaments in a cadaver model. *Journal of Shoulder and Elbow Surgery* 1992; **1**:140–150.

Borsa PA, Sauers EL, Herling DE. Patterns of glenohumeral joint laxity and stiffness in healthy men and women. *American Journal of Sports Medicine* 2000; **32**:1685–1690.

Broshek DK, Kaushik T, Freeman JR, Erlanger D, Webbe F, Barth JT. Sex differences in outcome following sports-related concussion. *Journal of Neurosurgery* 2005; **102**(5):856–863.

Burkhart SS, Morgan CD. The peel-back mechanism: Its role in producing and extending posterior type II SLAP lesions and its effect on SLAP repair rehabilitation. *Arthroscopy* 1998; **14**:637–640.

Burkhart SS, Morgan CD, Kibler WB. The disabled throwing shoulder: Spectrum of pathology. Part I: Pathoanatomy and biomechanics. *Arthroscopy* 2003; **19**:404–420.

Buschbacker RM, Prahlow ND, Shashank JD. *Sports Medicine and Rehabilitation: A Sport-specific Approach.* Philadelphia: Lippincott Williams & Wilkins, 2008, p. 249.

Byrne S, McLean N. Elite athletes: Effects of the pressure to be thin. *Journal of Science and Medicine in Sport/Sports Medicine Australia* 2002; **5**:80–94.

Cabarrus M, Ambekar A, Lu Y, Link T. MRI and CT of insufficiency fractures of the pelvis and the proximal femur. *American Journal of Roentgenology* 2008; **191**:995–1001.

Cain EL Jr., Dugas JR, Wold RS et al. Elbow injuries in throwing athletes: A current concepts review. *American Journal of Sports Medicine* 2003; **31**(4):621–635.

Cameron KL, Duffey ML, DeBerardino TM, Stoneman PD, Jones CJ, Owens BD. Association of generalized joint hypermobility with a history of gelnohumeral joint instability. *Journal of Athletic Training* 2010; **45**(3) 253–258.

Chen FS, Rokito AS, Jobe FW. Medial elbow problems in the overhead-throwing athlete. *Journal of the American Academy of Orthopaedic Surgeons* 2001; **9**:99–113.

Comstock RD. High School Sports-Related Injury: Recent Trends and Research Findings. *4th Annual Youth Sports Safety Summit – National Action Plan for Sports Safety.* 2013; Washington, DC.

Coronado VG, McGuire LC, Sarmiento K et al. Trends in traumatic brain injury in the U.S. and the public health response: 1995–2009. *Journal of Safety Research* 2012; **43**:299–307.

Cosman F, Ruffing J, Zion M et al. Determinants of stress fracture risk in United States Military Academy cadets. *Bone* 2013; **55**:359–366.

Covassin T, Elbin RJ, Harris W, Parker T, Kontos A. The role of age and sex in symptoms, neurocognitive performance, and postural stability in athletes after concussion. *American Journal of Sports Medicine* 2012; **40**(6):1303–1312.

Dick RW. Is there a gender difference in concussion incidence and outcomes? *British Journal of Sports Medicine* 2009; **43** Suppl 1:i46–50.

Eckner JT, Oh YK, Joshi MS, Richardson JK, Ashton-Miller JA. Effect of neck muscle strength and anticipatory cervical muscle activation on the kinematic response of the head to impulsive loads. *The American Journal of Sports Medicine* 2014; **42**:566–576.

Field J. Complex regional pain syndrome: A review. *The Journal of Hand Surgery, European volume* 2013; **38**:616–626.

Fredericson M, Jennings F, Beaulieu C, Matheson GO. Stress fractures in athletes. *Topics in Magnetic Resonance Imaging: TMRI* 2006; **17**:309–325.

Fulkerson JP, Arendt EA. Anterior knee pain in females. *Clinical Orthopedics and Related Research* 2000:69–73.

Gielen E, Boonen S, Vanderschueren D et al. Calcium and vitamin D supplementation in men. *Journal of Osteoporosis* 2011. Available at http://dx.doi.org/10.40 61/2011/875249.

Giza CC, Hoyda DA. The neurometabolic cascade of concussion, *Journal of Athletic Training* 2001; **36**(3):228–235.

Griffin LY, Agel J, Albohm MJ et al. Noncontact anterior cruciate ligament injuries: risk factors and prevention strategies. *Journal of the American Academy of Orthopedic Surgery* 2000; **8**:141–150.

Hecht PJ, Lin TJ. Hallux valgus. *The Medical Clinics of North America* 2014; **98**:227–232.

Hewett TE, Lindenfeld TN, Riccobene JV, Noyes FR. The effect of neuromuscular training on the incidence of knee injury in female athletes. A prospective study. *American Journal of Sports Medicine* 1999; **27**:699–706.

Hewett TE, Zazulak BT, Myer GD. Effects of the menstrual cycle on anterior cruciate ligament injury risk: a systematic review. *American Journal of Sports Medicine* 2007; **35**(4):659–668.

Hewett T, Zazulak B, Myer G, Ford K. A review of electromyographic activation levels, timing differences, and increased anterior cruciate ligament injury incidence in female athletes. *British Journal of Sports Medicine* 2005; **39**(6):347–350.

Homan KJ, Norcross MF, Goerger BM, Prentice WE, Blackburn JT. The influence of hip strength on gluteal activity and lower extremity kinematics. *Journal of Electromyography and Kinesiology* 2013; **23**(2):411–415.

Iguchi J, Tateuchi H, Taniguchi M, Ichihashi N. The effect of sex and fatigue on lower limb kinematics, kinetics, and muscle activity during unanticipated side-step cutting. *Knee Surgery, Sports Traumatology, Arthroscopy* 2014; **22**:41–48.

Ireland ML, Ott SM. Special concerns of the female athlete. *Clinical Sports Medicine* 2004; **23**(2):281–298.

Irick, E. NCAA *Sports Sponsorship and Participation Rates Report: 1981–1982 - 2010–2011.* Indianapolis, IN: National Collegiate Athletics Association, 2011, p. 69.

Jørgensen L, Jenssen T, Ahmed L, Bjørnerem Å, Joakimsen R, Jacobsen B. Albuminuria and risk of nonvertebral fractures. *Archives of Internal Medicine* 2007; **167**(13):1379–1385.

Jobe CM. Posterior superior glenoid impingement: Expanded spectrum. *Arthroscopy* 1995; **11**:530–536.

Kanis JA. Diagnosis of osteoporosis and assessment of fracture risk. *Lancet* 2002; **359**:1929–1936.

Kiebzak GM, Beinart GA, Perser K, Ambrose CG, Siff SJ, Heggeness MH. Undertreatment of osteoporosis in men with hip fracture. *Archives of Internal Medicine* 2002; **162**:2217–2222.

Kim YH, Choi Y, Kim JS Comparison of standard and gender-specific posterior cruciate retaining high-flexion total knee replacements: A prospective, randomized study. *Journal of Bone and Joint Surgery Br* 2010; **92**(5):639–645.

King N. Permanent post concussion symptoms after mild head injury: A systematic review of age and gender factors. *NeuroRehabilitation* 2014; **34**:741–748.

Kuhn JE, Huston LJ, Soslowsky LJ, Shyr Y, Blasier RB. External rotation of the glenohumeral joint: Ligament restraints and muscle effects in the neutral and abducted positions. *Journal of Shoulder and Elbow Surgery* 2005; **14**:S39–S48.

Kvitne RS, Jobe FW, Jobe CM. Shoulder instability in the overhand or throwing athlete. *Clinics in Sports Medicine* 1995; **14**:917–935.

Liang-Yu Chen, Chien-Liang Liu, Li-Ning Peng, Ming-Hsien Lin, Liang-Kung Chen. Associative factors of existing fragility fractures among elderly medical inpatients: A hospital-based study. *Journal of Clinical Gerontology and Geriatrics* 2012; **3**:94–96.

Loucks AB, Heath EM. Induction of low-T3 syndrome in exercising women occurs at a threshold of energy availability. *The American Journal of Physiology* 1994; **266**:R817–823.

Lynch SA. Assessment of the injured ankle in the athlete. *Journal of Athletic Training* 2002; **37**(4):406–412.

Marottoli RA, Berkman LF, Cooney LM Jr. Decline in physical function following hip fracture. *Journal of the American Geriatric Society* 1992; **4**(9):861–866.

Macy, S. *Winning Ways: A Photohistory of American Women in Sports.* New York: Henry Holt and Company, 1996.

McFarland EG, Campbell G, McDowell J. Posterior shoulder laxity in asymptomatic athletes. *American Journal of Sports Medicine* 1996; **24**:468–471.

Mehin R, Burnett RA, Brasher PM. Does the new generation of high-flex prostheses improve the post-operative range of movement?: A meta-analysis. *Journal of Bone and Joint Surgery Br* 2010; **92**(10):1429–1434.

Merry BJ, Holehan AM. Onset of puberty and duration of fertility in rats fed a restricted diet. *Journal of Reproductive Fertility* 1979; **57**:253–259.

Miller R, Ashar B, Cohen J, Camp M, Coombs C, Johnson E, Schneyer C. Disparities in osteoporosis screening between at-risk African-American and white women. *Journal of General Internal Medicine* 2005; **20**(9):847–851.

Nazem TG, Ackerman KE. The female athlete triad. *Sports Health* 2012; **4**(4):302–311.

Nguyen TV, Center JR, Eisman JA. Osteoporosis: Underrated, underdiagnosed and undertreated. *The Medical Journal of Australia* 2004; **180**:S18–22.

Nguyen US, Hillstrom HJ, Li W, Dufour AB, Kiel DP, Procter-Gray E, Gagnon MM, Hannan MT. Factors associated with hallux valgus in a population based study of older women and men: The MOBILIZE Boston Study. *Osteroarthrits Cartilage* 2010; **18**(1):41–46,

NIH Consensus Statement Osteoporosis Prevention, Diagnosis, and Therapy. 2000; 17:1–45.

Otis CL, Drinkwater B, Johnson M, Loucks A, Wilmore J. American College of Sports Medicine position stand. The Female Athlete Triad. *Medicine and Science in Sports and Exercise* 1997; **29**:i–ix.

Penedo FJ, Dahn JR. Exercise and well-being: a review of mental and physical health benefits associated with physical activity. *Current Opinion in Psychiatry* 2005; 18:189–193.

Perera AM, Mason L, Stephens MM. The pathogenesis of hallux valgus. *The Journal of Bone and Joint Surgery* American volume 2011; **93**:1650–1661.

Peskun CJ, Chahal J, Steinfeld ZY, Whelan DB. Risk factors for peroneal nerve injury and recovery in knee dislocation. *Clinical Orthopaedics and Related Research* 2012; **470**:774–778.

Pitts SR, Niska RW, Jinamin X, Burt CW. National Hospital Ambulatory Medical Care Survey: 2006 Emergency Department Summary. *National Health Statistics Reports*, No. 7, August 6, 2008.

Raukar N, Hoffman E, Zink D, Baird J. Future physicians not ready for Concussion Crisis, First Annual American Academy of Neurology Sports Concussion Conference, Chicago, Illinois, July 12, 2014.

Renstrom P, Ljungqvist A, Arendt E, Beynnon B, Fukubayashi T, Garrett W, Georgoulis T, Hewett T, Johnson R, Krosshaug T, Mandelbaum B, Micheli L, Myklebust G, Roos E, Roos H, Schamasch P, Shultz S, Werner S, Wojtys E, Engebretsen L. Non-contact ACL injuries in female athletes: An International Olympic Committee current concepts statement. *British Journal of Sports Medicine* 2008; **42**:394–412.

Roger AL, Sutton LD, Pierre G. Osteoporosis in men: An underrecognized and undertreated problem. *IBCMJ* 2011; **53**:535–540.

Rose MZ, Maffulli N et al. Special Gynecological Problems of the Young Female Athlete. In: N Maffulli et al., eds. *Sports Medicine for Specific Ages and Abilities*. London: Churchill Livingstone, 2001:139–147.

Rosen DS, Hough DO. Pathogenic weight-control behavior of female college gymnasts. *The Physician and Sportsmedicine* 1988;**16**:141–144.

Russo A, Holmquist L, Elixhauser A. U.S. Hospitalizations Involving Osteoporosis and Injury, 2006. In: HCUP, ed. Agency for Healthcare Research and Quality, 2009.

Shekelle P, Munjas B, Liu H, Paige N, Zhou A. *Screening Men for Osteoporosis: Who & How* (Prepared by the Greater Los Angeles Veterans Affairs

Healthcare System/Southern California/RAND Evidence-based Practice Center). Washington, DC: U.S. Department of Veterans Affairs, 2007.

Shine IB. Incidence of hallux valgus in a partially shoe-wearing community. *British Medical Journal* 1965; 1:1648–1650.

Shultz SJ, Schmitz RJ, Cone JR, Henson RA, Montgomery MM, Pye ML, Tritsch AJ. Changes in fatigue, multiplanar knee laxity, and landing biomechanics during intermittent exercise. *Journal of Athletic Training* 2015; **50**(5):486–497.

Skolnick AA. "Female athlete triad" risk for women. *JAMA: The Journal of the American Medical Association* 1993; **270**:921–923.

Stoneback JW, Owens BD, Sykes J, Athwal GS, Pointer L, Wolf JM. Incidence of elbow dislocations in the United States population. *Journal of Bone and Joint Surgery Am* 2012; **94**(3):240–245.

Thomsen MG, Husted H, Bencke J, Curtis D, Holm G, Troelson A. Do we need a gender-specific total knee replacement? A randomized controlled trial comparing a high-flex and gender-specific posterior design. *Journal of Bone and Joint Surgery Br* 2012; **94**:787–792.

Traumatic Brain Injury information webpage (online). Available at http://www.cdc.gov/traumaticbraininjury/get_the_facts.html (Accessed November 10, 2015).

Treasure J, Serpell L. Osteoporosis in young people. *Research and Treatment in Eating Disorders. The Psychiatric Clinics of North America* 2001; **24**:359–370.

Troy K, Hoch AZ, Stavrakos JE. Awareness and comfort in treating the Female Athlete Triad: are we failing our athletes? *WMJ: Official Publication of the State Medical Society of Wisconsin* 2006; **105**:21–24.

Walch G, Boileau P, Noel E, Donell ST. Impingement of the deep surface of the supraspinatus tendon on the posterosuperior glenoid rim: An arthroscopic study. *Journal of Shoulder and Elbow Surgery* 1992; 1:238–245.

Waterman BR, Belmont PJ, Jr., Owens BD. Patellar dislocation in the United States: Role of sex, age, race, and athletic participation. *The Journal of Knee Surgery* 2012; **25**:51–57.

White JJ, Titchener AG, Fakis A, Tambe AA, Hubbard RB, Clark DI. An epidemiological study of rotator cuff pathology using The Health Improvement Network database. *The Bone & Joint Journal* 2014.

World Health Organization. Assessment of fracture risk and its application to screening for postmenopausal osteoporosis. *WHO Technical Report Series* 1994; **843**:1–129.

Wilcox B. *Head Impact Exposure: The Biomechanics of Sports-Related Concussion*. Providence, RI: Brown University, 2013.

Wojtys EM, Huston LJ, Boynton MD, Spindler KP, Lindenfeld TN. The effect of the menstrual cycle on anterior cruciate ligament injuries in women as determined by hormone levels. *American Journal of Sports Medicine* 2002; **30**(2):182–188.

Wunderle K, Hoeger KM, Wasserman E, Bazarian JJ. Menstrual phase as predictor of outcome after mild traumatic brain injury in women. *The Journal of Head Trauma Rehabilitation* 2013. Available at www.ncbi .nlm.nih.gov/pubmed/24220566.

Are Women More Sensitive? Sex and Gender Differences in Pain Perception, Clinical Evaluation and Treatment

James Miner

Opening Case

A 43-year-old patient presents to the Emergency Department reporting severe leg pain after a 3-foot fall from a ladder. The patient presented to the Emergency Department's triage, reporting that she has been unable to bear weight since falling off the third step of a kitchen ladder and landing with her left leg twisted underneath her. The patient reports the pain is around and just below her left knee. Her initial vital signs are a heart rate of 122, blood pressure of 110/65 mmHg, respiratory rate of 14 and an oxygen saturation of 100%. She reports her pain to be 9/10.

On first appearance, the patient appears in pain and is sitting anxiously upright on an examination bed. Examination reveals a normal healthy patient, visibly agitated and in moderate distress due to pain. Examination of the left leg reveals swelling and ecchymosis to the knee and lower leg. There is guarding and pain with palpation and with any range of motion attempts. Neurologic examination reveals pain with light touch distal to the injury, with intact two-point sensation. Pulses and capillary refill distal to the injury are intact.

The patient had an IV placed to receive parenteral morphine, and an X-ray was ordered. She was given 0.1 mg/kg of morphine IV, for a total of 7 mg, and had an X-ray ordered of her knee and lower leg. The patient tolerated the initial dose of morphine well, but after 15 minutes reported pain that persisted at 8/10. She was given an additional 3.5 mg of morphine IV 15 minutes after the first dose. After the second dose, the patient reported her pain was more tolerable and rated it 4/10. She had developed nausea from the pain medication and did not want any further medication. The patient went to X-ray.

After returning from X-ray, the patient was noted to have an oxygen saturation of 88%. She

was noted to be somnolent, but her oxygen saturation and mental status improved after stimulation. She reported continued pain in her leg and nausea from the pain medication.

The patient's X-ray revealed a tibial plateau fracture that would require surgical treatment. Preparations were made for admission, and for the placement of a Robert-Jones splint on the affected leg. Although it was assumed that the splint placement would be painful, the decision was made to give no further pain medication because of the patient's hypoventilation and decreased mental status after the initial morphine doses. Immediately prior to the placement of the splint, the patient appeared comfortable but continued to have mild decreases in oxygen saturation (93%–95%) when left unstimulated. During the placement of the splint, the patient had severe pain in the leg and became distressed due to the pain. Her vital signs remained normal, and she was given an additional 3.5 mg of morphine, from which the patient reported no pain relief. After 5 minutes, the patient was given an additional 3.5 mg of morphine, which improved her pain from 10/10 to 8/10. She was then given a further 3.5 mg of morphine, which reduced her pain from 8/10 to 6/10. After this dose, the patient developed nausea and vomiting and was given odansetron 4 mg IV. This improved the vomiting, but the patient had persistent 6/10 pain. The decision was made to not give further pain medications despite the patient's continued pain because of the vomiting and the patient's earlier response of hypoventilation after the morphine. The patient was admitted to orthopedics with continuing 6/10 pain.

Introduction

Even though there are a wide variety of safe and effective pain treatments, the treatment of pain remains challenging, and often inadequate.[1–8] The early, accurate recognition and assessment of a patent's pain are the most important aspects of effective pain management.[9] When pain is not adequately treated, an inaccurate assessment of the patient's pain is very likely the underlying cause of the problem.[4] Numerous studies have shown that this inaccurate pain assessment results in imprecise and ineffective pain management.[10] Patients' perception of their treatment in the ED is greatly influenced by the way in which their pain is addressed. Satisfaction with emergency care often depends on the accurate assessment and effective treatment of pain, as well as the discharge plans for pain relief.[11, 12]

A variety of epidemiologic studies have found an increased risk of more severe pain for females across a range of conditions.[2, 13–15] Women have been shown to exhibit greater pain sensitivity, greater pain facilitation and less pain inhibition when compared with men.[16, 17] Furthermore, evidence suggests sex differences in responses to pain treatments.[14, 18] The magnitude of these differences varies across studies, but multiple mechanisms are hypothesized to contribute to these sex differences in pain, including endogenous opioid function, genetic factors, pain coping and catastrophizing, gender roles, and sex hormones. Many of these sex differences have been noted to only exist after puberty, suggesting a role of sex hormones and development [1, 13].

Gender differences have also been identified in clinical pain trials.[2, 5, 12, 15, 19–22] Women have been found to have lower pain thresholds (the degree of stimulus at which pain is reported) and lower pain tolerance than men. There are a variety of explanations for this. First, pain is a subjective experience both in the degree of misery it causes to a person and in a person's outward expression of his or her pain. It is possible that there is no difference in the experience of pain between men and women, but it may be expressed differently as result of differences in communication, reporting thresholds, or expressive differences influenced by social expectations. Alternatively, it is possible that men and women experience pain differently, and that there is a difference in the degree of perceived pain from a given noxious stimuli that is reflected in the differences seen in reports.

The inadequate treatment of pain is commonly referred to as oligoanalgesia.[2, 23–36] The risk of oligoanalgesia is not evenly distributed among patients, and factors such as ethnicity,[1, 2, 15, 37] age,[38] and socioeconomic status[2, 9] have been described as playing a role. Sex has also been described as a factor. While the fact that sex is a risk factor has been established, the background knowledge to explain why and account for it properly is lacking.[38, 39]

Studies in the ED have shown that women are more unlikely than men to receive pain medication.[40] It is likely that a significant portion of the lack of pain therapy given to women is related to the inaccurate assessment of pain. While adequate data on the role of gender in pain are generally lacking, it appears that gender plays a role both in how a patient expresses that pain and in the response to therapeutic interventions.[39] It is likely that a large portion of the undertreatment of pain in women is due to the inaccurate assessment of pain and a lack of appreciation of differences in the response to treatments.

Poorly treated acute pain is associated with both the development of chronic pain and vegetative symptoms, as well as an increase in the need for pain management over the course of an illness.[41–48] Pain during serial medical procedures may increase if successful analgesia was not provided during initial procedures.[49] It is also likely that a patient's experience of pain increases the ability to perceive pain from similar stimuli in the future.[50] This means that if a painful injury is not adequately treated initially, it will likely require more treatment over the course of the treatment than an injury that is adequately treated initially. The role of gender in this has not been well established, but it can be assumed that given the differences in pain sensitivity, pain treatment response, and emotional responses to pain, the effect of untreated pain is different based on gender, and that specific tailored approaches will decrease the progression of untreated pain.

The differences in reported pain between genders are probably due to both differences in the way pain is expressed and measured by providers and in the way it is perceived, but the degree to which these aspects play a role is not known.[39] The appropriate treatment of pain is more dependent on its accurate assessment than on its actual intensity, however. The apparent solution then, based on current knowledge, is to account for the role of gender in the assessment of pain, both in terms of a person's sensitivity to pain and expression of pain and in terms of the response to therapeutic interventions, and to modify assessments and interventions accordingly.

Pain Perception

Women exhibit greater sensitivity to noxious stimuli in laboratory settings,[51–53] and are more likely to report pain.[13, 51, 54] Women report more severe pain, more frequent pain, and longer duration of pain than men. Evidence indicates this difference in sensitivity is due to different pain thresholds and tolerances.[55–61] These differences originate from a variety of biological (nociceptive pathways, physiology, perceptual sensitivity) and psychosocial (cognitive or emotional appraisal of pain, pain behaviors, different social roles of men and women) differences affecting pain processing and pain behavior. In one study, [60] men and women were exposed to a similar painful stimulus from a cold pressor task (placing the hand in cold water). When the subject was only with the investigators during the exposure, there was no difference in the pain reported between genders. The exposure was repeated with the subjects having a same gender friend in the room, and the women complained of a higher degree of pain when a friend was present, but there was no change in the report from men due to the presence of a friend. This simple study indicated that reported differences could have some basis in relationship and communication styles.

Another study [61] found that pain from a cold pressor task was decreased if patient's exercised intensely prior to the exposure, and this post-exercise analgesia persisted longer in women than in men. A variety of other similar experimental exposure studies have shown pain reports to be similar between genders but have detected a difference in the threshold of perception of the stimuli. Other studies have shown a higher degree of temporal summation (increasing pain with repeat exposures) and secondary hyperalgesia (increased pain reports for a second stimulus than for the first).[14, 17] While the basic report of pain appears similar between men and women, modifying factors have varying effects on the pain report from a similar stimulus. Although most of the specifics have not been identified, it can be deduced from what is known that the while baseline pain is likely similar between the genders, changes in this report are not and differ by factors that are not well defined.

Pain perception can be divided into four processes: pain detection (transduction), pain transmission, pain modulation, and pain expression (Figure 9.1). Receptors responsible for the detection of pain are termed "nociceptors." Nociceptors include sensory nerves that are capable of detecting mechanical, thermal, or chemical stimulation.

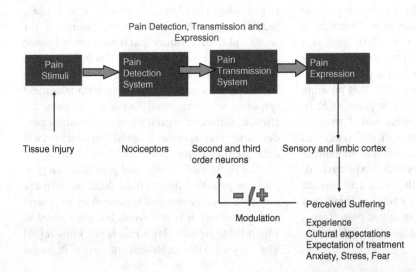

Pain Detection, Transmission and Expression

Figure 9.1 Pain detection, transmission, and expression

Several subtypes of nociceptors are present in cutaneous tissues, including mechanoreceptors, polymodal nociceptors (PMNs), and a variety of thermoreceptors.[62] Most nociceptive input is derived from inflammatory mediators through PMNs, in response to intense chemical, thermal, and mechanical stimuli.

The threshold of activation of a nociceptor can be modulated (increased or decreased) by a variety of chemical mediators including prostaglandin, cyclic adenosine monophosphate, leukotrienes, bradykinins, serotonin, substance P, thromboxanes, platelet-activating factor, and endorphins. This change in nociceptor activation thresholds is termed "peripheral sensitization." Trigger points, for example, are areas of frequent or constant low-level sensory stimulation (e.g., scar tissue or a degenerative joint) that have developed peripheral sensitized nociceptors that perceive pain from otherwise innocuous stimuli.

Once detected, pain transmission begins in peripheral nerve fibers, which are made up of the axons of sensory neurons. Once a nociceptor is activated, the signal travels up the peripheral nerve fiber to the cell body located in the dorsal root ganglia. From there, the signal travels to the dorsal horn on the spinal cord. The dorsal horn is an area of gray matter that is responsible for the initial integration of a painful stimulus with other signals. Here the signal is filtered, attenuated, or amplified depending on other sensory and afferent input, and then it is relayed to other spinal segments and the cortex. The dorsal horn processes information from visceral, muscle, bone, and cutaneous nerves into an integrated painful stimulus. The differentiation between painful and non-painful stimuli also occurs in the dorsal horn through cells called wide dynamic range neurons (WDRNs). WDRNs receive input from a variety of sources including efferent stimuli from the cortex, opioids, substance P, and inflammatory factors.

Nerve fibers carrying processed pain signals excite the dorsal horn and ascend to the brain through the spinothalamic, spinomesencephalic, and spinoreticular tracts. The spinothalamic tract transfers most sensation information through the thalamus to the sensory cortex. The spinoreticular tract ends in the reticular formations of the medulla, pons, midbrain, and thalamus, which then transfer the stimuli to the limbic forebrain. These signals directly stimulate the reticular activating system (alertness) and stress responses to pain. The spinomesencephalic tracts end in the midbrain and activate descending serotonergic and noradrenergic pain inhibitory signals.

The variety of inputs and intersecting points in the detection, transmission, and modulation of pain are only loosely understood and leave the degree of pain stimulation an individual experiences from a given physiologic stimuli highly variable. Sex and gender differences in these systems have not been well defined, but most evidence indicates differences that influence the perception of pain from a given stimulus.

Stress-induced analgesia is the phenomenon of reduced pain sensitivity in response to stress exposure. It has been poorly understood but likely is due to alpha-2 adrenergic stimulation at various sites in the pain transmission process. It has been difficult to quantify, as stress-induced hyperalgesia also occurs in reaction to acute stress. This is also poorly defined but is likely due to both cognitive and emotional aspects of pain perception and to decreased pain thresholds of nociceptors in the presence of inflammatory factors.[63–66]

Catecholamines are known to both inhibit and promote pain, and the mechanisms are not well understood. Pain is increased by alpha-1 stimulation peripherally and centrally and has been associated with increased pain during periods of anxiety and stress. Stress-induced analgesia has been shown to be alpha-2 mediated centrally and at the level of the spinal cord and is associated with analgesia during high catecholamine states. Factors influencing the development of increased pain or decreased pain due to stress are not well understood but have been shown to be different between men and women. The net effect of sympathetic outflow is a result of a balance between descending alpha-2 mediated inhibition and sympathetic outflow that can increase pain. Stress-induced analgesia has been shown to be increased by both estrogen and testosterone and to be diminished when either hormone is absent. This effect has been demonstrated through estrogen level cycles.[63–66]

After the processed pain signal reaches the cortex, the subjective emotional experience of pain develops (pain expression). There are multiple aspects to this development other than the magnitude of the pain signal, and the relationship between the pain signal and the experience of pain is not well understood beyond a general relationship between the magnitude of the pain signal and the degree of experienced pain. In addition to the processed pain signal, the experience of pain includes such factors as a person's cultural expectations, personality, experiences, and his or her underlying emotional state. Many of these factors can be influenced by a person's gender. If there is a true difference in pain perception between men and women, however, it has not been quantified or defined adequately.[59]

The processing of the pain signal can generally be divided into two areas, nociceptive, or the detection of pain stimuli, and neurogenic, which includes modulation of transmitted pain signals and the development of the cortical response. Many places along these pathways likely have sex- and gender-related differences that result in a variety of the differences that have been noted.

The Endorphin System

The endorphin system is the neuroendocrine system responsible for the modulation of pain and stress responses. It consists of a wide variety of poorly defined neurons and neuroendocrine cells that produce three main types of opioids: beta-endorphins, enkephalins, and dynorphins. These opioids function as neuromodulators by stimulating opioid receptors.

After a person has responded to a painful or stressful stimulus, the normal function of the endorphin system is to decrease the response to the pain and stress. This system is dynamic and can increase or decrease its effect to promote the appropriate response to a painful or stressful event. Like other neuroendocrine systems, it contains a feedback loop, and high levels of endorphins inhibit the further stimulation of the system. As a result of this feedback loop, when a pain signal is prolonged or intense or in the setting of exogenous opioid therapy, the system can become less responsive to pain, and less effective in controlling the pain response.

Endogenous opioid system responses differ between the sexes,[53, 67] accounting for some of the variation in responses to pain and pain treatments. Differences in the endorphin system would lead to differences in the response to pain

after its initial perception, as has been found in many pain studies. This could account for differences in the response to pain over time, and in differences in the response to therapy.

Clinical Evaluation

The degree to which a person experiences pain is a complex and subjective interaction between the perception of the physical stimulus and the patient's cognitive and emotional state. The experience of pain is not directly determined by the extent of a person's injury, and patients with identical injuries often display completely different amounts of pain.[9] This has frustrated attempts to uniformly recommend specific pain therapies based solely on the nature of the patient's illness of injury. The treatment must be based on the subjective assessment of the patient's pain.

The assessment of pain depends on the person's ability to communicate the nature of the pain to the physician, and the physician's ability to interpret the communication. No objective test or physiologic index measures pain reliably. Objective observations, such as hypertension, diaphoresis, or tachycardia, do not correlate well with the degree of pain present.[6, 68, 69] This leaves the assessment of pain dependent on communication, interpretation, and empathy, making the assessment of pain particularly vulnerable to the effects of a patient's gender[69–76] and a provider's gender.[77] Other factors, such as anxiety, which correlate well with the degree of pain present,[17] are just as difficult to measure as pain due to their subjective nature.[8, 22, 77–82]

Pain Measurement

Pain is typically measured using numeric rating scales, using a wide range of variations of a verbal 0 to 10 score ranking pain from none to worst imaginable.[83] Visual analogue scales, usually consisting of a 10-cm straight line with anchors at either extreme are frequently used in research to provide continuous data for analysis. These scales offer little practical advantage over verbal reports in the clinical setting.[70, 74, 84–86] Routine pain assessment encourages clinicians to communicate with patients to assess their pain and to evaluate responses to analgesic intervention attempts.[25, 87]

Whichever pain scale is used, it essentially serves as a communication tool between the patient and the physician to describe pain. The score a patient uses to describe pain may have as much to do with how the patient desires the health care provider(s) to respond to the pain complaint as it does a description of the pain relative to previous experiences. As a patient undergoes treatment, changes in the pain scores may represent a number of factors including satisfaction from analgesic interventions, a desire for further treatment, and actual changes in experienced pain. Generally, the significance of a change is pain in related more to the percentage change in a score than its absolute change.[88]

Differences in pain scale scores for identical painful stimuli by sex have been reported, with higher scores assigned to the stimuli by women.[61] Differences between the measurement of changes in pain scales with changes in described pain by sex have been reported as well,[20] with a larger change in pain scales associated with a change in verbally described pain for women than for men. The minimum clinically significant difference in pain scores or the change in score associated with a verbal description of a difference in pain was not detected between genders.[21, 88] Differences in the way a patient expresses pain, changes in pain, and desire for intervention that are not detected by the measurement tool are lost if that is the primary method of pain assessment. The active assessment of pain to determine the precision of a pain score is necessary for the score to be useful in clinical decision making. The measurement tools, however, provide a reference point for both the patient and the provider during repeat assessments. Available studies indicate that pain scores in women are more likely to vary relative to verbally described pain, but they similarly describe the presence, absence, or changes in pain. Standardizing the assessments and then using the information in conjunction with other historical information are likely to increase the accuracy of these scales and decrease differences in pain treatment due to assessment.[8]

The accurate diagnosis of the underlying cause of pain is the primary concern of the treating physician, but for the patient it is often secondary to the desire for adequate pain relief. The assessment of pain is closely related to the effectiveness of pain treatment, but an accurate interpretation of the degree of physiologic stimulation based on a patient's pain assessment is an important piece of information in the determination of the cause of the pain. If a patient has focal guarding and rebound tenderness in the right lower quadrant and appears in pain, it does not matter if the patient reports the pain score as a 2/10 or a 10/10, the patient will likely be evaluated for appendicitis. The patient with the higher pain score, however, may be expressing the desire for intervention by conveying that the pain is distressing, whereas the patient with the lower pain score may be attempting to downplay the pain to avoid the necessity of treatment. Understanding and accounting for pain scales in the context of gender requires recognition of these scales as communication tools rather than as a measurement of physiologic status.

Acute Versus Chronic Pain

Chronic pain can be described as any pain that persists after the tissue injury initially associated with the pain has healed as much as expected. This pain can be from injuries that are not expected to heal (e.g., degenerative joint disease) or from pain transmission system dysfunction (neurogenic pain). Chronic pain conditions are more frequently reported among women than men.[89] Chronic pain has also been associated with reported pain intensity and the adequacy of initial pain treatment. Women report higher degrees of pain than men and are more likely to be undertreated, accounting for some portion of the increased prevalence of chronic pain among women. Other factors are likely not yet defined, such as differences in the endorphin system responsiveness, differences in neuromodulation of pain signals, and differences in the effectiveness of treatments, that remain to be defined.

Treatment

The optimal current approach for treating moderate to severe acute pain is to titrate IV opioid analgesics effective levels for each individual patient.[1, 2] Research indicating that there are sex differences in pain and analgesia hold out the promise that pain treatment can be guided by a patient's sex.

Clinical studies of sex differences in response to μ-opioid agonists have had mixed results. Clinical studies have shown that gender does not appear to effect the likelihood of receiving opioids.[90] Clinical studies have also demonstrated that morphine is more effective in women than men, both in terms of the quantity needed to achieve pain relief with patient controlled analgesia (PCA)[91] and in terms of the analgesic effect of a given dose. A meta-analysis performed in 2010, however, found no overall sex differences in response to IV μ-opioid analgesics. There was substantial heterogeneity of findings, with about equal numbers of studies indicating superior female response, male response, and equal response. There has been evidence of greater efficacy of mixed-action opioid agonist-antagonists (pentazocine, nalbuphine, and butorphanol) in women than men in clinical studies, but no experimental studies have been done to determine the nature of this. In contrast to efficacy, evidence is more supportive that women experience more adverse responses to IV opioids than men, particularly nausea and vomiting and affective disorders associated with opioid use.[12, 18, 63–66, 89, 92–94]

Opioids are commonly used for the treatment of pain. Two percent of the US adult population uses some form of opioid each month.[95] Of these, women are more likely to be regular as well as long-term users.[96, 97] While most opioid prescriptions written for patients reporting pain are appropriate, patients seeking opioid analgesics for nonmedical use are common and represent a risk when pain is treated.[98] Data from the US DEA in 2012 showed that the annual retail sales of prescription opioids for nonmalignant pain have increased sevenfold between 1997 and 2006. The number of fatal overdoses from prescription opioids has also quadrupled during this period, exceeding those from cocaine or heroin and predominantly involves men. The estimated annual cost of prescription opioid abuse in the United States is $11 billion.[97]

The relationship between sex and vulnerability to opioids is therefore important to understand. Data show that women progress from use to dependence more quickly than men, suffer more severe emotional and physical consequences of opioid use as compared to men, and yet underutilize rehabilitation options. In addition, more women are prescribed opioids, have higher dosages prescribed relative to their body weight, and are more likely to have multiple and overlapping prescriptions, putting them at risk of abuse.[99] Both the higher risk of progression to dependence in women and the higher risk of fatal overdose in men must be accounted for in decisions about opioid therapy, especially in patients who appear at risk of dependence.

Stabilizing Secondary Pain Factors

The psychological response to acute pain depends on both the social and cultural context in which the pain occurs, the person's psychological predispositions, and the current health of the individual experiencing the pain.[100] Evidence from a variety of sources suggests that adverse acute psychological responses to pain, such as high levels of anxiety, distress, and depression, vary with gender.[101] Anxiety has been shown to be associated with pain to a greater degree in women than men.[17] Acute psychological responses to pain are important not only because they facilitate the severity of acute pain but also because they may affect risk of progression to chronic pain.[102–104]

Psychological responses to pain represent potential targets for intervention. Decreasing adverse psychological responses to pain will typically result in decreased reported pain and likely result in better pain relief over the course of an illness or injury. The interventions and treatments that are most effective in limiting these responses are likely to differ by gender.[105–108] As part of the effective treatment of pain, adverse psychological responses should be addressed. Interventions can range from patient education and reassurance and addressing fears about future pain to the symptom-targeted use of sedatives and antipsychotics. Controlling the psychological response to acute pain can be effective for both acute pain and the improvement of long-term outcomes.[106, 109]

Follow-Up and Prognosis of Disease

A large number of ED patients have underlying chronic pain syndromes, which are common in the US population, with rates as high as 40% noted [2]. The key step to the prevention of chronic pain appears to be the adequate treatment of acute pain. Acute pain usually occurs in response to tissue injury and resolves when the injury heals. It serves an adaptive purpose in that it stimulates protection of the injured area, the request for help, avoidance of future similar injuries, and increased blood pressure and respirations. As the injury heals, these adaptive purposes become maladaptive, as limited movement causes a decreasing range of motion, and pain facilitation can become so pronounced that the patient develops pain from otherwise non-painful stimuli.

It can be difficult to determine at what point pain changes from adaptive to maladaptive, or from acute to chronic. Acute and chronic pain call for different treatment approaches, both in terms of the approach to the patient and to the medications used. The maladaptive components of chronic pain can push patients toward behaviors that can hinder their recovery (lack of abnormal use of painful extremities, inactivity) and impact their mood, social interactions, and lifestyle. These issues must be addressed simultaneously with the physical perception of pain to blunt the negative impact of the pain on the patient. In terms of medical therapy, the principal difference between acute and chronic pain is that it cannot be assumed that chronic pain will resolve; therefore, sustainable treatment regimens with manageable side effects and negative impact should be selected.

Discussion

It has become increasingly apparent that women suffer a disproportionate amount of pain compared to men. A growing number of studies have suggested a variety of causes for this sex difference, on both a physiologic and a psychosocial basis. Many studies have demonstrated that the sexual differentiation of pain appears to occur at the same time as the sexual differentiation in puberty, implicating gonadal steroid hormones as important parts of this differentiation. Because these hormones affect the function and development of the nervous, immune, skeletal, and cardiovascular systems, the effects are complex, multifaceted, and still largely undefined.[110]

One of the great challenges we face in trying to determine the place of sex and gender in the treatment of pain is that our assessment of pain remains subjective. A person expresses his or her suffering

from pain according to learned behaviors and in accordance with the perceived role of medical care in the social milieu. We do not have an objective measure of pain and therefore must rely on physician assessment to attempt to measure it. The expression of pain is a combination of multiple factors; the physical stimuli, the threshold at which the stimuli are detected as pain, the degree to which the detected pain causes suffering to the individual, and the way in which that person expresses the suffering to observers, and finally the way those expressions are interpreted by the observers. Each of these factors is likely to be affected by the person's gender. These effects are likely a combination of both the effect of external gender roles and physiologic differences in the pain expression system. We are as yet unable to determine which of these is affecting these differences, and which is more important at what level of pain.

We do not yet have sufficient evidence on gender differences in pain detection thresholds and pain severity to accurately improve diagnosis and treatment in the clinical setting. It seems likely that the simplest step to improve the accurate assessment of pain is to measure it accurately and with a system that is robust to both differences in the detection of pain and the expression of pain. An accurate measurement would be robust to differences in threshold, since the total degree of suffering would be accounted for by an accurate pain measurement without regard to the degree of stimuli and its relative effect on the individual. The challenge is to employ pain measurement systems that accurately detect the degree of suffering an individual faces and any changes that occur over time and with intervention.

Accurate pain measurement requires appreciation of the effect of gender on the expression of pain. Although we do not have accurate information on the effects of gender on pain measurement, it is not a stretch to assume that gender will affect the way patients express their pain to another person. It is likely that the simple statement of a patient-derived pain rating will not take this into account, and that a pain score on a typical patient-derived 10-point scale could not be universally applied between men and women as equivalent. When a patient expresses pain, however, it can be assumed that he or she wants treatment. In using a pain measurement device, we need to pay more attention to the changes in the measurement rather than the degree of the measurement. For example, if a woman and a man with identical injuries present with pain, they would likely have different initial reported pain levels. If the women reports her pain is an "8" and the man reports a "6," it does not mean they have different levels of pain. It only means that both patients are not at zero and have given us a number that represents that they probably expect us to appreciate that they are in pain. If we give these two patients 0.1 mg/kg of morphine and then ask them to give us a new number, if the man has a score that goes to "3" and the woman has a score than goes to "4," they have both had their pain report improve by one-half and have probably had similar responses to the pain medication. If one patient's score went to 1 or 0, we can assume that patient perceives the treatment as adequate. If one patient's score only decreases by one point, does not change, or increases, the patient is expressing the need for more treatment and communicating that the treatment was not sufficient and that more therapy is expected. The actual values are not the principal determining factor in how much therapy is needed but rather the effect of the therapy given on the initial report. This sort of approach enables us to communicate in a fashion that allows for the inaccuracies of our current pain medication practices and avoids treatment failures, in terms of both undertreatment and overtreatment due to the inaccurate assessment of pain.

Conclusion

Men and women exhibit differences in measured pain and the response to pain treatment. We do not know the relative important of pain detection, pain expression, or pain measurement in differences in pain report, but by appreciating that such differences exist, we can implement more precise and accurate assessments and more effective therapy.

Case Conclusion

The presented case demonstrated many of the common pitfalls of pain management without the benefit of focus from gender differences in pain assessment and treatment. This patient's presentation, with tachycardia, a pain score of nine, and associated anxiety, exhibits characteristics of acute pain presentation more pronounced in women than in men. The patient had an IV placed and morphine titrated appropriately with adequate relief of pain and then developed nausea, which is also more common in women than men. The patient then developed hypoxia 15 minutes after the dose. Opioids are more efficacious in women than men, and the combination of this with the higher pain report in this case resulted in a large bolus being given. In addition, much of the effect of the first 0.1 mg/kg of morphine is on a patient's cognitive and emotional state, and it is likely here that the initial dose of morphine had a larger effect on the patient's anxiety than the underlying pain, resulting in the second dose having a more pronounced effect than the first because of the absence of underlying agitation from anxiety.

After the patient recovered from the large bolus, further treatment was withheld during splinting to avoid further complications. A better approach would be to give a smaller dose than the initial bolus, accounting for the pronounced effect but not limiting analgesia. The splinting procedure was started without further treatment, resulting in agitation and pain on the patient's part. Subsequent attempts to treat required multiple doses of morphine that had limited success in relieving pain relative to if adequate analgesia had been given prior to the splinting procedure. The patient then developed vomiting due to the large doses of morphine, which further complicated her care and led to the her being discharged without adequate pain relief.

This case demonstrates the complications and complexity of pain care, and that simply initiating treatment does not ensure adequate pain relief. This patient had poor pain relief despite aggressive and timely initial morphine dosing. Focusing on what we know about gender in this case would have improved the care. Knowing that opioids have increased efficacy in women and that pain and anxiety can be more common in women may have led to more accurate assessment of the patient's initial pain and more precise decision on the morphine dose. Understanding that the opioids effect can be more pronounced in women would have made it clearer that initial overmedication was due to the size of the dose rather than a predisposition to complications from opioids, which may have allowed for adequate pain medication for the splinting procedure. Adequate pain relief for the splinting procedure would have resulted in less subsequent need for opioids, limiting the degree of nausea the patient experienced and its associated complication of the patient's ongoing pain management.

This case exemplified the notion that the key to the management of pain is not the therapy chosen, but the accuracy of the assessment of pain, both initially and in response to therapy. Understanding differences associated with gender are central to the accuracy of pain assessments and the effective treatment of pain.

Gaps in Knowledge/Research Questions

If there is a difference in the reporting of pain that is principally due to the manner in which the measurement is taken, further work refining measurement tools to either be robust or to calculate gender differences should be developed to allow the comparison of pain and changes in pain between the genders. This would allow for the development of more accurate research accounting for the differences between men and women. If there is a true difference in the perception of pain between men and women, this difference should be quantified to allow for the development of pain trials that account for this difference and measure differences in pain effects of various noxious stimuli and pain treatments between men and women. Further studies of the measurements used to assess pain in the ED and of changes in pain in ED patients that account for gender differences are required to better advance knowledge on the treatment of pain in the ED.

References

1. Green, C.R. et al., *The unequal burden of pain: Confronting racial and ethnic disparities in pain.* Pain Medicine, 2003. **4**(3): 277–94.

2. Todd, K.H. et al., *Pain in the emergency department: Results of the Pain and Emergency Medicine Initiative (PEMI) multicenter study.* Journal of Pain, 2007. **8**(6): 460–6.

3. Arendts, G. and M. Fry, *Factors associated with delay to opiate analgesia in emergency departments.* Journal of Pain, 2006. **7**(9): 682–6.

4. Bijur, P.E., et al., *Lack of influence of patient self-report of pain intensity on administration of opioids for suspected long-bone fractures.* Journal of Pain, 2006. **7**(6): 438–44.

5. Fosnocht, D.E., E.R. Swanson, and E.D. Barton, *Changing attitudes about pain and pain control in emergency medicine.* Emergency Medicine Clinics of North America, 2005. **23**(2): 297–306.

6. Neighbor, M.L., S. Honner, and M.A. Kohn, *Factors affecting emergency department opioid administration to severely injured patients.* Academic Emergency Medicine, 2004. **11**(12): 1290–6.

7. Todd, K.H., et al., *Survey of pain etiology, management practices and patient satisfaction in two urban emergency departments.* Canadian Journal of Emergency Medicine, 2002. **4**(4): 252–6.

8. Uri, O., et al., *No gender-related bias in acute musculoskeletal pain management in the emergency department.* Emergency Medicine Journal, 2013, doi:10.1136/emermed-2013-202716.

9. Miner, J., et al., *Patient and physician perceptions as risk factors for oligoanalgesia: A prospective observational study of the relief of pain in the emergency department.* Academic Emergency Medicine, 2006. **13**(2): 140–6.

10. Jackson, T., Y. Wang, and H. Fan, *Associations between pain appraisals and pain outcomes: Meta-analyses of laboratory pain and chronic pain literatures.* Journal of Pain, 2014. **15**(6): 586–601.

11. Fosnocht, D.E., M.B. Hollifield, and E.R. Swanson, *Patient preference for route of pain medication delivery.* Journal of Emergency Medicine, 2004. **26**(1): 7–11.

12. Fosnocht, D.E., E.R. Swanson, and P. Bossart, *Patient expectations for pain medication delivery.* American Journal of Emergency Medicine, 2001. **19**(5): 399–402.

13. Robinson, M.E., et al., *Gender role expectations of pain: Relationship to sex differences in pain.* Journal of Pain, 2001. **2**(5): 251–7.

14. Bodnar, R.J. and B. Kest, *Sex differences in opioid analgesia, hyperalgesia, tolerance and withdrawal: Central mechanisms of action and roles of gonadal hormones.* Hormones and Behavior, 2010. **58**(1): 72–81.

15. Sobel, R.M. and K.H. Todd, *Risk factors in oligoanalgesia.* American Journal of Emergency Medicine, 2002. **20**(2): 126.

16. Robinson, M.E., et al., *Altering gender role expectations: Effects on pain tolerance, pain threshold, and pain ratings.* Journal of Pain, 2003. **4**(5): 284–8.

17. Robinson, M.E., et al., *Influences of gender role and anxiety on sex differences in temporal summation of pain. Journal of Pain*, 2004. **5**(2): 77–82.

18. Niesters, M., et al., *Do sex differences exist in opioid analgesia? A systematic review and meta-analysis of human experimental and clinical studies. Pain*, 2010. **151**(1): 61–8.

19. Todd, K.H., et al., *Chronic or recurrent pain in the emergency department: National telephone survey of patient experience. Western Journal of Emergency Medicine*, 2010. **11**(5): 408–15.

20. Fosnocht, D.E., et al., *Correlation of change in visual analog scale with pain relief in the ED. American Journal of Emergency Medicine*, 2005. **23**(1): 55–9.

21. Kelly, A.M., *Does the clinically significant difference in visual analog scale pain scores vary with gender, age, or cause of pain? Academic Emergency Medicine*, 1998. **5**(11): 1086–90.

22. Raftery, K.A., R. Smith-Coggins, and A.H. Chen, *Gender-associated differences in emergency department pain management. Annals of Emergency Medicine*, 1995. **26**(4): 414–21.

23. Brown, J.C., et al., *Emergency department analgesia for fracture pain. Annals of Emergency Medicine*, 2003. **42**(2): 197–205.

24. Crandall, M., et al., *The pain experience of adolescents after acute blunt traumatic injury. Pain Management Nursing*, 2002. **3**(3): 104–14.

25. Decosterd, I., et al., *Oligoanalgesia in the emergency department: Short-term beneficial effects of an education program on acute pain. Annals of Emergency Medicine*, 2007. **50**(4): 462–71.

26. Ducharme, J. and J. Gutman, *Pain management in the emergency department. Academic Emergency Medicine*, 1995. **2**(9): 850–2.

27. Jantos, T.J., et al., *Analgesic practice for acute orthopedic trauma pain in Costa Rican emergency departments. Annals of Emergency Medicine*, 1996. **28**(2): 145–50.

28. Jones, J.S., K. Johnson, and M. McNinch, *Age as a risk factor for inadequate emergency department analgesia. American Journal of Emergency Medicine*, 1996. **14**(2): 157–60.

29. Marquie, L., et al., *Pain rating by patients and physicians: Evidence of systematic pain miscalibration. Pain*, 2003. **102**(3): 289–96.

30. Nguyen, N.L., et al., *The importance of initial management: A case series of childhood burns in Vietnam. Burns*, 2002. **28**(2): 167–72.

31. Perry, S. and G. Heidrich, *Management of pain during debridement: A survey of U.S. burn units. Pain*, 1982. **13**(3): 267–80.

32. Perry, S.W., *Undermedication for pain on a burn unit. General Hospital Psychiatry*, 1984. **6**(4): 308–16.

33. Pines, J.M. and A.D. Perron, *Oligoanalgesia in ED patients with isolated extremity injury without documented fracture. American Journal of Emergency Medicine*, 2005. **23**(4): 580.

34. Rupp, T. and K.A. Delaney, *Inadequate analgesia in emergency medicine. Annals of Emergency Medicine*, 2004. **43**(4): 494–503.

35. Silka, P.A., M.M. Roth, and J.M. Geiderman, *Patterns of analgesic use in trauma patients in the ED. American Journal of Emergency Medicine*, 2002. **20**(4): 298–302.

36. Wilson, J.E. and J.M. Pendleton, *Oligoanalgesia in the emergency department. American Journal of Emergency Medicine*, 1989. **7**(6): 620–3.

37. Todd, K.H., *Influence of ethnicity on emergency department pain management. Emergency Medicine (Fremantle)*, 2001. **13**(3): 274–8.

38. Banz, V.M., et al., *Gender, age and ethnic aspects of analgesia in acute abdominal pain: Is analgesia even across the groups? Internal Medicine Journal*, 2012. **42**(3): 281–8.

39. Hurley, R.W. and M.C. Adams, *Sex, gender, and pain: An overview of a complex field. Anesthesia & Analgesia*, 2008. **107**(1): 309–17.

40. Chen, E.H., et al., *Gender disparity in analgesic treatment of emergency department patients with acute abdominal pain. Academic Emergency Medicine*, 2008. **15**(5): 414–8.

41. Bayer, B.M., et al., *Enhanced susceptibility of the immune system to stress in morphine-tolerant rats. Brain, Behavior, and Immunity*, 1994. **8**(3): 173–84.

42. Beilin, B., et al., *The effects of postoperative pain management on immune response to surgery. Anesthesia & Analgesia*, 2003. **97**(3): 822–7.

43. Charmandari, E., et al., *Pediatric stress: Hormonal mediators and human development. Hormone Research*, 2003. **59**(4): 161–79.

44. Koga, C., et al., *Anxiety and pain suppress the natural killer cell activity in oral surgery outpatients. Oral Surgery, Oral Medicine, Oral Pathology, Oral Radiology, and Endodontology*, 2001. **91**(6): 654–8.

45. Lyte, M. and M.T. Bailey, *Neuroendocrine-bacterial interactions in a neurotoxin-induced model of trauma. Journal of Surgical Research*, 1997. **70**(2): 195–201.

46. Lyte, M., et al., *Stimulation of Staphylococcus epidermidis growth and biofilm formation by catecholamine inotropes. Lancet*, 2003. **361**(9352): 130–5.

47. Morrison, R.S., et al., *The impact of post-operative pain on outcomes following hip fracture. Pain*, 2003. **103**(3): 303–11.

48. Taddio, A., et al., *Effect of neonatal circumcision on pain responses during vaccination in boys. Lancet*, 1995. **345**(8945): 291–2.

49. Weisman, S.J., B. Bernstein, and N.L. Schechter, *Consequences of inadequate analgesia during painful procedures in children. Archives of Pediatrics and Adolescent Medicine*, 1998. **152**(2): 147–9.

50. Nichols, M.L., et al., *Transmission of chronic nociception by spinal neurons expressing the substance P receptor. Science*, 1999. **286**(5444): 1558–61.

51. Berkley, K.J., *Sex differences in pain. Behav Brain Sci*, 1997. **20**(3): 371–80; discussion 435–513.

52. Riley, J.L., 3rd, et al., *Sex differences in the perception of noxious experimental stimuli: a meta-analysis. Pain*, 1998. **74**(2–3): 181–7.

53. Frew, A.K. and P.D. Drummond, *Negative affect, pain and sex: The role of endogenous opioids. Pain*, 2007. **132 Suppl 1**: S77–85.

54. Fillingim, R.B., et al., *Sex, gender, and pain: A review of recent clinical and experimental findings. Journal of Pain*, 2009. **10**(5): 447–85.

55. McClelland, L.E. and J.A. McCubbin, *Social influence and pain response in women and men. Journal of Behavioral Medicine*, 2008. **31**(5): 413–20.

56. Moettus, A., D. Sklar, and D. Tandberg, *The effect of physician gender on women's perceived pain and embarrassment during pelvic examination. American Journal of Emergency Medicine*, 1999. **17**(7): 635–7.

57. Ozawa, M., et al., *Effect of gender and hand laterality on pain processing in human neonates. Early Human Development*, 2011. **87**(1): 45–8.

58. Pokhrel, B.R., et al., *Effect of sub-maximal exercise stress on cold pressor pain: A gender based study. Kathmandu University Medical Journal (KUMJ)*, 2013. **11**(41): 54–9.

59. Racine, M., et al., *A systematic literature review of 10 years of research on sex/gender and pain perception – Part 2: Do biopsychosocial factors alter pain sensitivity differently in women and men? Pain*, 2012. **153**(3): 619–35.

60. Ravn, P., et al., *Prediction of pain sensitivity in healthy volunteers. Journal of Pain Research*, 2012. **5**: 313–26.

61. Walton, D.M., et al., *A descriptive study of pressure pain threshold at 2 standardized sites in people with acute or subacute neck pain. Journal of Orthopaedic and Sports Physical Therapy*, 2011. **41**(9): 651–7.

62. Gilman, S. In Manter, J. and Gates, A. (eds), *Clinical Neuroanatomy and Neurophysiology, 10th ed. Pain and Temperature*. Philadelphia: FA Davis, 1992, pp. 48–55.

63. Donello, J.E., et al., *A peripheral adrenoceptor-mediated sympathetic mechanism can transform stress-induced analgesia into hyperalgesia. Anesthesiology*, 2011. **114**(6): 1403–16.

64. Romero, M.T. and R.J. Bodnar, *Gender differences in two forms of cold-water swim analgesia. Physiological Behavior*, 1986. **37**(6): 893–7.

65. Romero, M.T., et al., *Modulation of gender-specific effects upon swim analgesia in gonadectomized rats. Physiology and Behavior*, 1987. **40**(1): 39–45.

66. Ryan, S.M. and S.F. Maier, *The estrous cycle and estrogen modulate stress-induced analgesia. Behavioral Neuroscience*, 1988. **102**(3): 371–80.

67. Smith, Y.R., et al., *Pronociceptive and antinociceptive effects of estradiol through endogenous opioid neurotransmission in women. Journal of Neuroscience*, 2006. **26**(21): 5777–85.

68. Bartfield, J.M., J.S. Janikas, and R.S. Lee, *Heart rate response to intravenous catheter placement. Academic Emergency Medicine*, 2003. **10**(9): 1005–8.

69. Marco, C.A., et al., *Self-reported pain scores in the emergency department: Lack of association with vital signs. Academic Emergency Medicine*, 2006. **13**(9): 974–9.

70. Bellamy, N., J. Campbell, and J. Syrotuik, *Comparative study of self-rating pain scales in rheumatoid arthritis patients. Current Medical Research and Opinion*, 1999. **15**(2): 121–7.

71. Bossart, P., D. Fosnocht, and E. Swanson, *Changes in heart rate do not correlate with changes in pain intensity in emergency department patients. Journal of Emergency Medicine*, 2007. **32**(1): 19–22.

72. Davies, G.M., D.J. Watson, and N. Bellamy, *Comparison of the responsiveness and relative effect size of the Western Ontario and McMaster Universities Osteoarthritis Index and the short-form Medical Outcomes Study Survey in a randomized, clinical trial of osteoarthritis patients. Arthritis Care Research*, 1999. **12**(3): 172–9.

73. Huiku, M., et al., *Assessment of surgical stress during general anaesthesia. British Journal of Anaesthesia*, 2007. **98**(4): 447–55.

74. Miner J.R. and K.C. Kapella, *Variations in perceived pain measurements within and between subjects using a standard painful stimulus. Academic Emergency Medicine* 2007. **14**(5): s283.

75. Todd, K.H., et al., *Clinical significance of reported changes in pain severity. Annals of Emergency Medicine*, 1996. **27**(4): 485–9.

76. Gj, H., *Assesment, measurement, history, and examination.* In Rowbotham, DJ, and Macintyre PE (eds), *Clinical Pain Management: Acute Pain.* New York: Oxford University Press, 2003: 93–112.

77. Safdar, B., et al., *Impact of physician and patient gender on pain management in the emergency department – a multicenter study. Pain Medicine*, 2009. **10**(2): 364–72.

78. Coll, M.P., et al., *The role of gender in the interaction between self-pain and the perception of pain in others. Journal of Pain*, 2012. **13**(7): 695–703.

79. Gardner, R.L., et al., *Does gender influence emergency department management and outcomes in geriatric abdominal pain? Journal of Emergency Medicine*, 2010. **39**(3): 275–81.

80. Leresche, L., *Defining gender disparities in pain management. Clinical Orthopaedics and Related Research*, 2011. **469**(7): 1871–7.

81. Marco, C.A., et al., *Pain perception among Emergency Department patients with headache: Responses to standardized painful stimuli. Journal of Emergency Medicine*, 2007. **32**(1): 1–6.

82. McClish, D.K., et al., *Gender differences in pain and healthcare utilization for adult sickle cell patients: The PiSCES Project. Journal of Womens Health (Larchmont)*, 2006. **15**(2): 146–54.

83. Daoust, R., et al., *Estimation of pain intensity in emergency medicine: A validation study. Pain* 2008. **61**(11): 88–91.

84. Berthier, F., et al., *Comparative study of methods of measuring acute pain intensity in an ED. American Journal of Emergency Medicine*, 1998. **16**(2): 132–6.

85. Bijur, P.E., C.T. Latimer, and E.J. Gallagher, *Validation of a verbally administered numerical rating scale of acute pain for use in the emergency department. Academic Emergency Medicine*, 2003. **10**(4): 390–2.

86. Bijur, P.E., W. Silver, and E.J. Gallagher, *Reliability of the visual analog scale for measurement of acute pain. Academic Emergency Medicine*, 2001. **8**(12): 1153–7.

87. Silka, P.A., et al., *Pain scores improve analgesic administration patterns for trauma patients in the emergency department. Academic Emergency Medicine*, 2004. **11**(3): 264–70.

88. Emshoff, R., S. Bertram, and I. Emshoff, *Clinically important difference thresholds of the visual analog scale: A conceptual model for identifying meaningful intraindividual changes for pain intensity. Pain*, 2011. **152**(10): 2277–82.

89. Fillingim, R.B., et al., *Clinical characteristics of chronic back pain as a function of gender and oral opioid use. Spine* 2003. **28**(2): 143–50.

90. Platts-Mills, T.F., et al., *More educated emergency department patients are less likely to receive opioids for acute pain. Pain*, 2012. **153**(5): 967–73.

91. Schnabel, A., et al., *Sex-related differences of patient-controlled epidural analgesia for postoperative pain. Pain*, 2012. **153**(1): 238–44.

92. Fosnocht, D.E., N.D. Heaps, and E.R. Swanson, *Patient expectations for pain relief in the ED. American Journal of Emergency Medicine*, 2004. **22**(4): 286–8.

93. Behzadnia, M.J., H.R. Javadzadeh, and F. Saboori, *Time of admission, gender and age: Challenging factors in emergency renal colic – a preliminary study. Trauma Monthly*, 2012. **17**(3): 329–32.

94. Zun, L.S., et al., *Gender differences in narcotic-induced emesis in the ED. American Journal of Emergency Medicine*, 2002. **20**(3): 151–4.

95. Hudson, T.J., et al., *Epidemiology of regular prescribed opioid use: Results from a national, population-based survey. Journal of Pain Symptom Management*, 2008. **36**(3): 280–8.

96. Campbell, C.I., et al., *Age and gender trends in long-term opioid analgesic use for noncancer pain. American Journal of Public Health*, 2010. **100**(12): 2541–7.

97. Parsells Kelly, J., et al., *Prevalence and characteristics of opioid use in the US adult population. Pain*, 2008. **138**(3): 507–13.

98. Logan, D.E. and J.B. Rose, *Gender differences in post-operative pain and patient controlled analgesia use among adolescent surgical patients. Pain*, 2004. **109**(3): 481–7.

99. Logan, J., et al., *Opioid prescribing in emergency departments: The prevalence of potentially inappropriate prescribing and misuse. Medical Care*, 2013. **51**(8): 646–53.

100. Sjors, A., et al., *An increased response to experimental muscle pain is related to psychological status in women with chronic non-traumatic neck-shoulder pain. BMC Musculoskeletal Disorders*, 2011. **12**: 230.

101. Lewis, G.C., et al., *Incidence and Predictors of Acute Psychological Distress and Dissociation after Motor Vehicle Collision: a Cross-Sectional Study. Journal of Trauma and Dissociation*, 2014. **76**(3): 561–75.

102. Severeijns, R., et al., *Pain catastrophizing predicts pain intensity, disability, and psychological distress independent of the level of physical impairment. The Clinical Journal of Pain*, 2001. **17**(2): 165–72.

103. Pincus, T., et al., *A systematic review of psychological factors as predictors of chronicity/disability in prospective cohorts of low back pain.* Spine, 2002. **27**(5): E109–20.

104. Feyer, A.M., et al., *The role of physical and psychological factors in occupational low back pain: A prospective cohort study.* Occupational and Environmental Medicine, 2000. **57**(2): 116–20.

105. Anderson, E.A., *Preoperative preparation for cardiac surgery facilitates recovery, reduces psychological distress, and reduces the incidence of acute postoperative hypertension.* Journal of Consulting and Clinical Psychology, 1987. **55**(4): 513–20.

106. Holbrook, T.L., et al., *Morphine use after combat injury in Iraq and post-traumatic stress disorder.* New England Journal of Medicine, 2010. **362**(2): 110–7.

107. Greenspan, J.D., et al., *Studying sex and gender differences in pain and analgesia: A consensus report.* Pain, 2007. **132 Suppl** 1: S26–45.

108. Keogh, E., L.M. McCracken, and C. Eccleston, *Do men and women differ in their response to interdisciplinary chronic pain management?* Pain, 2005. **114**(1–2): 37–46.

109. Burton, A.K., et al., *Information and advice to patients with back pain can have a positive effect. A randomized controlled trial of a novel educational booklet in primary care.* Spine, 1999. **24**(23): 2484–91.

110. Craft, R.M., *Modulation of pain by estrogens.* Pain, 2007. **132 Suppl** 1: S3–12.

Chapter 10

Digesting Sex and Gender: Gastroenterology

David J. Desilets

Case 1: Helen G. is a 47-year-old female who presented to the Emergency Department (ED) with right upper quadrant pain, nausea, and vomiting of three days duration. She did not take her temperature but felt that she may have been febrile for the past day. She had not had any recent travel or sick contacts, nor eaten food outside of her home. She had a past medical history notable for essential hypertension, obesity, depression, glucose intolerance, and low back pain. She had two vaginal deliveries and one Cesarean section. Her medications included hydrochlorothiazide, bupropion HCl, and over-the-counter ibuprofen. She did not smoke or drink alcohol. Her family history was notable for breast cancer in her mother; her review of systems was negative for weight loss, chest pain, cough, dyspnea, rash, itching, dark urine, dysuria, urinary frequency, headache, or dizziness. She was slightly tachycardic at 100 bpm; her temperature was 100.6 F, BP 136/87, and her respiratory rate was 20. She was alert and oriented to person, time, place, and situation. Her exam was remarkable for abdominal tenderness in the epigastrium and right upper quadrant, without rebound. Her bowel sounds were normal, as was the remainder of her exam except for obesity. There was no palpable liver or spleen. The WBC was 16,000, lipase 67, AST 121, ALT 256, alkaline phosphatase 186, and the total bilirubin was 2.1 with a direct fraction of 1.2.

What was this patient's most likely diagnosis? What else should have been in the differential? Does her sex change the way we rank order the differential diagnosis? What is the next test that should have been ordered?

Case 2: Roy G. is Helen's husband. He is a 47-year-old man who presented to the ED with right upper quadrant pain, nausea, and vomiting of three days duration. He did not take his temperature but felt that he may have been febrile for the past day. He denied any recent travel or sick contacts and had not eaten food outside of his home. He had a past medical history notable for essential hypertension, depression, glucose intolerance, and low back pain. He had had two ED visits in the past for broken ribs after a fall and an episode of idiopathic pancreatitis. He has had a previous appendectomy. Roy takes hydrochlorothiazide, bupropion HCl, and over-the-counter ibuprofen. He smokes one pack/day and drinks alcohol socially. His father had prostate cancer. His review of systems was negative for weight loss, chest pain, cough, wheezing, rash, itching, dark urine, dysuria, urinary frequency, headache, or dizziness. He was mildly tachycardic at 100 bpm and had a temperature of 100.6 F, BP 136/87, and a respiratory rate of 20. He was alert and oriented to person, time, and place but seemed confused about the situation. He was thin and had temporal wasting. He also had abdominal tenderness in the epigastrium and right upper quadrant, without rebound with a tender liver palpable four finger breadths below the right costal margin. Bowel sounds were active. His exam was otherwise normal. His WBC was 16,000, lipase 67, AST 256, ALT 121, alkaline phosphatase 186, and total bilirubin 2.1 with a direct fraction of 1.2.

What is the most likely diagnosis? What else is in the differential? Does the fact that Roy is a man change the order of the differential? What is the next best test?

Introduction

These case vignettes illustrate how two patients of different sexes with gastrointestinal illnesses can present with identical symptoms, identical vital signs, and similar labs, and yet the differential diagnosis, and indeed the main working diagnosis, may be entirely different. These differences are not just because of small variations in the lab results, but because clinicians tend to think along different lines for these two patients primarily because of their different sexes.

There were more than 122 million Emergency Department visits in the United States in 2007, and 15 million of these patients (12%) had a primary gastrointestinal (GI) diagnosis (Myer, 2013). The leading primary GI diagnoses were abdominal pain (4.7 million visits), nausea and vomiting (1.6 million visits), and functional GI disorders (0.7 million visits). For each of the three leading categories, women far outnumber men in visits to the ED (Table 10.1). In fact, when looking at all age groups except the early childhood years and all GI diagnoses, women have more ED visits than men (Figure 10.1).

Table 10.1 Number of ED Visits by Gender in the United States in 2007

	Women	Men
Abdominal pain	3,089,684	1,572,162
Nausea and vomiting	940,160	615,149
Functional GI disorders	417,022	309,635

Adapted from Myer, 2013.

The patient's sex should influence the clinician's approach to the patient in the acutecare or ED setting. However, it is not intuitively obvious that men and women are different when it comes to GI illnesses. Both sexes have the same digestive organs in the same arrangement and with the same function. It is not so obvious as it is, for example, in urological matters, that "boys and girls are different." And yet it is the careless physician who forgets, at his or her own risk that sex informs most diagnoses.

This chapter reviews how sex differences influence gastrointestinal disease and provides a foundation for a sex-based approach to the patient with GI complaints. We proceed anatomically, from the mouth to the anus, covering all the digestive organs along this route, outlining where men and women are different, and how these differences can influence the differential diagnosis presentations of illness. Each section begins with differences in normal physiology and then focuses on how selective disease states are influenced by sex. Women tend to have considerably more visceral hypersensitivity than men; so, a recurrent theme of this chapter is that functional disorders predominate among women, at least in the industrialized West. The chapter concludes with a discussion of the "top 5" GI illnesses where sex matters.

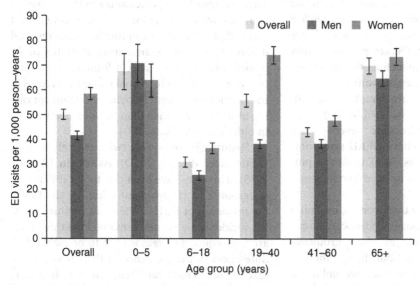

Figure 10.1 Emergency department visits with primary gastrointestinal diagnoses by age and gender. In all the age groups, except for age group 0–5 years, women had more ED visits than men

Normal Physiology

Tongue

Sex differences start with the tongue. More women than men can be classified as "super tasters," tasting both bitter and sweet foods more intensely (Bartoshuk, 1994). Put another way, more women can detect certain tastes at lower concentrations than men. This fundamental difference in physiology, a hypersensitivity to sensory input, is reprised throughout the GI tract. That is, women are more likely than men to have a visceral hypersensitivity. This hypersensitivity seen in the tongue continues throughout the remainder of the GI tract. For example, women tend to have a lower pain threshold than men during balloon inflation in the esophagus (Nguyen, 1995).

Esophagus

There are only minor differences in esophageal motility between the sexes (Dantas, 1998). Women tend to have longer peristaltic wave duration with swallowing than men, but slower wave velocity. There was no difference in the amplitude of contractions, duration of lower esophageal sphincter relaxation, sphincter tone, or in the number of failed swallows, multipeaked swallows, or simultaneous contractions.

Globus sensation (feeling of a lump in the throat) can result from a hypertensive upper esophageal sphincter (UES). Men and women are equally likely to have globus due to a hypertensive UES; however, patients who experience globus without a hypertensive UES, are predominantly women (Corso, 1998), reflecting the increased visceral hypersensitivity seen in women.

Men and women who are symptomatic with gastroesophageal reflux disease (GERD) have similar patterns of endoscopic severity, but women are more likely to have GERD symptoms without esophagitis (55% vs. 38%), while symptomatic men are more likely to have Barrett's esophagus (Lin, 2004).

Men are far more likely than women, by a ratio of 6–8 to 1, to develop esophageal adenocarcinoma, which generally develops in the chronically inflamed Barrett's esophagus, but the specific factors influencing this sex difference are unknown (Lofdahl, 2008). Men are also far more likely to have esophageal squamous cell carcinoma, probably as a result of men's greater prevalence of tobacco use and heavier drinking (Pandeya, 2013). Furthermore, women age 55 and older who do develop loco-regional esophageal squamous-cell carcinoma, and women less than age 55 with metastatic esophageal squamous-cell carcinoma, tend to have better outcomes than men (Bohanes, 2012).

Stomach

Gastric emptying is slower in women. When measured with scintigraphy, men and women demonstrate similar lag periods in their mean solid-phase gastric emptying curves, but men show faster linear gastric emptying rates, shorter half-emptying times, and lower residual radioactivity after two hours (Hermansson, 1996). Others researchers (Datz, 1987) have duplicated these findings using ingested liquids and solids. Remembering that women have greater visceral hypersensitivity than men, it is easy to infer that women's reporting of a greater frequency of symptomatic bloating ("I have gas!") and non-ulcer dyspepsia may reflect their "normal" physiology.

Women with type II diabetes tend to have a greater body mass index and hemoglobin A1c levels than men. The prevalence of nausea, early satiety, loss of appetite, and the severity of these symptoms were all significantly greater in women, especially obese women (Dickman, 2014).

Gastric cancer is twice as prevalent in men. There is almost no gastric cancer in the absence of concomitant H. pylori infection; consequently, it seems that men's gastric epithelium may respond differently to the inflammatory stimulus of H. pylori. Investigators have confirmed this correlation as atrophy and intestinal metaplasia scores in the gastric corpus with H. pylori infection appearing more severe in men than in women, especially in older patients (Kato, 2004).

Historically, men were twice as likely to have peptic ulcer disease (PUD) as women (Kurata, 1985). This may have been due to sex differences in response to H. pylori infection. By the 1980s, the incidence of PUD in men had declined while the incidence in women remained flat;thus, rates are now equal. For reasons yet to be elaborated, differences in the incidence of PUD between the sexes seems to have vanished, and there is no sex-based difference in incidence.

Duodenum and Small Bowel

For all histological types, rates of duodenal and small bowel malignant neoplasms are higher in men than in women, including small bowel adenocarcinomas, neuroendocrine tumors, sarcomas, and lymphomas (Qubaiah, 2010). The reasons for this difference are unknown.

As has been demonstrated with gastric transit, delayed small bowel transit is also more common in women (Bennett, 2000). Patients with delayed small bowel transit are more likely to be diagnosed with functional bowel disorders; therefore, women carry these diagnoses more frequently than men. Although the causes have not yet been elucidated, the sex-specific delay in small bowel transit time may be one explanation of the higher frequency of irritable bowel syndrome (IBS) in women in the Western world. IBS is sometimes treated with selective serotonin reuptake inhibitors. It has been shown that women with IBS respond better to SSRIs than men do (Khan, 2005). This improved response may reflect a direct effect of SSRIs on delayed bowel transit and its associated symptoms or may it be a result of the relationship of IBS to depression. The therapeutic effects of SSRIs on depression may be manifest in the individual patient as a decrease in IBS (somatic or functional) symptoms.

Liver

Liver metabolism is markedly sexdimorphic. This dimorphism is based on sexual differences in a superfamily of nuclear receptors that governs the expression of liver metabolism genes by responding to the plasma concentrations of lipid-soluble hormones and circulating dietary lipids (Rando, 2011). As a result of this variance, the prevalence of liver diseases is different between the sexes. The increased prevalence of liver disease in women is especially true in pregnancy, as will be discussed in the section on "Pregnancy-Related GI Disorder," although women are believed to be more resistant to some liver diseases than men (Rando, 2011).

Men more commonly have malignant liver masses, primary sclerosing cholangitis, and viral hepatitis (Guy, 2013). Women are more commonly afflicted with autoimmune hepatitis, nonalcoholicsteatohepatitis (NASH), Wilson's disease, primary biliary cirrhosis, acute liver failure, and toxin-mediated hepatotoxicity. There is no difference in survival between men and women in alcohol-related liver disease, but women have improved survival from hepatocellular carcinoma. Men have an increased rate of decompensated cirrhosis with hepatitis C virus infection (Guy, 2013). Men are twice as likely to die from chronic liver disease and cirrhosis than are women, and more likely to need and receive a liver transplant. Interested readers may refer to the excellent summary by Guy and Peters (2013) for a more in-depth review of sex differences in chronic liver disease.

There are also sex differences in liver-dependent pharmacokinetics and drug metabolism, resulting in part from women's predominant expression of CYP3A4, the most important cytochrome P450 catalyst of drug metabolism in the human liver (Waxman, 2009). The sex difference in the expression of genes regulating the synthesis of cytochrome P450s and other catabolic enzymes is probably controlled by divergence in the timing of pituitary growth hormone secretion between sexes. These variations in the rate of drug metabolism may affect response to antibiotics, anti-inflammatories, and other pharmaceuticals.

Gallbladder and Biliary Tract

It is estimated that 20.5 million people have gallstone disease in the United States, affecting 14.2 million women and 6.3 million men, a ratio of 2.25 to 1 (Everhart, 1999). Everhart defined "gallstone disease" as the presence of gallstones on ultrasonography of a select sample of the general population or an absent gallbladder indicating prior cholecystectomy, presumably for symptomatic cholelithiasis or cholecystitis. Other work demonstrates that during the reproductive years, women have a fourfold higher incidence of gallstones (Dua, 2013).

Surprisingly though, men with cholelithiasis have more complications of gallstone disease than women with stones. For example, the percentage is 65% female, or a male-to-female ratio of only 1.5-to-1 (Dua, 2013). The expected ratio of patients hospitalized with acute cholecystitis based on the prevalence of cholelithiasis would range from 2.25:1 to 4:1; however, actually 65% of these patients are women, a ratio of 1.5:1. Fourteen percent of men with gallstones in one study developed gallstone pancreatitis, as opposed to 6% of women (Taylor, 1991). Men have a larger cystic duct diameter, allowing larger stones to exit the gall bladder, stones that subsequently become lodged more distally inciting pancreatic inflammation. At the author's institution, Baystate Medical Center in Springfield, Massachusetts, in a QA database of more than 3,500 ERCPs, the ratio of women to men referred for the treatment of common bile duct stones is 1.5:1, a ratio that is not reflective of the underlying prevalence of cholelithiasis by sex. Based on this prevalence, the ratio of women to men undergoing ERCP would be expected to have been at least 2.5:1 or even 4:1 if patients developed this complication with equal frequency.

Pancreas

Men and women appear to secrete equal amounts of pancreatic enzymes and bicarbonate, although slight but clinically insignificant differences between the sexes can be seen with age (Keller, 2005). Nevertheless, there is variance across studies; overall, there is a paucity of research focusing on sex-specific differences in pancreatic function.

More men than women develop alcoholic acute pancreatitis, while gallstone pancreatitis affects more women than men because more women than men by far have gallstone disease (Lankisch, 2001). However, with minor exceptions, the severity of acute pancreatitis is generally the same in both sexes. Because alcoholic acute pancreatitis affects males predominantly, and because nonhereditary chronic pancreatitis is thought to be caused mainly by repeated episodes of alcoholic acute pancreatitis, chronic pancreatitis also has a male predilection (Yadav, 2010). The actual sex-based prevalence of chronic pancreatitis in men and women, like the sex-based prevalence of alcoholic pancreatitis, varies widely based on the geographic location of the study. This is likely the result of regional differences in alcohol consumption between men and women.

Complications of biliary pancreatitis differ by sex. In a study from Taiwan, men with severe acute biliary pancreatitis had a mortality rate of 11% compared to a mortality rate of 7.5% in women (p<0.001) (Shen, 2013). Whether this is due to a direct sex effect or to comorbidities that are traditionally higher in men, such as smoking, alcohol use, and cirrhosis, is unclear.

Men are 30% more likely to develop pancreatic cancer than women (American Cancer Society, 2014). However, this difference is likely the result of confounding risk factors that were historically more prevalent among men such as smoking and alcoholism. As prevalence of smoking and alcohol consumption increase in women, the sex gap in pancreatic cancer is rapidly closing.

Colon and Rectum

In addition to having a more rapid gastric and small bowel transit than women, men also have a more rapid colonic transit (Degen, 1996; Meier, 1995). Women's delayed colonic transit may contribute to chronic constipation seen more commonly in women than in men. Women are far more likely to report symptoms of constipation than men. A cross-sectional study conducted at a tertiary referral center reported that 79% of women versus 21% of men seeking treatment in a specialty clinic reported symptoms of constipation, and higher adjusted odds ratios for all symptoms of constipation than men (Table 10.2) (McCrea, 2009).

Using rectal balloon inflation in healthy volunteers, men have been shown to have larger rectal volumes at a given pressure than women (Sloots, 2000). Men also have greater compliance at maximum tolerable pressure and so are presumed to tolerate episodes of diarrhea better than women. This finding may also explain why diarrhea-predominant irritable bowel syndrome is more common in women. The diagnosis of IBS can only be made if the patient seeks medical care. The increased incidence (apparent) in

Table 10.2 Adjusted Odds Ratios, Female to Male, for Symptoms of Constipation

Symptom	AOR
Infrequent bowel movements	2.97
Abnormal stool consistency	3.08
Longer duration of symptoms	2.00
Increased frequency of abdominal pain	2.22
Bloating	2.65
Unsuccessful attempts at evacuation	1.74
Anal digitation to evacuate stool	3.37
Adapted from McCrea, 2009.	

women may reflect their choice to seek care, unable to tolerate symptoms that may be less irksome in men because of their rectal physiology.

Men generally have higher resting anal tone than women, and resting tone declines with age in both sexes (McHugh, 1987). However, aging affects resting tone more in women. Despite this, in the aging population, men are more likely to self-report fecal incontinence than women (ratio 1.5:1) (Talley, 1992).

Although ulcerative colitis does not demonstrate a sex preference, Crohn's disease occurs more commonly in women, with ratios ranging from 1.2:1 to 1.4:1 in various studies. This greater incidence among women is tempered by the presence or absence of risk factors such as geography, tobacco use, and race (the African American female-to-male ratio is 2.2).

Although colon cancer has long been said to affect the sexes equally, sex differences exist in both incidence and mortality (Brenner, 2007). For a given age, men have higher incidence of, and higher mortality from, colorectal cancer (Figure 10.2). Colon cancer catches up with women who reach equivalent levels of incidence and mortality four to eight years later than men. Given that women tend to live longer than men, if age is discounted, then the incidence and mortality show a similar distribution by sex without predilection for either sex.

Top Five GI Illnesses Where Sex Matters

1. Non-ulcer Dyspepsia

Non-ulcer dyspepsia (NUD) is characterized by a sensation of epigastric discomfort associated with bloating, fullness, and sometimes early satiety. There is often considerable symptom overlap with GERD. Patients with non-ulcer dyspepsia are predominantly female (Mahadeva, 2006). The actual proportion of men to women varies widely across published studies, as geography seems to affect epidemiology of this disease; nevertheless, women tend to be afflicted with this NUD more often than men. Compared to men, women with NUD tend to have significantly more impairment and lower quality of life (Welen, 2008). The causes of NUD are not well understood, and the treatment is difficult. Eradication of H. pylori, chronic acid suppression, and dietary modifications yield little benefit.

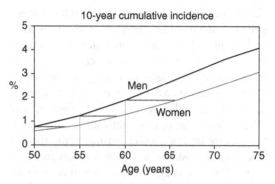

Figure 10.2A Ten-year cumulative incidence of colorectal cancer in subsequent 10 years among men and women at various ages. The dotted lines indicate the age differences at comparable levels of cumulative incidence between women and men

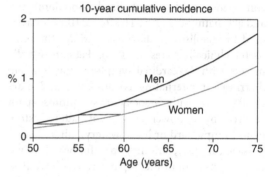

Figure 10.2B Ten-year cumulative mortality from CRC in subsequent 10 years among men and women at various ages. The dotted lines indicate the age differences at comparable levels of cumulative mortality between women and men

If endoscopy or radiography shows no evidence of peptic ulcer disease, gastritis, or esophagitis, then management includes a supportive physician-patient relationship, avoidance of culprit foods, stress reduction, and reassurance.

2. Irritable Bowel Syndrome

Women in industrialized societies seek health care for, and likely are more often affected by, IBS (Heitkemper, 2008). The ratio of affected women to men is about 2:1. The illness usually affects younger women, who often describe lifelong difficulty with bowel habits. They tend to have multiple life stressors, including prior history of physical or mental abuse, unstable social situation, stressful employment, and so on, and they often have functional comorbid illnesses such as fibromyalgia, chronic pelvic pain, or migraine headaches. IBS is a poorly understood disturbance in the sensitivity and motility of the whole gut, which is most likely to be multifactorial. Symptoms can be centered anywhere in the digestive tract and can mimic other disorders such as GERD, peptic ulcer disease, biliary colic, inflammatory bowel disease, and others. Treatment of IBS is difficult because a unifying cause and/or a common target for therapy has never been identified. Sex differences also exist in response to drug therapies for this disorder (Waxman, 2009; Chang, 2002), which may be a reflection of sex-specific pathophysiology or pharmacokinetics and drug metabolism. Some drugs for IBS were initially only tested in, and approved for, women.

There are three broad categories of IBS: constipation-predominant, diarrhea-predominant, and alternating-type IBS. The Rome III criteria are used to establish the diagnosis and are the most useful clinically (Tresca, 2012). Patients usually present with the cardinal symptom (constipation, diarrhea, or alternating constipation and diarrhea) along with associated symptoms: pain relieved by a bowel movement, altered stool form (lumpy/hard or loose/watery), altered stool passage (urgency, straining, painful bowel movements, sensation of incomplete evacuation), passage of mucus, and bloating. Symptoms must be present most days for at least three months. The pain and the diarrhea (when present) are often postprandial. Patients with these symptoms are frequent visitors to the Emergency Department, convinced that "something is wrong" with their digestive tract.

Evaluation of these patients consists of recording a detailed history, eliciting the diagnostic features noted earlier, performing a physical exam, and carrying out basic lab testing. The physical exam should be normal except for abdominal tenderness. Tachycardia, fever, rebound tenderness, gross blood on digital rectal exam, and palpable masses all suggest other diagnoses. A normal complete blood count, sedimentation rate or C-reactive protein, and liver-associated enzymes are all reassuring. Thyroid-stimulating hormone should always be checked to rule out hypothyroidism (constipation) or hyperthyroidism (diarrhea).

The typical patient is a young female (but remember that a third are male) with abdominal pain relieved by bowel movements, who has either constipation or diarrhea, or both. She should be without weight loss and blood per rectum and should have normal labs. Frequent visits to the PCP or the ED are often found on review of the medical record. Many of these patients go on to get abdominal plain films or a CT scan (sometimes multiple scans on multiple different visits) without findings. In a patient with the classic history, CT scanning or other imaging is unnecessary and should be avoided unless an organic disorder is strongly suspected. Patients with diarrhea-predominant IBS are sometimes difficult to distinguish from those with ulcerative colitis or Crohn's disease. Given that adolescence and young adulthood are typically times when inflammatory bowel disease presents, these patients may need to be referred to a gastroenterologist for possible flexible sigmoidoscopy or colonoscopy.

The mainstays of therapy are reassurance, a nonjudgmental physician–patient relationship, stress reduction (with vigorous aerobic exercise if possible), a high-fiber diet, and fiber supplements if necessary. Many patients seek alternative medicine remedies. This is sometimes beneficial, if only for the placebo effect engendered, as long as cost is not extreme. Narcotic analgesics should be avoided because of the high potential for abuse, and because tachyphylaxis renders them rapidly ineffective often leading to dose escalation. Anxiolytics/benzodiazepines are occasionally helpful and can be used in moderation in the short term, but the abuse potential is great as well. Antispasmodics (hyoscyamine, dicyclomine, donnatol) along with anti-diarrheals can help with the diarrhea-predominant subtype. The constipation-predominant type is treated with fiber supplements and osmotic (nonirritant) laxatives. The alternating type of IBS is more difficult to treat, as anti-spasmodics or anti-diarrheals can make patients quite constipated, and a single dose of laxative can give diarrhea lasting days. Judicious titration of these medications by the patient is the best approach. Fiber supplements can be helpful. Occasionally, low-dose, bedtime amitriptyline is helpful. A number of newer medications are available; however, patients requiring higher-order pharmacotherapy for persistent symptoms should be referred for evaluation by a gastroenterologist.

3. Pregnancy-Related GI Disorders

Numerous GI illnesses are more frequent, more severe, or only appear in pregnancy. Gastroesophageal reflux is exacerbated by pregnancy because of the rising fundal height in the third trimester, causing increased mechanical displacement of the viscera and gastric compression. Progesterone is present at high levels later in pregnancy and acts as a smooth muscle relaxer; it reduces lower esophageal sphincter resting tone and contributes to the development or exacerbation of GERD.

Gallstone formation and complications of gallstones are more common in pregnancy or immediately after parturition. Gallstone formation is facilitated by high estrogen turnover in pregnancy, with resultant increased secretion of cholesterol and decreased secretion of chenodeoxycholic acid into bile (Mendez-Sanchez et al., 2006). Gallstone formation is also precipitated by stagnation of bile due to progesterone-mediated smooth muscle relaxation with concomitant decrease in gallbladder emptying (Everson, 1992). Because of this increase in gallstone formation, complications of gallstone disease in pregnant women tend to be more common during and shortly after pregnancy compared with women who are not or have never been pregnant, and certainly also in comparison to men.

The so-called HELLP syndrome (hemolysis, elevated liver enzymes, and low platelets) is thought to be a complication of pregnancy-induced hypertension or preeclampsia, which usually begins in the third trimester but can occur earlier and, also, immediately after parturition. Prepartum HELLP syndrome is treated by prompt delivery of the infant. Acute fatty liver of pregnancy also occurs in the third trimester and is treated with supportive care and prompt delivery.

Anorectal disorders and disorders of defecation are common complications of pregnancy and parturition and range from anal sphincter and continence problems to chronic obstipation. Anorectal pathology and disorders of defecation can result from postpartum complications, including fourth-degree tears or episiotomies, rectoceles, cystoceles, and vaginoceles.

4. Chronic Abdominal Pain

More women than men report chronic abdominal pain, and pain of higher intensity. Surprisingly though, men with chronic pain, especially chronic abdominal pain, consistently report a lower quality of life than women (Rustøen, 2004). Functional abdominal pain syndrome (FAPS) is more common in women, with a female:male ratio of 3:2 (Clouse, 2006). This disorder is generally thought to be of lower prevalence than IBS and is not associated with changes in bowel habits or food ingestion. There is also a higher frequency of psychiatric comorbidities with FAPS as compared to IBS. FAPS may actually be a heterogeneous group of disorders.

Patients with chronic, functional abdominal pain are frequent visitors to the ED and primary care providers. They often have underlying organic diseases such as recurrent acute pancreatitis or multiple prior surgeries. They are frequently given a diagnosis of "chronic pancreatitis" or "symptomatic postoperative adhesions." Many such patients seek narcotic analgesia because the pain is real. However, when no etiology is found, patients are labeled as "drug seeking," which is true if one considers that seeking pharmacologic pain relief is drug-seeking behavior. Some patients go on to develop narcotic bowel syndrome, which is a subset of opioid bowel dysfunction that is characterized by chronic or frequently recurring abdominal pain that worsens with continued or escalating dosages of narcotics (Grunkemeier, 2007). Indeed, narcotic bowel syndrome should be considered in the differential diagnosis for patients with chronic abdominal pain who have received opiates.

The treatment of FAPS is multifactorial. A therapeutic (and nonjudgmental) physician-patient relationship and the judicious use of tricyclic antidepressants have been shown to decrease the symptoms and the patient's frequent use of health care facilities. Goalsetting, mental health referral as needed, and occasionally involvement of a multidisciplinary pain management team are all components of effective therapy. Psychotherapy and complementary therapies (acupuncture, massage, etc.) may help. Surgery should be avoided unless there is compelling evidence supporting the need for adhesiolysis.

5. Gallbladder and Biliary Tract Disorders, and Solution to the Case Vignettes

In the clinical vignettes described at the beginning of this chapter, Helen G. illustrates the classic "four Fs" of gallstone disease: "fat, female, fertile, and forty." She is an obese woman who has had three children, and is over 40. Gallstone disease is highly prevalent in this group of patients. She has leukocytosis, elevated liver enzymes and bilirubin, and right upper quadrant and epigastric pain. Acute cholecystitis should be the leading differential. Other diagnostic considerations should include acute cholangitis and metabolic liver disease (steatohepatitis). The next best diagnostic test would be a right upper quadrant ultrasound to determine if gallstones are present, to assess gallbladder wall thickness, to look for pericholecystic fluid, to measure the diameter of the common bile duct (a dilated duct might be indicative of biliary obstruction/cholangitis), and to assess for a sonographic Murphy sign (pain elicited by pressing the sonographic transducer over the gallbladder in acute cholecystitis).

Given her obesity and glucose intolerance, nonalcoholic steatohepatitis (NASH) is in the differential as well; NASH should be considered because it is more common in women, although it would not explain her leukocytosis and low-grade fever. An ultrasound can support this diagnosis if there are no gallstones and if the liver has increased echodensity suggesting fatty infiltration. NASH can cause pain that results from stretching of the liver capsule. It can also be painless. Thus Helen might still have NASH along with another disorder accounting for her fever and elevated white blood cell count. Her clinician might order a hepatobiliaryiminodiacetic acid (HIDA) scan, but this test would not provide information about common bile duct diameter or fatty infiltration of the liver, and a HIDA scan is much more expensive than a bedside ultrasound.

Although Roy G. presents similarly to his wife, he is far less likely to have gallstones than Helen; thus sex considerations shift our differential immediately and change our approach to this patient. His tender hepatomegaly and his reversed AST/ALT ratio are suggestive of prior or recent alcohol use despite his assertion that he only drinks socially. This level of denial is more common in men who drink. His prior history of "idiopathic" pancreatitis and rib fractures attests to possible prior alcohol abuse. His confusion and tachycardia all lend support to a diagnosis of acute alcoholic hepatitis. The next best diagnostic test for him would be a simple blood alcohol level. If elevated, then no further testing is needed. Given his wasting, the differential diagnosis includes infectious causes such as viral hepatitis or HIV and neoplasm, such as pancreatic or hepatocellular carcinoma. If Roy's blood alcohol level is undetectable, the clinician should order a CT scan of the abdomen.

The differential diagnosis for Helen includes acute cholecystitis, cholangitis, NASH, or NASH coincident with another infectious or inflammatory disorder; the astute clinician should order an abdominal ultrasound for further evaluation. Roy's differential includes alcoholic hepatitis, infectious hepatitis/HIV, or neoplasm. The clinician should do a simple and inexpensive blood alcohol level before embarking on more expensive or invasive testing. These cases that initially presented with similar signs and symptoms clearly illustrate how sex-specific considerations by the astute clinician will affect the differential diagnosis and diagnostic work-up of women and men seeking treatment for gastroenterological complaints in the acute care setting.

Summary

Women tend to seek out health care more frequently than men (Bertakis, 2000), thus many studies demonstrating sex differences in the presentation of many diseases may be affected by selection bias. Nevertheless, it is clear that at least from the time of puberty, and possibly earlier, the GI tract in men is different from the GI tract in women; visceral hypersensitivity is significantly more prevalent in women than in men. Sex differences can be seen in the types and frequencies of acute GI illnesses in patients who present to the Emergency Department or to their primary care providers. Although men and women certainly may suffer from the same afflictions, sex-specific differences in the epidemiology, presentation, and work-up of these diseases must be understood and kept in mind when formulating a differential diagnosis and diagnostic plan for each patient.

References

American Cancer Society information webpage (online). Available at www.cancer.org/cancer/pancreaticcancer/detailedguide/pancreatic-cancer-risk-factors (Accessed March 29, 2014).

Bartoshuk, l.M., Duffy, V.B., and Miller, I.J. (1994). PTC/PROP Tasting: Anatomy, Psychophysics, and Sex Effects. *Physiology & Behavior*, **56**, 1165–71.

Bennett, E.J., Evans, P., Scott, A.M., Badcock, C-A., Shuter, B., et al. (2000). Psychological and Sex Features of Delayed Gut Transit in Functional Gastrointestinal Disorders. *Gut*, **46**, 83–7.

Bertakis, K.D., Azari, R., Helms, L.J., Callahan, E.J., and Robbins, J.A. (2000). Gender Differences in the Utilization of Health Care Services. *Journal of Family Practice*, **49**, 147–52.

Bohanes, P., Yang, D., Chhibar, R.S., Labonte, M.J., Winder, T., et al. (2012). Influence of Sex on the Survival of Patients with Esophageal Cancer. *Journal of Clinical Oncology*, **30**, 2265–72.

Brenner, H., Hoffmeister, M., Arndt, V., and Haug, U. (2007). Gender Differences in Colorectal Cancer: Implications for Age at Initiation of Screening. *British Journal of Cancer*, **96**, 828–31.

Chang, L., and Heitkemper, M.M. (2002). Gender Differences in Irritable Bowel Syndrome. *Gastroenterology*, **123**, 1686–701.

Clouse, R.E, Emeran, A.M., Qasim, A., Drossman, D.A., Dumitrascu, D.L., et al. (2006). Functional Abdominal Pain Syndrome. *Gastroenterology*, **130**, 1492–7.

Corso, M.J., Pursnani, K.G., Mohiudin, M.A., et al. (1998). Globus Sensation Is Associated with Hypertensive Upper Esophageal Sphincter but Not with Gastroesophageal Reflux. *Digestive Diseases and Sciences*, **43**, 1513–17.

Dantas, R.O., Ferriolli, E., and Souza, M.A.N. (1998). Gender Effects on Esophageal Motility. *Brazilian Journal of Medical and Biological Research*, **31**, 539–44.

Datz, F.L., Christian, P.E., and Moore, J. (1987). Gender-Related Differences in Gastric Emptying. *Journal of Nuclear Medicine*, **28**, 1204–7.

Degen, L.P., and Phillips, S.F. (1996). Variability of Gastrointestinal Transit in Healthy Women and Men. *Gut*, **39**, 299–305.

Dickman, R., Wainstein, J., Glezerman, M., Niv, Y., and Boaz, M. (2014). Gender Aspects Suggestive of Gastroparesis in Patients with Diabetes Mellitus: A Cross-Sectional Survey. *BMC Gastrology*, **14**, 34 (online). Available atwww.biomedcentral.com/1471-230X/14/34 (Accessed March 15, 2014).

Dua, A., Dua, A., Desai, S.S., Kuy, S., Sharma, R., et al. (2013). Gender Based Differences in Management and

Outcomes of Cholecystitis. *American Journal of Surgery*, **206**, 641–6.

Everhart, J.E., Khare, M., Hill, M., and Maurer, K.R. (1999). Prevalence and Ethnic Differences in Gallbladder Disease in the United States. *Gastroenterology*, **117**, 632–39.

Everson, G.T. (1992). Gastrointestinal Motility in Pregnancy. *Gastroenterology Clinics of North America*, **21**, 751–76.

Grunkemeier, D.M., Cassara, J.E., Dalton, C.B., and Drossman, D.A. (2007). The Narcotic Bowel Syndrome: Clinical Features, Pathophysiology, and Management. *Clinical Gastroenterology and Hepatology*, **5**, 1126–39.

Guy, G., and Peters, M.G. (2013). Liver Disease in Women: The Influence of Gender on Epidemiology, Natural History, and Patient Outcomes. *Journal of Gastroenterology and Hepatology*, **9**, 633–9.

Heitkemper, M.M., and Jarrett, M.E. (2008). Update on Irritable Bowel Syndrome and Gender Differences. *Nutrition in Clinical Practice*, **23**, 275–83.

Hermansson, G., and Sivertsson, R. (1996). Gender-Related Differences in Gastric Emptying Rate of Solid Meals. *Digestive Diseases and Sciences*, **41**, 1994–8.

Kato, S., Matsukura, N., Togashi, A., Masuda, G., Matsuda, N., et al. (2004). Sex Differences in Mucosal Response to Helicobacter pylori Infection in the Stomach and Variations in Interleukin-8, COX-2 and Trefoil Factor Family 1 Gene Expression. *Alimentary Pharmacology & Therapeutics*, **Suppl 1**, 17–24.

Keller, J., and Layer, P. (2005). Human Pancreatic Exocrine Response to Nutrients in Health and Disease. *Gut*, **54**, 1–28.

Khan, A, Brodhead, A.E., Schwartz, K.A., Kolts, R.L., and Brown, W.A. (2005). Sex Differences in Antidepressant Response in Recent Antidepressant Clinical Trials. *Journal of Clinical Psychopharmacology*, **25**, 318–24.

Kurata, J.H., Haile, B.M., and Elashoff, J.D. (1985). Sex Differences in Peptic Ulcer Disease. *Gastroenterology*, **88**, 96–100.

Lankisch, P.G., Assmus, C., Lehnick, D., Maisonneuve, P., and Lowenfels, A.B. (2001). Acute Pancreatitis: Does Gender Matter? *Digestive Diseases and Sciences*, **46**, 2470–74.

Lin, M., Gerson, L.B., Lascar, R., Davila, M., and Triadafilopoulos G. (2004). Features of Gastroesophageal Reflux Disease in Women. *American Journal of Gastroenterology*, **99**, 1442–7.

Lofdahl, H.E., Lu, Y., and Lagergren, J. (2008). Sex-Specific Risk Factor Profile in Oesophageal Adenocarcinoma. *British Journal of Cancer*, **99**, 1506–10.

Mahadeva, S., and Goh, K-L. (2006). Epidemiology of Functional Dyspepsia: A Global Perspective. *World Journal of Gastroenterology*, **12**, 2661–6.

McCrea, G.L., Miaskowski, C., Stotts, N.A., Macera, L., Paul, S.M., et al. (2009). Gender Differences in Self-Reported Constipation Characteristics, Symptoms, and Bowel and Dietary Habits among Patients Attending a Specialty Clinic for Constipation. *Gender Medicine*, **6**, 259–71.

McHugh, S.M., and Diamant, N.E. (1987). Effect of Age, Gender, and Parity on Anal Canal Pressures. *Digestive Diseases and Sciences*, **32**, 726–36.

Meier, R., Beglinger, C., Dederding, J.P., Meyer-Wyss, B., Fumagalli, M., et al. (1995). Influence of Age, Gender, Hormonal Status and Smoking Habits on Colonic Transit Time. *Neurogastroenterology & Motility*, **7**, 235–8.

Mendez-Sanchez, N., Chavez-Tapia, N.C., and Uribe, M. (2006). Pregnancy and Gallbladder Disease. *Annals ofHepatology*, **5**, 227–30.

Myer, P.A., Mannalithara, A., Singh, G., Pasricha, P.J., and Ladabaum, U. (2013). Clinical and Economic Burden of Emergency Department Visits due to Gastrointestinal Diseases in the United States. *American Journal Gastroenterology*, **108**, 1496–1507.

Nguyen, P., Scott, M.D., and Castell, D.O. (1995). Evidence of Gender Differences in Esophageal Pain Threshold. *American Journal Gastroenterology*, **90**, 901–5.

Pandeya, N., Olsen, C.M., and Whiteman, D.C. (2013). Sex Differences in the Proportion of Squamous Cell Carcinoma Cases Attributable to Tobacco Smoking and Alcohol Consumption. *Cancer Epidemiology*, **37**, 579–84.

Qubaiah, O., Devesa, S.S., Platz, C.E., Huycke, M.M., and Dores, G.M. (2010). Small Intestinal Cancer: APopulation-Based Study of Incidence and Survival Patterns in the United States, 1992–2006. *Cancer Epidemiology, Biomarkers, & Prevention*, **19**, 1908–18.

Rando, G., and Wahli, W. (2011). Sex Differences in Nuclear Receptor-Regulated Liver Metabolic Pathways. *Biochimicaet Biophysica Acta*, **1812**, 964–73.

Rustøen, T., Wahl, A.K., Hamestad, B.R., Lerdal, A., Paul, S., and Miaskowski, C. (2004). Gender Differences in Chronic Pain – Findings from a Population-Based Study of Norwegian Adults. *Pain Management Nursing*, **5**, 105–17.

Shen, H-N.,Wang, W-C., Lu, C-L., and Li, C-Y. (2013). Effects of Gender on Severity, Management and Outcome in Acute Biliary Pancreatitis. *PLoS ONE* **8**(2): e57504. doi: 10.1371/journal.pone.0057504.

Sloots, C.E., Felt-Bersma, R.J., Questa, M.A., and Meuwissen, S.G. (2000). Rectal Visceral Sensitivity in Healthy Volunteers: Influences of Gender, Age and Methods. *Neurogastroenterology & Motility*, **12**, 361–8.

Talley, N.J., O'Keefe, E.A., Zinsmeister, A.R., and Melton, L.J. 3rd. (1992). Prevalence of Gastrointestinal Symptoms in the Elderly: A Population-Based Study. *Gastroenterology*, **102**, 895–901.

Taylor, T.V., Rimmer, S., Holt, S., Jeacock, J., and Lucas, S. (1991). Sex Differences in Gallstone Pancreatitis. *Annals of Surgery*, **214**, 667–70.

Tresca, A.J. (2012). The Rome Criteria for IBS.About .com (online). Available at http://ibdcrohns.about.com/cs/ibs/a/romecriteria.htm (Accessed April 7, 2014).

Waxman, D.J., and Holloway, M.G. (2009). Sex Differences in the Expression of Hepatic Drug Metabolizing Enzymes. *Molecular Pharmacology*, **76**, 215–28.

Welen, K., Faresjo, A., and Faresjo, T. (2008). Functional Dyspepsia Affects Women More than Men in Daily Life: A Case-Control Study in Primary Care. *Gender Medicine*, **5**, 62–73.

Yadav, D., and Whitcomb, D.C. (2010). The Role of Alcohol and Smoking in Pancreatitis. *Nature ReviewsGastroenterology & Hepatology*, **7**, 131–45.

Overcoming Resistance: Importance of Sex and Gender in Acute Infectious Illnesses

Erica Hardy, Mitchell Kosanovich and Arvind Venkat

Opening Cases

A 25-year-old female patient – gravida 1, para 0, 26 weeks pregnant – presents to the Emergency Department with a fever of 101°F and myalgias. Her symptoms began 72 hours prior to presentation and include vomiting and shortness of breath. She has noted no change in fetal movement, contractions, vaginal bleeding, or rush of amniotic fluid. The triage nurse documents that the patient is tachycardic, tachypneic, and hypoxic with an oxygen saturation of 85% on room air. On your examination, you note that the patient has crackles at the right lung base. What historical factors are critical in evaluating this patient?

A 21-year-old female, gravida 0, presents to the emergency room with vaginal discharge. She is sexually active with one male partner with whom she does not use barrier contraception. Although she does note some dysuria, she has no pelvic pain and has noticed no vaginal lesions. In addition, she has not noted any systemic symptoms such as fevers or chills. On your examination, you note that she has erythema of the external vaginal canal and cervix, with homogenous thin white discharge. Based on her demographics, what sexually transmitted infection (STI) is she most likely to have? What are the implications of an STI diagnosis based on her gender?

Introduction

Infectious disease represents an important domain where gender differences are present in acute care presentation, diagnosis, and treatment. Most emergency physicians have an instinctive awareness of differences in which infectious disease can present more commonly or, in some cases, exclusively in either male or female patients. For example, numerous studies confirm that urinary tract infections are more common in female rather than male patients (Magliano, 2012; McLaughlin, 2004). What is less understood is that differences between male and female patients in infectious disease range beyond the epidemiology of presentation to host responses to various microbial pathogens, the resultant severity of illness, and the need for tailored approaches to therapy. Without such knowledge, emergency physicians may not appropriately manage both male and female patients who present with infectious disease.

Infectious diseases also are unique in the acute care setting in that their manifestation can directly relate to a means of transmission between male and female patients, namely STIs. Microbial pathogens that are transmitted sexually can manifest in a gender-specific manner, both related to clinical symptoms and severity. The additional social and behavioral factors that govern sexual transmission of infectious disease are directly relevant to ED practice as well. These epidemiologic factors affect the means of diagnosis, the duration of treatment, and the need to counsel patients on the risk of transmission to their sexual partner(s). Again, gender-specific knowledge on the nature of STIs is critical to proper management in the ED.

In this chapter, we review the existing evidence on gender-related differences and similarities in infectious disease epidemiology, diagnosis, and management. We present the literature that shows that variations in severity and treatment exist between men and women for specific pathogens. Given the robust literature on gender differences in STIs, this chapter is divided in its discussion between non-sexually transmitted and sexually transmitted infectious diseases. Finally, we discuss where there are gaps in the existing literature on gender differences in the acute management of infectious disease.

Epidemiologic Differences between Males and Females in Infectious Disease

As with many medical disorders, the differences between males and females in infectious diseases have a combination of genetic and behavioral explanations. Overall, males appear more susceptible to infectious diseases than females, and this susceptibility extends beyond humans to other species (Guerra-Silveira, 2013). Two hypotheses are proposed for why males may be more susceptible. The first hypothesis, termed the "physiologic hypothesis," is based on genetic and hormonal differences between males and females. In this theory, the relationship between sex-specific hormones and immune system development affects how males and females respond to infectious pathogens. The second hypothesis, termed "the behavioral hypothesis," focuses on varying gender-assigned roles in the past (e.g., hunter-gatherer for men, family nurturer for women) as a possible explanation for the male predominance in infectious disease presentations. In this theory, behavior-driven activities such as roles in hunting-gathering versus lack thereof may have led to evolutionary changes that drive susceptibility to particular pathogens (Guerra-Silveira, 2013).

To be valid, the physiologic hypothesis would predict that sex differences in infectious diseases would appear in infancy and in puberty, both times in development when changes in levels of sex hormones occur. In contrast, the behavioral hypothesis would not predict differences in infancy, as major variations between the genders in activities related to infectious disease susceptibility do not occur until later in life. The preponderance of evidence supports the physiologic rather than the behavioral hypothesis. A study of the epidemiology of 10 major pathogens in Brazil over three years found that the prevalence of these disorders, including leishmaniasis, schistosomiasis, and leprosy, follow the predictions of the physiologic hypothesis (Guerra-Silveira, 2013). Similarly, an Israeli study found that the prevalence of infectious diseases such as viral hepatitis, viral meningitis, salmonellosis, and shigellosis were higher among

Table 11.1 Physiologic versus Behavioral Hypotheses to Explain Gender Differences in Infectious Disease Epidemiology

Physiologic Hypothesis – Based on observations that infectious disease epidemiology differs between males and females at stages of life where behavior is similar. Relies on the role of sex hormones on immune response and genetic variations between the sexes.
Behavioral Hypothesis – Based on observations that infectious disease epidemiology differs between males and females who have different occupations and roles in society. Relies on variations in gender-assigned behavior in traditional societies leading to differentiated exposures to microbiologic pathogens.

male children younger than age five than among female children, a finding that could not be explained by behavioral differences (Green, 1992). Yet both studies suggest that there are behavioral factors that are gender based that may increase the risk of infectious disease, especially in communities where presumed societal roles are ascribed based on traditional beliefs. Overall, the current state of the literature suggests that the physiologic hypothesis is stronger, but that behavioral-related susceptibilities exist in explaining the higher prevalence of infectious diseases among males when compared to females. Table 11.1 summarizes the differences between the physiologic and behavioral hypotheses; Table 11.2 provides an overview of gender differences in non-sexually transmitted infectious diseases discussed in this chapter.

Respiratory Infections

Respiratory infections, ranging from viral upper respiratory pathogens to bacterial pneumonias, are the fourth most common primary diagnosis given to patients from the ED and represent the cause of 3.2% of all ED visits in the United States (Centers for Disease Control, 2010). This high incidence has allowed a number of studies to evaluate the differing epidemiology between males and females in respiratory infectious diseases. A longitudinal study of Danish children and adolescents observed that hospitalizations for respiratory infectious diseases were approximately 1.5 times more common in males than

Table 11.2 Overview of Gender Differences in Non-sexually Transmitted Infectious Diseases

Infectious Diseases without Evidence for Gender Differences in Presentation or Severity

Staph aureus Bacteremia
Methicillin-resistant Staph aureus Colonization
Salmonella
Shigella
Campylobacter
Diarrheal Ova and Parasites
Cellulitis
Diabetic Foot Infections

Infectious Diseases with Evidence for Male Predominance or Severity

Upper Respiratory Infections (Childhood)
Pneumonia
Tuberculosis
Aortic Native Valve Endocarditis
Traveler's Infections – Febrile Illnesses, Vector-
  Borne Illnesses, Viral Hepatitis
Hepatitis C (less likelihood of spontaneous
  clearance)
Leptospirosis
Lyme Disease – United States and Lyme
  neuroborreliosis and Lyme arthritis
Q Fever
Cryptococcal Meningitis

Infectious Diseases with Evidence for Female Predominance or Severity

Upper Respiratory Infections (Adolescence)
Influenza
Urinary Tract Infection
Mitral Prosthetic Valve Endocarditis
Clostridium difficile diarrhea (postpartum)
Traveler's Infections – Diarrheal Illnesses, Upper
  Respiratory Infections, and Urinary Tract
  Infections
Malaria (weak evidence)
Lyme Disease – Europe and Cutaneous
  Manifestations
Onchocerciasis (societal factors in treatment)

females in early childhood. At later ages, the ratio reversed, with males being hospitalized for respiratory ailments at a ratio of 0.8 to 1 female. This reversal in hospitalization ratio extended across respiratory ailments, including viral upper respiratory infections, influenza, and otitis media. The authors note that the nature of Danish child care, with most children being cared for in similar types of day care situations, makes it unlikely that behavioral differences would explain the gender difference observed. Rather, the previously

discussed physiologic changes that occur in infancy and puberty in males and females are more likely factors that contribute to this changing epidemiology (Jensen-Fangel, 2004).

Studies of the nature of respiratory infectious diseases in males and female also indicate that the type of ailments that most commonly affect each population differs based on gender. A review of available studies on the subject found that female patients are more likely to present with upper respiratory infections, while male patients were more likely to present with lower respiratory infections, including pneumonia. These differences in the anatomical location of respiratory infectious diseases may also explain the observation that males have worse outcomes than females when afflicted by respiratory pathogens, given that pneumonia is generally more virulent than upper respiratory infections. Other potential mechanisms for the worse outcomes in male patients with respiratory infections include sex hormone differences and their role in host immune response and behavioral factors, such as workplace environmental exposures (Falagas, 2007).

Male patients also appear more likely to experience pneumonia after trauma. Data from 26 trauma centers in Pennsylvania showed that for moderate and severely injured patients (Injury Severity Score >15), males were more likely to develop pneumonia than females. However, the same study found no evidence that there were mortality differences in post-injury pneumonia between the genders (Gannon, 2004).

Overall, the literature on pneumonia shows evidence that males are more likely to be diagnosed with pneumonia than females. Evidence on outcomes from pneumonia is less robust; males may have poorer outcomes when afflicted with community-acquired pneumonia but may have equal outcomes to females when diagnosed with nosocomial pneumonia (Falagas, 2007; Gannon, 2004).

Tuberculosis is another respiratory disease for which gender epidemiologic differences have been observed. Observational evidence from passive reporting (based on patient presentation to health care services as opposed to active surveillance that evaluates for the presence of cases outside the health care system) suggests that beginning in adolescence, males are more likely than females to develop clinically evident tuberculosis. The criticism of this evidence is that it might be attributable to national health resources in underdeveloped nations being disproportionately accessible to males than females (Holmes, 1998). However, studies based on sputum positivity have also found that males are more likely to develop pulmonary tuberculosis than females with age (Borgdorff, 2000).

Influenza represents the most commonly encountered respiratory pathogen for which female gender is associated with a more severe clinical presentation. It is well established that pregnant women represent a patient population with a particular susceptibility to morbidity and mortality from influenza. Prior to the advent of H1N1 influenza in 2009, epidemiologic survey evidence had confirmed that seasonal influenza from 1998 to 2005 in the United States affected pregnant women in a manner that warranted their labeling as a high-risk population that should be targeted for immunization (Callaghan, 2010). The H1N1 influenza pandemic was particularly virulent among pregnant women, who represented 5% of all deaths attributable to that pathogen. For emergency physicians and other acute care practitioners, these studies suggest that pregnant women with influenza should be treated aggressively with antiviral medications, even if presenting beyond the traditional 24 to 48 hours from symptom onset when these treatments are considered most effective.

Urinary Tract Infection

Infections of the urinary tract represent an extremely common reason for patients to present to the ED. Estimates suggest that 1 million visits to the ED annually are attributable to this disease process. Urinary tract infections also are a prototypical example of how the epidemiology of infectious diseases can vary between sexes. Under age 1 and above age 60, males and females have a similar incidence in urinary tract infections. However, between these two age groups, females are up to 40 times more likely to present with urinary tract infections. Half of all women experience a urinary tract infection during their lifetime. Anatomical (proximity of genitourinary tract to the rectum, shorter urethra), physiologic (gender variations in

uroepithelial receptors for pathogenic bacteria), and behavioral (use of spermicidal contraception) factors all contribute to the female predominance in observed presentations for urinary tract infections (McLaughlin, 2004).

For emergency physicians, the higher prevalence in female patients of urinary tract infections can create a danger of overdiagnosis. A retrospective analysis of women age 70 and older diagnosed with urinary tract infections in the ED found that 43% had negative cultures. Obtaining a urine sample by straight catheterization rather than clean catch reduced the likelihood of a false positive diagnosis of urinary tract infection (Gordon, 2013).

Epidemiology varies between males and females with regard to urinary tract infections. Asymptomatic bacteriuria and acute cystitis in men are rare outside of the extremes of age (neonates and the elderly); when it occurs, it is often due to urinary tract anatomic abnormalities. The data on treatment of urinary tract infections in men are limited and often extrapolated from treatment studies in women. The emergency physician should be familiar with current treatment guidelines as well as local antimicrobial resistance patterns when prescribing empiric treatment for acute cystitis. Current expert treatment guidelines, written by the Infectious Diseases Society of America and the European Society for Microbiology and Infectious Diseases, and cosponsored by the American Congress of Obstetricians and Gynecologists, the American Urological Association, the Association of Medical Microbioplogy and Infectious Diseases – Canada, and the Society for Academic Emergency Medicine, take into consideration both efficacy as well as collateral damage in the form of community antimicrobial resistance and the ecological adverse effects of antimicrobial therapy such as *clostridium difficile* colitis and colonization with multidrug-resistant organisms when recommending first-line empiric treatment for urinary tract infection in women. Current guidelines recommend first-line therapy with nitrofurantoin, trimethoprim/sulfamethoxizole, or fosfomycin for uncomplicated cystitis. Trimethoprim/sulfamethoxozole should not be chosen empirically if the local community resistance is greater than 20%, and neither nitrofurantoin nor fosfomycin should be chosen if early pyelonephritis is suspected since the tissue levels of these agents are not sufficient. The quinolones are effective, but second-line options due to the propensity for ecological adverse effects secondary to the broad spectrum nature of these agents (Infectious Diseases Society of America and the European Society for Microbiology and Infectious Diseases, 2011).

Endocarditis and *Staph aureus* Bacteremia/Colonization

Unlike urinary tract infections, endocarditis and *Staph aureus* bacteremia are two infectious conditions for which gender differences in epidemiology and treatment are either not apparent or attributable to other disease-specific factors. In endocarditis, investigators suggested that women were more likely to die from this disease, probably due to a decreased likelihood of receiving surgical treatment (Sambola, 2010). However, as confounding factors such as diabetes mellitus, receiving hemodialysis, or being immunosuppressed are considered, gender differences in outcomes and surgical treatment seem to fall away (Aksoy, 2007). This suggests that observed gender variations in endocarditis are more a function of other patient-specific factors rather than biases due to sex.

Where differences do exist in endocarditis between the sexes is in the heart valves affected. In registry studies, both genders had a similar percentage of cases in native valves (70%) versus prosthetic valves (20%) with the remainder being unidentified. However, among patients with native endocarditis, men were more likely than women to be affected in their aortic valve. Among patients with prosthetic valve endocarditis, women were more likely to be affected in their artificial mitral valve (Sevilla, 2010). These predilections are of relevance to emergency physicians when assessing patients who are at risk for endocarditis. Knowledge of gender variations in the potential location of endocarditis may allow physical examination findings to guide a risk assessment of the presence of endocarditis in males versus females. Diagnostic criteria and modalities for endocarditis are similar between the genders.

Gender differences have not been found in the incidence of *Staph aureus* bacteremia (Hanses, 2010) or methicillin-resistant *Staph aureus* colonization in hospitalized patients (Forster, 2013). For emergency physicians, the evidence to date does not suggest that patient sex should serve as a risk assessment factor for the diagnosis of these conditions.

Diarrheal Illness, Traveler's Infectious Diseases, and Malaria

There is a paucity of literature on the subject of gender differences in pathogens that cause infectious diarrhea. Among the organisms for which gender as a risk factor has not been assessed in a widespread fashion are Salmonella, Shigella, Campylobacter, and ova and parasites. For emergency physicians, there is essentially no evidence to guide whether male versus female patients may be at higher risk for diarrhea due to these conditions.

In contrast, emerging evidence suggests that women who are postpartum are at risk for *Clostridium difficile* infections. Case control studies have found that otherwise healthy postpartum females who received prophylactic antibiotics, especially ampicillin, gentamicin, or clinidamycin, or delivered by caesarean section were most at risk for this condition. Given that emergency physicians generally consider *C. difficile* infections to be more present in either hospitalized or debilitated patients, this observed association in generally healthy and young postpartum women is an important epidemiologic risk factor that should be considered in assessing this patient population in the ED (Garey, 2008; Unger, 2011).

Traveler's infections are an area where gender differences have been established, in terms of both pathogens and symptom presentation. In a large retrospective study of more than 58,000 patients worldwide who presented to traveler's clinics over a decade, women were more likely to present with diarrheal symptoms, upper respiratory infections, and urinary tract infections. In contrast, men were more likely to present with febrile illnesses, vector-borne illnesses, STIs, and viral hepatitis. Again, however, no evidence suggests that once a particular traveler's infectious disease diagnosis is made that management should vary between male and female patients (Schlagenhauf, 2010).

Malaria is one of the most common infectious diseases globally. Unfortunately, despite its widespread prevalence, there are few studies on gender differences in the presentation or complications related to malaria. One single center study from Thailand found that women were more likely to develop shock in *Plasmodium falciparum* malaria at rate of 77% versus 35% in males (Arnold, 2013). However, a smaller earlier single center study from Europe did not find such a difference (Bruneel, 1997). Further studies are needed to establish whether gender differences in either the presentation or management of malaria exist.

Hepatitis C

Hepatitis C is a viral infection whose acute phase is often asymptomatic, but in up to 75% of patients may lead to chronic infection with risk for liver fibrosis or cirrhosis. For emergency physicians, there are no established protocols for prophylaxis or acute treatment. However, evidence suggests that women are more likely to spontaneously clear the virus in comparison to males. This is especially evident in Caucasian women with an IL28B genetic polymorphism rs12979860 (van den Berg, 2011; Grebely, 2013). In Asian women, the evidence suggests that different IL28B genetic polymorphisms are synergistic with hepatitis C viral clearance (Rao, 2012). This research does indicate that female gender and particular genetic factors can be used to provide risk counseling on the likelihood of spontaneous hepatitis C clearance after exposure, although this will likely occur in referral to subspecialty evaluation after ED evaluation.

Cutaneous Infections

Cellulitis and diabetic foot infections are two common cutaneous infections. The danger with cellulitis is that the patient will not respond to typical antibiotics and will develop an abscess or other systemic infection. For diabetic foot infections, the danger is the development of a deeper space infection requiring surgical debridement or amputation. Although the evidence is limited to retrospective analyses, for both conditions, no data suggest that gender alone is a factor associated with either poor outcome. Rather, for cellulitis, single-center evidence suggests that an apparent observed male predominance in development of abscess after cellulitis is better explained by alcohol use and delayed antimicrobial treatment (Picard, 2013). Similarly, for diabetic foot infections, initial increased ulcer size is the most clearly associated factor with poor outcome in comparison to gender, age, or degree of diabetic control (Oyibo, 2001). For emergency physicians, these studies suggest it is not necessary to consider gender as a separate epidemiologic factor associated with poor outcome.

Other Infectious Diseases

Leptospirosis is a zoonotic infectious disease caused by a spirochete-type bacterium. Humans typically acquire this disease through exposure to animal urine and experience initial flulike symptoms followed by a more severe second phase after apparent recovery. The second phase can cause meningitis or renal or liver failure. Worldwide, 80% to 90% of cases are reported in males. This was initially presumed to be due to behavioral hypothesis explanations, such as occupational tendencies and exposures. For example, males were assumed to be more at risk through traditional roles in farming and butchering. However, it is now clear from seroprevalence studies that women are as commonly exposed to leptospirosis as men but experience a less severe phenotype, supportive of a physiologic hypothesis explanation for gender differences in this disease. The decreased severity of leptospirosis in females may also lead to lower rates of reporting in this population relative to males. Existing evidence does not support the need for treatment differences between the genders, with doxycycline serving as first-line therapy (Jansen, 2007).

Lyme disease is another entity for which gender differences have been observed in both the incidence of illness and symptom manifestation, although the difference varies by geographic location. In the United States, there is a male predominance of cases; in Europe, there is a female predominance. It is unclear what the driving factors behind this differing incidence are. Possibilities include behavioral factors associated with tick vector exposure and likelihood of seeking treatment. Lyme disease also seems to show variability in how it manifests between males and females. In a 20-year retrospective study from

Slovenia, female patients were more likely to present with erythema migrans and acrodermatitis chronica atrophicans, early dermatologic manifestations of Lyme disease. In contrast, men were more likely to present with Lyme neuroborreliosis and Lyme arthritis, which are later manifestations of the disease. Again, it is unclear whether this difference is a function of behavioral factors, with male patients not seeking care until later symptoms manifest, or physiologic factors, such as gender-specific genetic background and host response (Strle, 2013). Some support for a physiologic hypothesis explanation comes from studies that show that males manifest a more severe form of Q fever, another spirochete disease, and that sex hormones play a role in its pathogenesis (Raoult, 2000; Leone, 2004).

Cryptococcal meningitis, caused by *Cryptococcus neoformans*, is another infectious disease for which gender differences in disease incidence and prevalence have been observed. Male AIDS patients experience this opportunistic infection at a higher rate than female AIDS patients. A seminal study of HIV patients from Botswana noted that this is not a function of worse HIV control. In fact, male patients in this study were found to have higher CD4 counts compared to female patients, but they still were more likely to experience cryptococcal meningitis. Instead, the investigators found that sex hormones and gender-specific macrophage activity were likely explanations, with testosterone leading to higher fungal activity and male macrophages experiencing more cell death (McClelland, 2013). For emergency physicians, knowledge of this pathophysiology supports the epidemiologic evidence of a male predominance in cryptococcal meningitis and should lead to a gender-specific risk assessment in AIDS patients suspected of manifesting this disease process.

Finally, onchocerciasis, or river blindness, represents an infectious disease for which gender differences are profound not in pathophysiology but in societal efforts in eradication. Caused by a parasitic nematode, river blindness is readily treated with ivermectin. However, eradication programs in endemic areas tend to follow patterns where males, especially older men, are in positions of authority. This leads to decreased female participation in these programs, which may have an effect on long-term adherence and sustainability (Clemmons, 2002). In general, there is a paucity of medical literature on the role that gender plays in treatment programs of endemic and epidemic infectious diseases.

Sexually Transmitted Infections and Gender

The relationship between gender, biomedical risk, and STIs is complex, with local epidemiology playing an equally important role. The emergency physician must take all of this into consideration when evaluating a patient for a potential STI. Women are uniquely at increased risk of STIs in several ways, including susceptibility to infection, severity of infection, and the difficulty in screening and diagnosis.

Women's increased susceptibility to STIs is illustrated by the case of the adolescent patient. While adolescents ages 15 to 24 make up only a quarter of the US population, they represent nearly half of the STIs (CDC surveillance data, 2012). This phenomenon is partially explained by the increased susceptibility of the female adolescent to STIs due to biomedical reasons. Squamous epithelial cells are more resistant to chlamydia and gonorrhea, whereas columnar epithelium supports their growth. The adolescent cervix normally contains an area of ectopy, where columnar cells are located on the exposed portion of the cervix. It has been hypothesized that the exposure of these columnar cells (which are more susceptible to some STIs) places the adolescent at increased risk of these infections, whereas on the mature cervix, the exposed columnar cells are slowly replaced by squamous epithelium (more resistant to infection). Cervical mucous, which plays a protective role in STI prevention, is more easily penetrated by these organisms in early adolescence (Vickery, 1968). And while playing an important role in preventing unwanted pregnancy, oral contraceptives alter the local immunity by increasing the size of this squamocolumnar junction, thereby increasing susceptibility to STIs (Park, 1995).

In addition to these local factors in the female genital tract, STIs are often more efficiently transmitted from a male to his female partner(s). Genital herpes transmission from male to female is 19% compared to 5% from female to male (Mertz, 1992). Gonorrhea is transmitted from an infected male to his female partner 60% to 90% of the time, compared to 20% to 30% of the time from female to male (Hooper, 1978). Some of the proposed mechanisms for this disparity have been more infectious innoculum as a result of pooled semen in the vagina as well as greater trauma to the genital tract tissues during sexual intercourse.

It is known that male circumcision decreases the risk of STIs such as the human immunodeficiency virus (HIV) as well as the human papilloma virus (HPV). Interestingly, circumcision in a male partner also decreases the risk of cervical cancer in the female partner (Castellsague, 2002).

In addition to the baseline increased infection risk, women are disproportionately affected by the sequelae of STIs. Pelvic inflammatory disease, chronic pelvic pain, ectopic pregnancy, and infertility, affecting only women, are the end result of STIs, and decreasing these serious sequelae is the ultimate goal of prevention programs. Each subsequent infection increases a women's risk for pelvic inflammatory disease and ectopic pregnancy. So breaking the chain of transmission is extremely important, and emergency medicine providers play an important role in interrupting this cascade.

Screening and diagnosis may also be more problematic in females, because infection in females is more likely to be asymptomatic. Gonorrhea and chlamydia infection are asymptomatic in up to 80% of females, compared to 10% to 20% of males, resulting in less diagnosis if only symptomatic individuals are tested for the disease (Zimmerman, 1990). Two things may occur as a result – asymptomatic infection may continue in women, placing them more at risk for serious sequelae, and screening programs focusing on women may fail to eliminate infection in men, which is then retransmitted to females partners, even after the woman has been treated. Prevention strategies such as expedited partner therapy, a strategy easily employed by the emergency medicine provider, have been proven in randomized controlled clinical trials to be effective at treating asymptomatic partners and decreasing the reinfection rate in females. Data have shown that men may be more likely to be tested for syphilis when an STI is suspected (Garfinkel, 1999), which has implications for a missed diagnosis in females, especially problematic given the serious sequelae of congenital syphilis.

Some have suggested that sexual behaviors, resulting from socialization into different gender roles, affected by culture, peer, and parental influences, may account for some of the gender differences in STIs. Males often have an earlier age at first sexual encounter (Institute of Medicine, 1997) and a higher rate of partner changes (Siegel, 1999). Women are more likely to have been forced into their first sexual encounter (Department of Health and Human Services, 1997). Women may be uncomfortable negotiating condom use, and dynamics of intimate partner violence against women may make it more difficult for women to advocate for themselves in protecting against STIs. If the provider is aware of these potential barriers to avoiding STIs in women, then screening is more likely to take place. Prevention programs that address gender roles have shown a significant reduction in STI rates (Kamb, 1998; Shain, 1999).

Chlamydia, Gonorrhea, Trichomonas

Chlamydia is the most common reportable, as well as the most prevalent, STI in the United States with more than 1.4 million chlamydial infections reported to the Centers for Disease Control (CDC) in 2012 (CDC surveillance data, 2012). Infections in women are usually asymptomatic, making screening especially important since infection, especially repeat infection, can lead to pelvic inflammatory disease (PID), resulting in infertility, ectopic pregnancy, and chronic pelvic pain. Since this gender-associated difference in prevalence as well as sequelae affects who should be tested for suspected infection, emergency physicians should be familiar with national and local screening guidelines. Because the largest burden of disease rests with women, the CDC recommends screening all sexually active women younger than age 26 for chlamydia at least annually (CDC Treatment Guidelines, 2011). Screening programs are highly effective, leading to as much as a 60% reduction in the incidence of PID (Scholes, 1996).

Chlamydia prevalence is estimated to be approximately 6.8% in sexually active females ages 14–19, approximately two times the case rate in males (CDC, MMWR, 2011). The increased case rate in females is probably largely due to the higher screening rate in females as well as missed opportunities to identify and treat the male sex partners of infected females (CDC, MMWR, 2012).

Some groups have evaluated gender and age disparities in the prevalence of chlamydia infection in the United States and found that age at first sexual experience was inversely related to chlamydial infection among males but not females. Unprotected sexual activity was associated with decreased rates of chlamydia infection in males but not females (Beydoun, 2010). This study did confirm that adults younger than age 25 are disproportionately affected by chlamydia infection and that adjusting for demographic, socioeconomic, and behavioral factors had little effect on age disparities, further supporting the age-based screening criteria currently recommended. Other STIs (including HIV) have been associated with alcohol, substance use, and risky sexual behaviors: a relationship documented in men who have sex with men, adolescents, heterosexual men and women, and psychiatric patients. These lifestyle factors were not associated with chlamydia prevalence in a recent study; however, the cross-sectional design, self-reported data, and small sample size limit the conclusions that can be drawn from these data (Beyoun, 2010).

Trichomonas is the most common protozoal infection in the developed world. While much has been written about gender prevalence rates in trichomonas infection, far less has been reported on the role gender plays in risk, disease outcomes, and treatment. Trichomonas is asymptomatic in 70% to 80% of cases, which may contribute to the lack of well-defined infection rates. Untreated trichomonas infection can have a serious effect on women's health outcomes, with sequelae such as preterm delivery, PID, and increased susceptibility to HIV infection. The pathogenesis of poor obstetric outcomes with trichomonas is yet to be understood fully, since treatment of trichomonas often fails to prevent these adverse outcomes (Klebanoff, 2001). More research is needed to define this complex relationship, given the serious sequelae of even asymptomatic infection. Some data suggest that oral contraceptives inhibit trichomonas infection, with obvious gender implications. However, one study did not show a protective effect of oral contraceptives after adjusting for covariables (Torok, 2009).

Syphilis

After being on the verge of elimination, many US states have experienced a resurgence of syphilis infection. The number of primary and secondary syphilis cases reported to the CDC nearly doubled between 2005 and 2013. The vast majority of these infections have been in men who have sex with men (nearly 84% of the infections in 2012) (Patton, MMWR, 2014). This is especially concerning given the high rates of coinfection with HIV seen in this population.

Data have shown that men may be more likely to be tested for syphilis when an STI is suspected (Garfinkel, 1999) which has implications for a missed diagnosis in females, especially problematic given the serious sequelae of congenital syphilis. While women undergo routine screening for syphilis in the first trimester of pregnancy, they may have ongoing risk later in pregnancy and should be retested based on risk and local prevalence in the third trimester. Men have no such screening recommendation. The emergency medicine provider must be knowledgeable about this risk group and test for HIV in those diagnosed with syphilis and vice versa.

Human Immunodeficiency Virus (HIV)

Gender is well known to be a significant factor in the transmission of HIV/AIDS and also influences treatment, care, and support (Gupta, 2000). It is important that emergency physicians are aware of these differences to increase HIV testing and identification of infections that might not otherwise have been diagnosed, even in a primary care setting. Women's vulnerability to HIV may be partially explained in some societies by the culture of silence that surrounds sexual activity, whereby "good" women are expected to be ignorant about sex and more passive in sexual interactions (Carovano, 1992). This may make it difficult for women to become informed about sex, sexual safety, and risk reduction, and for them to be proactive in negotiating for safer sex. In some countries, virginity places women at increased risk of HIV since males may believe that sex with a virgin cleanses them of infection. This false belief also places the women at risk for sexual coercion in countries where HIV is highly prevalent. There is also some data that women in countries where virginity is particularly valued practice non-vaginal sex, such as anal sex, which may in turn place them at increased risk for HIV infection (Weiss, Whelan, and Gupta, 2000).

A culture of silence also often surrounds sex, making access to sexually transmitted disease services challenging, especially for young women and girls. Seeking such services may be stigmatizing, making it less likely that they will be utilized. Emergency room providers are in a unique position to diagnose STIs including HIV, since young women may seek care for these issues in an ED, not wishing to disclose sensitive symptoms to their primary care physician or lacking access to care elsewhere.

Women's economic dependence in most cultures further increases their vulnerability to HIV. Research has shown that this may make it more likely for women to exchange sex for money, less likely to leave a relationship that may place them at increased risk for STI and less able to negotiate protection from STIs (Weiss and Gupta, 2000). Emergency room providers should be aware of this dynamic and allow for a confidential space for risk factor inquiry and empiric testing as recommended by national guidelines. Women in situations of vulnerability may not be aware of their own risks because of lack of disclosure of sexual behaviors by their partners and may not be aware of their own risk.

These gender differences, in turn, affect not only diagnostic opportunity but a woman's ability to access and adhere to treatment and therefore also affect disease outcomes. A group in Tanzania evaluated gender differences in HIV disease progression among HIV patients, one year after starting antiretroviral therapy. They hypothesized that there would be differences in disease progression based on gender, since previous studies had demonstrated different rates of disease progression as well as virologic and immunologic response to treatment among

HIV-infected women compared to men. They performed a cohort study following HIV-infected antiretroviral therapy (ART) naïve patients for one year (70% females) after being started on triple-drug ART. After one year on treatment, the virologic response was significantly better in females, but the mean CD4 increase was significantly higher in males. As has been seen in other studies, they found that males initiated care with more advanced disease than females. This could be partly due to the fact that women can enter treatment programs as part of PMTCT (Prevention of Mother to Child Transmission) services in many countries. However, this was not the case in this study. The study investigators found that males were better informed than females about the use of ART. They found that although women started the study and treatment at higher CD4 counts, for unclear reasons they lost their immunologic advantage over the course of the first year on treatment since at the end of the first year, men and women had similar clinical and immunologic conditions. The investigators suggest this could be due to the lower socioeconomic status of the women in the study compared to the men, or to unknown biological differences; however, more study is needed (Mosha, 2013).

The relationship between HIV disease progression and response to treatment and gender is complex. Some studies have shown that HIV-infected males on antiretroviral treatment have worse treatment outcomes and mortality (Druyts, 2012). Other studies have found that women may be less likely to start ART due to having less time to keep outpatient appointments because of family commitments, fears about pregnancy, or socioeconomic factors (Mocroft, 2000). Women have been shown to have lower rates of ART utilization, possibly because of competing needs such as food, housing, clothing, and transportation that disproportionately affect women (Cunningham, 1999). Despite higher rates of utilization, men have been shown to have a higher rate of loss to follow-up and nonadherence to ART (Hawkins, 2011).

Women with difficulty taking medications openly at home had approximately 20% lower probability of receiving ART than those who reported no difficulty (Sayles, 2006). Even having children, delaying one's own medical care because of being a caregiver to others, drug or alcohol dependence, and intimate partner violence did not explain the difference (Sayles, 2006). This is an important part of the history for the emergency medicine provider, since fear of disclosure may keep a patient from relaying a complete history to a provider and may also affect her ability to adhere to medication, increasing her risk of opportunistic infections.

Being engaged in HIV care does not seem to be protective, since even among women in the United States receiving care for HIV, female sex was associated with increased mortality, even after adjusting for ART use (Lemly, 2009). These data were retrospective, but compelling, and warrant further study. Health outcomes in international cohorts have been evaluated as well. In Vietnam, where an increasing number of women are affected by the AIDS epidemic, quality of life indicators were compared by gender, and women had more severe deterioration in morbidity and psychological functioning after their HIV/AIDS diagnosis but better perceived social support. Familial and working environments tended to be supportive to male but negative to female patients (Tran, 2012). The authors conclude that when developing HIV treatment programs and interventions, gender differences must be considered. Interestingly, and especially relevant for the emergency medicine provider, a study comparing mortality rates in the Multicenter AIDS Cohort study (men) and the Women's Interagency HIV Study found that rates of accident or injury-related death were higher among women and that risk factors for death among women with HIV included unemployment, higher level of alcohol use, and intravenous drug use (Hessol, 2007).

It is well known that male circumcision decreases the rate of female to male HIV transmission and has been evaluated as one potential HIV prevention strategy, especially in Sub-Saharan Africa, where women may have less power to negotiate safer sex practices, including condom use. However, the effectiveness of such programs is affected by gender disparities and behaviors. One group devised a mathematical model to evaluate the relationship between decrease in HIV transmission as a result of a circumcision program and change in risk behavior (such as decreased condom use) as well as the ability to negotiate condom use. This group found that although circumcision programs would result in an overall decrease in male HIV infection, and resultant indirect decrease in female infections, there could be a decrease in this benefit to women if men decreased condom use with the knowledge of their decreased HIV risk after circumcision (Andersson, 2011). This is yet another illustration of the effect of gender disparities on HIV transmission risk and an argument to incorporate behavioral manifestations of gender differences in research as well as clinical care. These results serve as a reminder for the emergency medical provider that there may be gender differences in the ability of one sexual partner to negotiate for safer sexual practices, which should inform counseling practices that occur in the ED.

The gender differences seen in HIV infection – access to care, treatment outcomes, and mortality – are varied and depend on the gender constructs of each population. The emergency medicine provider should be aware of these differences when evaluating the HIV-infected patient.

Sexual Violence and STIs

Violence against women also contributes to women's vulnerability to HIV and STIs. Heterosexual transmission of HIV accounts for the majority of new infections worldwide and disproportionately affects women in many areas such as Sub-Saharan Africa, where women represent 58% of those living with HIV (UNAIDS, 2012). Sexual violence is also a global problem. Reports reveal that in some African countries, nearly one in three girls and women ages 13 to 24 reported at least one incident of sexual violence before age 18 (UNICEF, 2010; UNICEF, 2011). In the United States, 17.6% of women surveyed reported being raped at some point during their lives, often by an intimate partner: 64% of women who reported being raped were victimized by a partner (Tjaden, 2000).

The relationship between sexual violence and HIV is multifactorial. The threat of violence inhibits a woman's ability to advocate for safer sex, and the experience of violence may increase sexual risk taking in later years (Hillis, 2001). There is evidence that male sexual assailants as a group have an increased seroprevalence of HIV, placing their victims at increased risk of HIV acquisition (Rich, 2002). Disruption of the mucosal epithelial barrier of the genital tract can increase the HIV transmission risk, and a preexisting STI or an STI acquired during the assault creates an inflammatory microenvironment that may increase the risk for HIV transmission (Myer, 2006). Studies have documented more cervico-vaginal mucosal damage (such as abrasions or lacerations) in the setting of sexual assault compared to consensual sex, placing the sexual assault survivor at a higher risk of HIV and other STI transmission (Lauber, 1982; McLean, 2011). Other cofactors such as age, hormonal contraception, pregnancy, substance use, and preexisting STI also play a role in HIV transmission risk, and there is even some suggestion that sexual violence in the form of intimate partner violence may result in immunosuppression, contributing ultimately to increased risk of HIV transmission (Schwartz, 2003; Sugar, 2004; Campbell, 2008).

Emergency providers should be aware of the increased risk of HIV in those who experience sexual violence, which disproportionately affects women. Studies have revealed that women are offered HIV post-exposure prophylaxis at lower rates than they are offered prophylaxis against chlamydia, gonorrhea, and undesired pregnancy (Merchant, 2008). This is especially troubling since the risk of HIV may be particularly high in this group.

There is a paucity of data on gender disparities in the provision of STI and HIV prophylaxis after sexual assault. The male sexual assault victim is less well studied. Males do utilize sexual assault services, but the actual prevalence is difficult to define and may be higher than reported. Reasons for underreporting may include fear of negative reactions such as doubts about their sexuality, disbelief, and blame (Davies, 2002). It has also been suggested that certain male groups, such as those who identify as gay, bisexual, or transgender, have mental health problems or developmental delay, work in the sex trade, live on the streets, are veterans and are in prison or jail, may experience higher rates of sexual assault (Hickson, 1994; Peterson, 2011; DuMont, 2013). Special care must be taken by the emergency medicine provider when evaluating these patient populations, since

the history of sexual assault may not be readily forthcoming on initial evaluation.

Conclusion

There is a complex interaction between gender and infectious disease epidemiology and pathophysiology. Whether due to physiologic differences, such as the relationship between sex hormones and immune response or behavioral/societal factors, such as perceived traditional gender roles in occupations or community responses to disease, infectious diseases exemplify how physicians cannot presume that males and females are at similar risk and should be treated similarly. Instead, knowledge of variations based on causative pathogens can aid emergency physicians in diagnosing or treating both males and females with infectious disease.

Case Conclusions

Case 1

The emergency physician recognized that despite the onset of symptoms 72 hours prior to presentation, the fact that this otherwise healthy woman was pregnant placed her at heightened risk for adverse outcome due to influenza. Chest radiography showed pneumonia, and although the patient's pneumonia severity index score was low, the patient was admitted and treated aggressively with an antiviral and standard antibiotics for community acquired pneumonia. The next day, the patient tested positive on PCR test for influenza A. Fortunately, early treatment led to a good outcome. The patient recovered and was discharged three days later.

Case 2

The emergency physician recognized that this young female patient was likely to have chlamydia based on her age and performed testing for that as well as other STIs, including HIV. She also utilized expedited partner therapy for the patient's heterosexual male partner, thereby decreasing the chance of reinfection in this patient. She counseled the patient on the long-term reproductive risks of repeat infection and encouraged condom use for prevention of STIs in the future. She tested her for pregnancy and screened for intimate partner violence, since both of these would necessitate referral to specialty services.

Gaps in Knowledge

In the area of infectious disease, a number of gaps in knowledge are apparent in the evaluation and treatment of male and female patients. First, the vast majority of studies that have looked at gender differences in infectious disease are retrospective and secondary data analyses; many may be underpowered to detect a difference. What are needed are prospective, observational longitudinal studies that evaluate whether gender differences in infectious disease are due to physiologic or behavioral/societal differences. Second, there are essentially no studies in non-STIs, with the exception of urinary tract infections, on whether treatment differences and responses vary between the genders. It may be that current treatment regimens for infectious disease are comparable in males and females, but the absence of supporting evidence is a ripe opportunity for investigation. Compared to non-STIs, there is more data on gender differences in STIs, and especially in gender differences in HIV outcomes. Despite the research in this area, the relationship to HIV outcomes and gender is complex. Much of the data are conflicting, reflecting that the multifactorial psychosocial and potential biomedical risk factors are still not well defined. The implications of these gender-associated STI and HIV risks are profound from both an individual and public health standpoint, and research in this area should continue despite the complexity of the relationship.

References

Aksoy, O, Meyer, LT, Cabell, CH, et al. (2007). Gender differences in infective endocarditis: Pre- and co-morbid conditions lead to different management and outcomes in female patients. *Scandinavian Journal of Infectious Diseases*. 39. 101–7.

Andersson, KM, et al. (2011). Scaling up circumcision programs in Southern Africa: The potential impact of gender disparities and changes in condom use behaviors on heterosexual HIV transmission. *AIDS Behavior*. 15. 938–48.

Arnold, BJ, Tangpukdee, N, Krudsood, S, et al. (2013). Risk factors of shock in severe falciparum malaria.

Southeast Asian Journal of Tropical Medicine and Public Health. **44**. 541–50.

Beydoun, HA, et al. (2010). Gender and age disparities in the prevalence of chlamydia infection among sexually active adults in the United States. *Journal of Women's Health*. **19**(12). 2183–90.

Borgdorff, MW, Nagelkerke, NJ, Dye, C, et al. (2000). Gender and tuberculosis: A comparison of prevalence surveys with notification data to explore sex differences in case detection. *International Journal of Tuberculosis and Lung Disease*. **4**. 123–32.

Bruneel, F, Gachot, B, Timsit, JF, et al. (1997). Shock complicating severe falciparum malaria in European adults. *Intensive Care Medicine*. **23**. 698–701.

Callaghan, WM, Chu, SY, Jamieson, DJ. (2010). Deaths from seasonal influenza among pregnant women in the United States, 1998–2005. *Obstetrics & Gynecology*. **115**. 919–23.

Campbell, JC, Baty, ML, Ghandour, RM, Stockman, JK, Francisco, L, Wagman, J. (2008). The intersection of intimate partner violence against women and HIV/AIDS: A review. *International Journal of Injury Control and Safety Promotion*. **15**(4). 221–31.

Carovano, K. (1992). More than mothers and whores: Redefining the AIDS prevention needs of women. *International Journal of Health Services*. **21**(1). 131–42.

Castellsague, X, et al. (2002). Male circumcision, penile human papilloma virus infection, and cervical cancer in female partners. *New England Journal of Medicine*. **346**(15). 1105–12.

Centers for Disease Control and Prevention. (2010). National Hospital Ambulatory Medical Care Survey: 2010 Emergency Department Summary Tables. Available at www.cdc.gov/nchs/data/ahcd/nhamcs_emergency/2010_ed_web_tables.pdf. Accessed February 5, 2014.

Centers for Disease Control and Prevention. (2010). Sexually Transmitted Diseases Treatment Guidelines. No. 59(RR-12):1–110. Erratum in MMWR Recomm Rep. 2011. 60(1). 18.

Centers for Disease Control Grand Rounds. (2011). Chlamydia Prevention: Challenges and Strategies for Reducing Disease Burden and Sequelae. *MMWR Morbidity and Mortality Weekly Report*. **60**(12). 370–3.

Centers for Disease Control. (2012). Sexually Transmitted Diseases Surveillance. Available at www.cdc.gov/std/stats12/chlamydia.htm. Accessed June 8, 2014.

Clemmons, L, Amazigo, UV, Bissek, AC, et al. (2002). Gender issues in the community-directed treatment with ivermectin (CDTI) of the African programme for onchocerciasis control (APOC). *Annals of Tropical Medicine and Parasitology*. **96**. s59–s74.

Cunningham WE, et al. (1999). The impact of competing subsistence needs and barriers on access to medical care for persons with HIV receiving care in the United States. *Medical Care*. **37**. 1270.

Davies, M. (2002). Male sexual assault victims: A selective review of the literature and implications for support services. *Aggression and Violent Behavior*. **7**. 203–14.

den Heijer, CD, Penders, J, Donker, GA, et al. (2013). The importance of gender-stratified antibiotic resistance surveillance of unselected uropathogens: A Dutch Nationwide Extramural Surveillance study. *PLoS One*. **8**. e60497.

Department of Health and Human Services. (1995). Fertility, family planning and women's health: New data from the National Survey of Family Growth. PHS97. United States DHHS. Series 23: Data from the National Survey of Family Growth.

Druyts, E, et al. (2012). Male gender and the risk of mortality among individuals enrolled in antiretroviral treatment programs in Africa: A systematic review and meta-analysis. *AIDS*, **26**.

DuMont J, et al. 2013. Male victims of sexual assault: a descriptive study of survivors' use of sexual assault treatment services. *Journal of Interpersonal Violence*. **28**(13). 2676–94.

Falagas, ME, Mourtzoukou, EG, Vardakas, KZ. (2007). Sex differences in the incidence and severity of respiratory tract infections. *Respiratory Medicine*. **101**. 1845–63.

Forster, AJ, Oake, N, Roth, V, et al. (2013). Patient-level factors associated with methicillin resistant Staphylococcus aureus carriage at hospital admission: Asystematic review. *American Journal of Infection Control*. **41**. 214–20.

Gannon, CJ, Pasquale, M, Tracy, JK, et al. (2004). Male gender is associated with increased risk for postinjury pneumonia. *Shock*. **21**. 410–4.

Garey, KW, Jiang, ZD, Yadav, Y, et al. (2008). Clostridium difficile infection: Case series and review of the literature. *American Journal of Obstetrics and Gynecology*. **199**. 332–7.

Garfinkel, M, et al. (1999). Gender differences in testing for syphilis in emergency department patients diagnosed with sexually transmitted diseases. *Journal of Emergency Medicine*. **17**(6). 937–40.

Gordon, LB, Waxman, MJ, Ragsdale, L, et al. (2013). Overtreatment of presumed urinary tract infection in older women presenting to the emergency department. *Journal of the American Geriatrics Society*. **61**. 788–92.

Grebely, J, Page, K, Sacks-Davis, R, et al. (2013). The effects of female sex, viral genotype, and IL28B genotype on spontaneous clearance of acute hepatitis C virus infection. *Hepatology*. (epub ahead of print).

Green, MS. (1992). The male predominance in the incidence of infectious diseases in children: A postulated

explanation for disparities in the literature. *International Journal of Epidemiology*. **21**. 381–6.

Guerra-Silveira, F, and Abad-Franch, F. (2013). Sex bias in infectious disease epidemiology: patterns and processes. *PLoS One*. **8**. e62390.

Gupta, GR. (2000). Gender, sexuality, and HIV/AIDS: The what, the why, and the how. *Canadian HIV/AIDS Policy & Law Review*. **5**(4). 86–93.

Hanses, F, Spaeth, C, Ehrenstein, BP, et al. (2010). Risk factors associated with long-term prognosis of patients with Staphylococcus aureus bacteremia. *Infection*. **38**. 465–70.

Hawkins, C, et al. (2011). Sex differences in antiretroviral treatment outcomes among HIV-infected adults in an urban Tanzania setting. *AIDS* **25**. 1189–97.

Heise, L, Ellsberg, M, Gottemoeller, M. (1999). Ending Violence Against Women. *Population Reports, Series L, No 11*. Baltimore: Johns Hopkins University School of Public Health, Population Information Program.

Hessol, NA, et al. (2007). Mortality among participants in the Multicenter AIDS Cohort Study and the Women's Interagency HIV Study. *Clinical Infectious Diseases*. **44**. 287–94.

Hickson, FCI, et al. (1994). Gay men as victims of nonconsensual sex. *Archives of Sexual Behavior*. **23**, 294.

Hillis, SD, Anda, RF, Felitti, VJ, Marchbanks, PA. (2001). Adverse childhood experiences and sexual risk behaviors in women: a retrospective cohort study. *Family Planning Perspectives*. **33**(5). 206–11.

Holmes, CB, Hausler, H, Nunn, P. (1998). A review of sex differences in the epidemiology of tuberculosis. *International Journal of Tuberculosis and Lung Disease*. **2**. 96–104.

Hooper, RR, et al. (1978). Cohort study of venereal disease: The risk of gonorrhea transmission from infected women to men. *American Journal of Epidemiology*. **108**(2). 136–44.

Infectious Diseases Society of America and the European Society for Microbiology and Infectious Diseases. (2011). International clinical practice guidelines for the treatment of acute uncomplicated cystitis and pyelonephritis in women: A 2010 update. *Clinical Infectious Diseases*. **52**(5). e103–e20.

Institute of Medicine. (1997). *The Hidden Epidemic Confronting Sexually Transmitted Diseases*. Washington, DC: National Academy Press.

Jansen, A, Stark, K, Schneider, T, et al. (2007). Sex differences in clinical leptospirosis in Germany: 1997–2005. *Clinical Infectious Diseases*. **44**. e69–e72.

Jensen-Fangel, S, Mohey, R, Johnsen, SP, et al. (2004). Gender differences in hospitalization rates for respiratory tract infections in Danish youth. *Scandinavian Journal of Infectious Diseases.* **36**. 31–6.

Jones, JS, Rossman, L, Wynn, BN, Dunnuck, C, Schwartz N. (2003). Comparative analysis of adult versus adolescent sexual assault: Epidemiology and patterns of anogenital injury. *Academic Emergency Medicine: Official Journal of the Society for Academic Emergency Medicine.* **10**(8). 872–7.

Kamb, ML, et al. (1998). Efficacy of risk-reduction counseling to prevent human immunodeficiency virus and sexually transmitted diseases: A randomized controlled trial. *Project RESPECT Study Group. JAMA.* **80**(13). 1161–7.

Klebanoff, MA, et al. (2001). Failure of metronidazole to prevent preterm delivery among pregnant women with asymptomatic trichomonas vaginalis infection. *New England Journal of Medicine.* **345**. 487–93.

Koeijers, JJ, Verbon, A, Kessels, AG, et al. (2010). Urinary tract infection in male general practice patients: Uropathogens and antibiotic susceptibility. *Urology.* **76**. 336–40.

Lauber, AA, and Souma, ML. (1982). Use of toluidine blue for documentation of traumatic intercourse. *Obstetrics and Gynecology.* **60**(5). 644–8.

Lemly, DC et al. (2009). Race and sex differences in antiretroviral therapy use and mortality among HIV-infected persons in care. *Journal of Infectious Diseases.* **199**. 991–8.

Leone, M, Honstettre, A, Lepidi, H, et al. (2004). Effect of sex on Coxiella burnetii infection: Protective role of 17 beta-estradiol. *Journal of Infectious Diseases.* **189**. 339–45.

Magliano, E, Grazioli, V, Deflorio, L, et al. (2012). Gender and age-dependent etiology of community-acquired urinary tract infections. *Scientific World Journal.* 349597.

McClelland, EE, Hobbs, LM, Rivera, J, et al. (2013). The role of host gender in the pathogenesis of Cryptococcus neoformans infections. *PLoS One.* **8**. e63632.

McGregor, JC, Elman, MR, Bearden, DT, et al. (2013). Sex- and age-specific trends in antibiotic resistance patterns of Escherichia coli urinary isolates from outpatients. *BMC Family Practice.* **14**. 25.

McLaughlin, SP, and Carson, CC. (2004). Urinary tract infections in women. *Medical Clinics of North America.* **88**. 417–29.

McLean, I, Roberts, SA, White, C, Paul, S. (2011). Female genital injuries resulting from consensual and non-consensual vaginal intercourse. *Forensic Science International.* **204**(1–3). 27–33.

Merchant, RC et al. (2008). Disparities in the provision of sexually transmitted diseases and pregnancy testing and prophylaxis for sexually assaulted women in Rhode Island Emergency Departments. *Journal of Womens Health.* **17**(4). 619–29.

Mertz, GJ, et al. (1992). Risk factors for the sexual transmission of genital herpes. *Annals of Internal Medicine.* **116**. 197–202.

Mocroft A, et al. (2000). Are there gender differences in starting protease inhibitors, HAART, and disease progression despite equal access to care? *Journal of Acquired Immune Deficiency Syndrome.* **24**. 475–82.

Mosha F, et al. (2013). Gender differences in HIV disease progression and treatment outcomes among HIV patients one year after starting antiretroviral treatment (ART) in Dar es Salaam, Tanzania. *BMC Public Health.* 13:38.

Myer, L, Wright, TC, Denny, L KL. (2006). Nested case-control study of cervical mucosal lesions, ectopy, and incident HIV infection among women in Cape Town, South Africa. *Sexually Transmitted Diseases.* **33**(11). 683–7.

Oyibo, SO, Jude, EB, Tarawneh, I, et al. (2001). The effects of ulcer size and site, patient's age, sex and type and duration of diabetes on the outcome of diabetic foot ulcers. *Diabetic Medicine.* **18**. 133–8.

Park B, et al. (1995). Contraceptive methods and the risk of Chlamydia trachomatis infection in young women. *American Journal of Epidemiology.* **142**(7). 771–8.

Patton, ME, et al. (2014). Primary and secondary syphilis – United States, 2005–2013. *Morbidity and Mortality Weekly Report.* **63**(18). 402–6.

Peterson, ZD, et al. 2001. Prevalence and consequences of adult sexual assault of men: Review of empirical findings and state of the literature. *Clinical Psychology Review.* **31**(1). 1–24.

Picard, D, Klein, A, Grigioni, S, et al. (2013). Risk factors for abscess formation in patients with superficial cellulitis (erysipelas) of the leg. *British Journal of Dermatology.* **168**. 859–63.

Rao, HY, Sun, DG, Jiang, D, et al. (2012). IL28B genetic variants and gender are associated with spontaneous clearance of hepatitis C virus infection. *Journal of Viral Hepatitis.* **19**. 173–81.

Raoult, D, Tissot-Dupont, H, Foucault, C, et al. (2000). Q fever 1985–1998. Clinical and epidemiologic features of 1,383 infections. *Medicine.* **79**. 109–23.

Rich, J. (2002). HIV seroprevalence of adult males incarcerated for a sexual offense in Rhode Island, 1994–1999. *The Journal of the American Medical Association.* **288**(2). 164.

Sambola, A, Fernández-Hidalgo, N, Almirante, B, et al. (2010). Sex differences in native-valve infective endocarditis in a single tertiary-care hospital. *American Journal of Cardiology.* **106**. 92–8.

Sayles, J, et al. (2006). The inability to take medications openly at home: Does it help explain gender disparities in HAART use? *Journal of Women's Health*. **15**(2). 173–81.

Schlagenhauf, P, Chen, LH, Wilson, ME, et al. (2010). Sex and gender differences in travel-associated disease. *Clinical Infectious Diseases*. **50**. 826–32.

Scholes, D, et al. (1996). Prevention of pelvic inflammatory disease by screening for cervical chlamydial infections. *New England Journal of Medicine*. **34**(21). 1362–6.

Siegel, DM, et al. (1999). Sexual behavior, contraception, and risk among college students. *Journal of Adolescent Health*. **25**(5). 336–43.

Sevilla, T, Revilla, A, López, J, et al. (2010). Influence of sex on left-sided infective endocarditis. *Revista Española de Cardiología*. **63**. 1497–500.

Shain, RN, et al. (1999). A randomized controlled trial of a behavioral intervention to prevent sexually transmitted disease among minority women. *New England Jouranl of Medicine*. **340**(2). 93–100.

Siston, AM, Rasmussen, SA, Honein, MA, et al. (2010). Pandemic 2009 influenza A (H1N1) virus illness among pregnant women in the United States. *Journal of the American Medical Association*. **303**. 1517–25.

Strle, F, Wormser, GP, Mead, P, et al. (2013). Gender disparity between cutaneous and non-cutaneous manifestations of lyme borreliosis. *PLoS One*. **8**. e64110.

Sugar, NF, Fine, DN, Eckert, LO. (2004. Physical injury after sexual assault: Findings of a large case series. *American Journal of Obstetrics and Gynecology*. **190**(1). 71–6.

Tjaden, P, Thoennes N. (2000). *Full Report on the Prevalence, Incidence, and Consequences of Violence against Women*. Washington, DC: U.S. Department of Justice.

Torok, MR, et al. (2009). The association between oral contraceptives, depo-medroxyprogesterone acetate, and trichomoniasis. *Sexually Transmitted Diseases*. **36**(6). 336–40.

Tran, BX, et al. (2012). Gender differences in quality of life outcomes of HIV/AIDS treatment in the latent feminization of HIV epidemics in Vietnam. *AIDS Care*. **24**(10). 1187–96.

Unger, JA, Whimbey, E, Gravett, MG, et al. (2011). The emergence of Clostridium difficile infection among peripartum women: A case-control study of a C. difficile outbreak on an obstetrical service. *Infectious Diseases in Obstetrics and Gynecology*. 267249.

UNICEF. (2010). *A National Study on Violence against Children and Young Women in Swaziland*. New York: Author.

UNICEF USC for DC and P and MU of H and AS. *Violence against children in Tanzania: findings from a national survey* 2009. Dar es Salaam, 2011.

van den Berg, CH, Grady, BP, Schinkel, J, et al. (2011). Female sex and IL28B, a synergism for spontaneous viral clearance in hepatitis C virus (HCV) seroconverters from a community-based cohort. *PLoS One*. **6**. e27555.

Vickery, BH et al., (1968). The cervix and its secretion in mammals. *Physiology Review*. **48**(1). 135–54.

Weiss, ED, Whelan, D, and Gupta GR. (2000). Gender, sexuality and HIV: making a difference in the lives of young women in developing countries. *Sexual and Relationship Therapy*. **15**(3). 233–45.

Zimmerman, HL, et al. (1990). Epidemiologic differences between chlamydia and gonorrhea. *American Journal of Public Health*. **80**(11). 1338–42.

Diagnostic Imaging: Focusing a Lens on Sex and Gender

Christopher L. Moore

Case

A 28-year-old woman who is otherwise healthy and taking no medications (including no oral contraceptives) presents to the emergency department with right-sided chest pain that is worse when she moves or takes a deep breath. The pain started this morning and is sharp, and she feels it is making her somewhat short of breath. Review of symptoms is otherwise negative. On examination her heart rate is 74, blood pressure is 125/70, respiratory rate is 12, and oxygen saturation is 100% on room air. Exam shows clear breath sounds bilaterally and some reproducible tenderness over the right rib cage. There is no lower extremity pain or swelling. Urine hCG is negative for pregnancy, and an EKG shows normal sinus rhythm. The resident taking care of the patient is concerned about pulmonary embolism and suggests that a d-dimer be obtained to determine whether a CT pulmonary angiogram should be obtained.

Introduction

Diagnostic imaging is an integral part of the evaluation of the Emergency Department (ED) patient. Numerous imaging modalities are now routinely available in the ED setting: plain radiography (X-ray), ultrasound, computed tomography (CT), and often magnetic resonance imaging (MRI) and nuclear studies. In many cases, several diagnostic imaging tests that be helpful in a given situation, and often a patient will have more than one diagnostic imaging study during an ED visit. Overall, nearly half (46.6% in 2008) of ED visits in the United States now involve an imaging study.[1] Plain X-rays are the most common imaging test obtained in the emergency setting, with CT scans being the second most common (Table 12.1). The challenges are to determine what (if any)

diagnostic imaging is appropriate and what the value of imaging is in a given situation. Women account for more than half of all ED visits, and gender often has, or should have, a role in determining appropriate imaging.

While some efforts have focused on appropriate use of plain X-rays (e.g., the Ottawa ankle rules), much more attention has been focused on advanced medical imaging (CT, MRI, and nuclear studies), partly because advanced medical imaging has seen explosive growth over the past two decades, resulting in nearly $100 billion in annual expenditures on imaging in the United States.[2,3] This growth might be justifiable if advanced imaging improved patient outcomes; however, in many cases it has not changed rates of diagnosis, intervention, or hospitalization.

In addition to increased costs, obtaining an imaging study also adds time to the ED visit, which may contribute to ED crowding, increasingly recognized as a public health issue in terms of access to timely care for true emergencies.[4,5] Imaging may also lead to incidental findings, which are occasionally helpful in the early detection of a cancer but much more commonly lead to further imaging, anxiety, and unnecessary intervention.[6,7]

Among appropriate use of advanced medical imaging modalities in the emergency setting, CT has received the most attention. CT is second only to X-rays in the frequency of imaging obtained in the ED,[4] yet it is both much more expensive and exposes the patient to substantially more ionizing radiation, which may cause cancer later in life. While CT, fluoroscopy, and nuclear medicine tests make up approximately 26% of imaging tests, they are responsible for 89% of radiation from medical sources.[8] It is estimated that radiation from medical sources – primarily CT –has doubled the average yearly radiation dose received

Table 12.1 Percentage of Emergency Department (ED) Visits When Imaging Type Is Obtained

Imaging Test	Percent
Plain radiography (X-ray)	35.5
Computed tomography (CT)	14.6
Head CT	7.2
CT other than head	7.6
Ultrasound (US)	3.1
Magnetic resonance imaging (MRI)	0.6
Other imaging	1.0
Any imaging	46.6

Source: National Ambulatory Medical Care Survey, 2008.

by individuals in the United States over the past several decades.

CT use in the United States peaked in 2011, with more than 80 million CT scans obtained during that year. Since then, CT use has actually declined about 5% per year, with approximately 76 million obtained in the United States in 2013.[9] Some of this may be due to efforts to curb over-utilization as well as a broader understanding of risks of radiation from CT scans. However, this still represents nearly one CT performed per year for every four residents of the United States, a rate that is nearly twice that of Canada.[10] It has been estimated that between 20% and 40% of CT scans may be "medically unnecessary."[11] The risk of ionizing radiation is potentially relevant to the influence of gender on appropriate imaging choice, as females face a greater risk of malignancy from CT scanning. In addition to radiation risks, contrast-induced nephropathy and anaphylactoid reactions to radiographic contrast media have also been shown to be more prevalent in the female population.[12,13] Although the risk of these reactions should be discussed with all patients, the emergency physician should have a heightened awareness in females as compared to their male counterparts.

Gender is an important consideration in selecting appropriate imaging. Prevalence and type of disease will vary by gender, as will diagnostic yield and risk from radiation. Cost, time, and radiation should not be an impediment to an appropriate imaging study that can help guide therapy regardless of gender. However, the art and science of appropriate use of diagnostic imaging can be better implemented if gender differences are understood.

"Appropriate" Imaging, "Value," and "Comparative Effectiveness"

Diagnostic imaging saves lives every day and is one of the major advances of modern medicine. However, as advanced imaging (CT, MRI, nuclear studies) has become much more readily available and more frequently used, both the physician community (such as the "too much medicine campaign" spearheaded by the *British Medical Journal*) and governmental organizations (such as the Medicare Payment Advisory Committee) have increasingly called for physicians to ensure imaging is appropriate.[3] What is "appropriate," however, has been called "elusive" and depends on the imaging procedure, the patient and his or her characteristics, and the setting where imaging is obtained.[14]

The Affordable Care Act ("Obamacare") passed in 2010 accelerated the development of so-called appropriateness criteria for imaging. The law suggested that one of the ways that the newly created Center for Medicare and Medicaid Innovation (CMI, under the Centers for Medicare and Medicaid Services or CMS) could "test innovative service and delivery models" is by

> Varying payment to physicians who order advanced diagnostic imaging services (as defined in section 1834(e)(1)(B)) according to the physician's adherence to appropriateness criteria for the ordering of such services, as determined in consultation with physician specialty groups and other relevant stakeholders.[15]

Appropriateness criteria have been published by organizations concerned with imaging, such as the American College of Radiology and the American Society of Echocardiography. However, while there are some differences in suggested appropriate imaging based on patient characteristics (typically pediatric and pregnant patients) for certain guidelines, in general the guidelines do not factor in gender when determining appropriateness. These appropriateness criteria may also be more focused on provider-centered issues, such as ensuring that studies are considered "appropriate for reimbursement" rather than truly representing "patient-centered imaging."[16]

Despite increased imaging, it is debatable whether patient-centered outcomes have been improved in relation to the increase in imaging. A study of ED visits between 2001 and 2005 representing more than 38 million visits for abdominal pain reported CT use in 17.8% of patients (an increase from 10.1% of visits in 2001 to 22.5% of visits in 2005) and found no difference in detection of surgical disease or a decrease in admissions with this increased use.[17] Similar studies looking at the effect of increasing CT in suspected kidney stone found no impact on patient-centered outcomes.[18,19]

This raises the challenge of determining "value" in imaging, an effort behind pushes for research in comparative effectiveness.[20,21] A recent study that used a Delphi process to elicit expert consensus opinion on the top five areas of practice improvement "to improve the value of emergency care" included four imaging studies, three of which involved CT (CT of the neck in trauma, CT in suspected pulmonary embolism, and CT in minor head trauma).[22]

Understanding areas where gender may influence both the risk and diagnostic yield of the test may help clinicians (and patients) make more informed decisions about appropriate imaging.

Understanding the Risks of Radiation from CT Scanning

A study published in 2004 suggested that physicians largely misunderstood and misestimated the risk of radiation from CT.[23] The past decade has seen increased awareness of the issue in both the medical and lay press, and now much of the public appreciates that there is some radiation risk from CT. However, quantifying the risk has remained difficult because of debates about the evidence as well as confusion about units of measurements. However, having a basic understanding of the concepts and the range of risks that may be involved can help inform decision making, particularly when imaging may involve little or no marginal benefit.

Reporting and Measuring Radiation from CT

Ionizing radiation is the type of radiation used by CT scans, plain radiographs (X-rays), and nuclear studies to obtain images. It is generally acknowledged that there is some small increased risk of cancer when ionizing radiation is applied to radiosensitive organs in a patient. However, the magnitude of this risk for an individual and on a population basis is incompletely understood; may be quite variable based on age, size, and gender; and remains controversial.[24,25]

The best way to get a working understanding of how radiation delivered by a CT scan is measured is to get in the habit of looking at the metrics displayed with each CT scan in actual patients (Figure 12.1). Most modern CT scanners will include an image at the end of a CT series that includes two measures: the CT dose index (CTDI or $CTDI_{vol}$, in milligray or mGy) and the dose-length-product (DLP, in mGy-cm). The $CTDI_{vol}$ can be considered the output of the scanner; the DLP is related more to overall absorbed radiation as it is equal to the $CTDI_{vol}$ × the length of the body scanned.

While DLP is the more frequently reported dose metric, it is important to understand that DLP is calculated based on a standardized phantom (i.e., simulated patient) and does not take patient size into account in terms of actual effective organ dose. To account for this, the American Association of Physicists in Medicine has recently proposed conversion factors for $CTDI_{vol}$ into a size specific dose estimate (SSDE), which utilizes conversion factors based on patient size.[26] The key concept here is that for a given $CTDI_{vol}$ or DLP, a larger patient will have relatively lower actual dose delivered to the radiosensitive organs because of absorption by non-radiosensitive tissue.

Regarding actual radiation dose delivered to a patient and the potential for organ damage, several metrics are in use, and ongoing controversy about the best reporting methods can make comparison and estimation of risk at the individual and population levels confusing. Both rad and gray (gray is the SI unit) refer to the amount of radiation absorbed, while rem and sievert (seivert is the SI unit) refer to the effective organ dose that should be most directly related to risk of malignancy. For CT scanning, the most commonly used units will be milligray (mGy) and millisieverts (mSv). As mentioned earlier, a CT report will provide the total dose delivered as the DLP in mGy-cm. Converting to effective dose can be estimated depending on what body part is scanned.[27] For example, the conversion factor for a CT of the

Patient Name:				Exam no:	
Accession Number:				Feb 10 2014	
Patient ID:				Discovery CT750 HD	
Exam Description: CT ABDOMEN PELVIS WO I					

Dose Report

Series	Type	Scan Range (mm)	CTDIvol (mGy)	DLP (mGy-cm)	Phantom cm
1	Scout	-	-	-	-
2	Helical	I115.500–I570.500	12.42	622.42	Body 32
		Total Exam DLP:		622.42	

1/1

Figure 12.1 Dose report from a non-contrast CT of the abdomen pelvis for suspected kidney stone. The two reported values are the CT dose index (CTDI$_{vol}$) and the dose length product (DLP). The DLP is equal to the CTDI$_{vol}$ × the scan length. In this case, the scan length from top of the kidneys was 50 cm, so the DLP of 622.4 mGy-cm is equal to the CTDI$_{vol}$ of 12.42 mGy × 50 cm. In terms of effective dose, using a conversion factor of 17 microseiverts per mGy-cm in the abdomen-pelvis would correspond to an effective dose of approximately 10.6 mSv (slightly below the national average dose of 11.2 mSv for renal colic protocol CTs)

abdomen and pelvis is ~15–17 microseiverts per milligray-centimeters, so a CT scan with a DLP of 622 mGy-cm (see Figure 12.1; Table 12.2) would be estimated to deliver an effective dose of approximately 10.6 mSv. To put this in perspective, the average yearly background radiation (without any medical radiation) in the United States is approximately 2–3 mSv (~6 mSv per year with medical radiation).[11]

The Risk of Radiation from CT

A dramatic paper published in 2009 estimated that there could be as many as 29,000 future malignancies resulting from CTs performed in the United States in the year 2007 alone.[28] Published population-based risks of developing a malignancy from CT scans depend on age, gender, and type of scan performed but have been estimated to range from approximately 1 in 150 for a 20-year-old female undergoing a CT angiogram to about 1 in 15,000 for a 60-year-old male undergoing a routine head CT (see Table 2).[29]

The estimates of risk were derived from the rates of malignancy in survivors of the atomic bomb attacks on Japan during World War II. The current generally accepted model is called the "no threshold linear model," meaning each increased radiation dose is directly related to the increased risk of malignancy, and there is no

single threshold amount that becomes more dangerous.[30] However, the number of people in these cohorts developing cancer after receiving smaller doses of radiation was small, and a recent study has called this model into question.[25] Larger epidemiologic studies are being conducted now on data from patients receiving CT scans that should yield more accurate estimates; some early studies show increased risks, although definitive estimates may take decades.[11,31]

Dose Variability from CT Scanning

Given the potential harms of ionizing radiation, radiological societies have endorsed the concept of using a dose that is "as low as reasonably achievable" (ALARA). While this is good in theory, in practice dosing may vary considerably for similar protocols between centers. In certain states (California, Texas, and Connecticut, to date), estimated radiation dose is a required element of the CT report. Additionally, the National Quality Forum (NQF) has endorsed "participation in a systemic dose index registry" as a quality measure, and the American College of Radiology founded the national Dose Imaging Registry (DIR, part of the National Registry of Diagnostic Radiology) in 2011.[32] However, there is no actual requirement to lower dosing for a given protocol, and although these protocols are typically set by

Table 12.2 Approximate Effective Dose, Equivalent Number of Chest Radiographs (PA), Conversion Factors from Dose Length Product to Effective Dose, and Estimated Number of CT Scans that Would Cause an Additional Malignancy

Imaging Modality	Approximate Delivered Dose (mSv)	Equivalent # of CXRs	Conversion Factor from DLP to Effective Dose in mSv per mGy-cm	Estimated Additional Lifetime Risk of Malignancy: 20 yo Female	Estimated additional lifetime risk of malignancy: 60 yo male
Chest X-ray, anteroposterior (AP)	0.02	1			
Chest x-ray (CXR) – AP and lateral	0.05–0.08	3			
Abdominal X-ray ("KUB")	1	50			
Yearly background radiation in U.S. without any medical imaging	2–3*	100–150			
Average yearly background radiation in U.S. including medical imaging	6	300			
Head CT	1–2	50–100	2.0–2.3	1 in 4,360	1 in 14,680
Cervical spine CT	4	200	5.1–5.9	1 in 2,390	1 in 8,030
Chest CT pulmonary angiography	7	350	17–19	1 in 330	1 in 1,770
CT coronary angiogram	12	600	17–19	1 in 150	1 in 790
Chest CT "triple rule-out"	17	850	17–19	1 in 320	1 in 840
Abdomen-pelvis CT	10	500	15–18	1 in 500	1 in 1,330
"Low dose" CT (for kidney stone)	2	100	15–18	1 in 5,000	1 in 10,000
"Pan scan" for trauma	32	1,600	variable	sum of risks of each scan	

* Higher at higher elevations, for example ~10 mSv per year in Denver CO.

manufacturers, they may be modified by radiologists and CT technicians. A recent report from the DIR found that dosing for CTs looking for kidney stones could vary by a factor of 10, with less than 2% done using the low-dose protocols (less than ~3 mSv) that have been shown to be effective in diagnosing kidney stones while lowering risk from radiation.[33,34] The range of doses used for a given study, therefore, can vary substantially from institution to institution.

Gender Considerations in Specific Clinical Situations

Imaging in Chest Pain and/or Dyspnea

Chest pain is the most common presenting ED chief complaint in adult males, and the second leading complaint in adult females, accounting for more than 5 million annual visits to U.S. EDs.[1] The ED evaluation of chest pain and dyspnea involving advanced medical imaging has risen from 3.4% in 1999 to 15.9% in 2008.[35] It is estimated that 40% of all medical radiation is related to cardiovascular imaging and intervention.[36]

Almost all chest pain evaluated in the ED will receive a plain chest X-ray. While the utility of this as a routine test has been questioned for more than 30 years,[37] it is a common and inexpensive test without much radiation and typically functions as a screen for pneumonia, heart failure, pneumothorax, and aortic pathology. Whether imaging beyond a chest X-ray is obtained will depend on the suspicion for serious pathology, with the three most serious pathologies being acute coronary syndrome (ACS), pulmonary embolism (PE), and thoracic aortic dissection (TAD).

Echocardiography offers an attractive modality with no ionizing radiation that can be helpful in evaluation of the ED patient with chest pain and/or dyspnea. While access to formal echocardiography is often restricted in the ED setting,[38] point-of-care ultrasound of the heart and lungs involves no radiation, is easily performed at the bedside, and can help provide diagnostic guidance in chest pain and dyspnea.[39,40] Bedside echocardiography can exclude pericardial effusion, provide information about left ventricular function (affected by coronary disease), right ventricular strain (seen in large PEs), and aortic root size (associated with TAD), although echocardiography in particular represents a user-dependent diagnostic technology and the accuracy for these conditions will vary based on the experience of the clinician performing it.

While chest X-ray and ultrasound can be helpful, definitive diagnosis in coronary disease, PE, or TAD is typically obtained using imaging modalities with ionizing radiation. For PE and TAD, the test of choice is a contrast-enhanced CT scan of the chest. For coronary disease, cardiac catheterization with coronary angiography is the reference standard. However, in both PE and ACS evidenced-based approaches allow effective exclusion of disease in a substantial proportion of patients without using ionizing radiation. Data suggest that testing occurs more than is warranted by the evidence, and thus ionizing radiation is used more than is necessary. When ionizing radiation of the chest is over utilized, women are disproportionally at risk due to the exposure of breast tissue to the potentially carcinogenic radiation.[41]

Chest Pain concerning for Coronary Artery Disease

Heart disease is the leading cause of death in the United States for both men and women, and efforts to minimize missed diagnoses have led to extensive diagnostic testing. While cardiac catheterization and coronary angiography are the gold standard for diagnosis of coronary disease, these are usually not immediately performed on patients with chest pain unless the history is convincing or there is a documented myocardial infarction or positive stress test. The majority of chest pain seen in the ED can be considered "low-risk chest pain," with a normal or nonspecific EKG and negative cardiac biomarkers.[42] About 2% to 4% of people presenting with low-risk chest pain will ultimately be found to have significant coronary disease.[43]

If the history is concerning, it is often standard care in the United States to evaluate the coronary arteries either with a CT angiogram or a stress test.[42] Options for a stress test include stress EKG, stress echo, and nuclear perfusion studies. More than 10 million nuclear stress tests are currently performed annually in the United States, accounting for about 20% of the medical radiation received by the population, equivalent to half the radiation from all non-cardiac CT scanning put together.[44] While nuclear stress tests are an effective tool for risk stratification, other options such as exercise echocardiography may be as effective and do not involve radiation. A recent survey of practitioners using nuclear stress tests found that only 7% were using a stress-first approach (i.e., only moving to a nuclear study if stress EKG or stress echocardiography were not conclusive) that could decrease radiation by as much as 75%.[45]

Increasingly, coronary CT angiogram (CCTA) is an option for detecting coronary disease.[46] However, the radiation involved is higher than that typically delivered for a CT of the abdomen and pelvis and includes irradiation of the breasts in female patients.[47] However, CCTA may allow clinicians to make an immediate disposition decision on a patient, avoiding lengthy observation admissions or stress testing, and can reduce negative cardiac catheterizations.[46] There is also the potential for using CT to do a "triple rule-out" of all serious causes of chest pain (coronary disease, PE, and TAD). A triple rule-out CT protocol typically adds nearly 5 mSv to the radiation dose, but a recent study showed minimal added diagnostic benefit.[48]

Our recommendation is that in younger, lower-risk patients (including younger females) if provocative testing for coronary artery disease is desired, stress EKG, stress echo, or CT/nuclear strategies that minimize radiation should be considered first, with nuclear studies and CCTA reserved for cases for which these tests will not provide adequate risk stratification.

Chest Pain and/or Dyspnea concerning for Pulmonary Embolism

PE is estimated to occur in as many as 600,000 patients annually in the United States. CT pulmonary angiogram (CTPA) is now considered the diagnostic gold standard; since its introduction, the diagnosis of PE has nearly doubled in the United States. However, with increased diagnosis, mortality from PE has only been minimally affected, while complications from anticoagulation have risen, suggesting that we are treating more and potentially less clinically significant PEs.[49] The authors of a study on breast irradiation from CT scanning for PE concluded that we should "encourage the judicious use of CT pulmonary angiography and lower doses and nonionizing radiation alternatives when appropriate."[41]

Several clinical decision rules can stratify patients with symptoms of PE below the testing threshold for CT scan, either using clinical presentation alone or with d-dimer testing.[50] The PE rule-out criteria (PERC) can stratify patients into a group that is low enough that a d-dimer or other imaging is likely to do more harm than good.[50,51] The Wells score indicates whether patients have a low enough pretest probability that if a d-dimer is negative further imaging is not needed.[52] Women are more likely to have a positive d-dimer (which is more likely to be falsely elevated), and this may contribute to the higher rate of imaging even if decision rules are followed.[53] However, it is estimated that as many as a third of CTPAs (in both genders) could be avoided by utilizing these evidence-based rules.[54] While women and men have an approximately equivalent incidence of PE, women undergo two-thirds of the CT scans for PE, and thus the diagnostic yield in women overall is substantially lower.[55]

Imaging in Abdominal Pain

Abdominal pain is the leading reason that adult females and the second leading reason that adult males visit the ED.[1] Abdominal pain is a symptom that arises from a myriad of pathologies that can range from benign to serious both inside and outside of the abdominal cavity. A substantial number of patients with abdominal pain will not have a definitive diagnosis established during their ED visit. Like chest pain, evaluation of abdominal pain in the Emergency Department setting has seen a marked rise in advanced medical imaging. There are approximately 7 million annual ED visits for abdominal pain, with use of advanced medical imaging in its evaluation increasing from 19.9% to 44.3% between 1999 and 2008.[35] Specifically, the use of CT for the evaluation of abdominal pain has seen the most dramatic rise, from 1.4% of visits in 1996 to 31.7% of visits in 2007.[56] Despite this rise in CT imaging, there has been no change in the diagnosis of appendicitis, diverticulitis, or gallbladder disease, and admission rates for patients with abdominal pain have not changed.[17] This suggests that utilization of CT for the evaluation of abdominal pain may not be adding value to patient-centered outcomes.

For some of the most common diagnosable causes of abdominal pain, use of ultrasound is a safe and effective alternative to CT, and the benefit: risk ratio may be higher for women. Biliary disease represents a disorder that is more common in women and is most effectively diagnosed with ultrasound. More than 20 million people in the United States suffer from biliary disease, and 70% of these are women.[57] Biliary disease accounts for as many as 9% of admissions for abdominal pain, and 700,000 cholecystectomies are performed annually in the United States.[58] While classically there is pain and tenderness in the right upper quadrant, midline epigastric pain is also consistent with biliary colic. Ultrasound is the initial test of choice if biliary disease is suspected. Point-of-care ultrasound has also been shown to be accurate for detection of biliary pathology and may be performed at the bedside by experienced practitioners.[59,60]

Appendicitis occurs in about 7% of the population in their lifetime. While appendicitis occurs more commonly in males (male-to-female ratio is 1.4:1), the diagnosis may be more challenging in women due to other etiologies of pain in the right lower quadrant.[61] CT scanning is often considered the test of choice for appendicitis and is highly accurate. However, ultrasound is typically the first-line approach for pediatric and pregnant patients. A recent analysis of an ultrasound-first approach for appendicitis estimated that adopting such an approach could potentially avoid about 180 excess cancer deaths per year along with substantial cost savings.[62] Such an approach would again be most effective in younger female patients.

The elderly with abdominal pain represent a special population for both genders, as they are more likely to harbor a serious diagnosis, particularly a vascular etiology.[63] Abdominal aortic aneurysm (AAA) causes about 15,000 deaths annually in the United States with twice as many deaths occurring in men.[64] While AAA is more common in men, women face an increased risk of rupture at smaller sizes.[65] Ultrasound screening for AAA is currently recommended by the U.S. Preventive Services Task Force for asymptomatic men between the ages of 65 and 75 who have ever smoked, but routine screening is not recommended for women.[66] Identification of AAA may be accomplished with bedside ultrasound in the ED.[67] While ultrasound may help discern the etiology of abdominal pain in elderly men or women, a non-diagnostic ultrasound should generally be followed by a CT scan due to the prevalence of serious causes of pain and the lower lifetime risk of radiation in this population.

Sex-specific causes of lower abdominal pain must also be considered. In men with lower abdominal pain, a testicular etiology should be considered and a testicular examination should be performed. If there are concerning testicular findings on physical examination, scrotal ultrasound is typically the test of choice. For women, pelvic etiologies should be considered in most cases of abdominal pain, and ultrasound remains the test of choice for examination of the ovaries and uterus.

As noted earlier, CT scanning is frequently performed in the evaluation of abdominal pain in the emergency setting and is an excellent test, particularly for ruling out serious bowel and vascular pathologies. A recent review in radiology concluded that "CT can therefore be considered the primary technique for the diagnosis of acute abdominal pain, except in patients clinically suspected of having acute cholecystitis," but it went on to note that "When costs and ionizing radiation are primary concerns, a possible strategy is to perform US as the initial technique in all patients with acute abdominal pain, with CT performed in all cases of nondiagnostic US."[68] Ultrasound as a primary or initial modality is used more frequently outside of the United States.

Imaging in Flank or Back Pain concerning for Renal Colic

Kidney stones are estimated to occur in about 10.6% of men and 7.1% of women during their lifetime.[69] Despite CT having a lower diagnostic yield and a higher risk of later malignancy in women, a recent large study in the United States showed that women were undergoing 53.9% of CTs for renal colic and that the average age of CT scanning for renal colic was 45.[33]

Two reasons are cited to obtain a CT in a patient with suspected renal colic: (a) to determine the size and location of a stone, helping with prognosis and need for intervention and (b) to ensure no other important diagnoses are mimicking renal colic. However, approximately 80% of kidney stones will pass spontaneously, and those that are unlikely to pass will be clinically evident over time. While there are several mimics of renal colic, acutely important alternate causes of symptoms occur uncommonly (<3%) in patients without typical symptoms or evidence of infection or typical symptoms.[70] A clinical prediction rule for ureteral stone (the "STONE score") has been derived and validated that includes gender as an element.[71] While women are still less likely to have a kidney stone, the incidence in women has been increasing, and women with a stone are more likely to be admitted.[72–74]

A recent position paper from the American College of Emergency Physicians (ACEP) asserts that "North American practice is to perform a noncontrast CT for new-onset flank pain/renal colic."[75] While this appears to be true in terms of practice patterns, the only evidence to support this practice is apparently a single study of 121 patients more than 10 years ago.[76] Larger epidemiologic studies have shown no difference in rate of diagnosis, intervention, or admission despite the large increase in CT scanning for this condition.[18,19] While low-dose CT protocols are recommended by both the ACR and the ACEP for evaluation of kidney stones, these are currently being used less than 2% of the time in the United States. The average effective dose in the United States for renal colic protocol CTs is approximately 11.2 mSv with a large variation in median institutional dose ranging from 3.5 to 19.8 mSv.[33,75,77] For CT scans in younger persons, a 10 mSv effective dose may lead to an additional malignancy for approximately every 1,000 scans, potentially causing malignancy while diagnosing a usually self-limited condition.

Ultrasound offers an effective method for diagnoses in younger women with flank pain.[78] While ultrasound may not always visualize a ureteral stone, it is effective in showing the presence of hydronephrosis, which is nearly always present with a ureteral stone that may require intervention.[79,80] For women in particular, several mimics of renal colic are readily diagnosable using ultrasound. Adnexal torsion in particular is an emergent condition more likely to occur in younger women that is poorly diagnosed by CT scan, and for which ultrasound is the test of choice.[81] Ovarian cysts without torsion or other pelvic pathologies represent possible mimics of renal colic as well. Appendicitis may be positively identified with ultrasound, although if the appendix is not visualized and the diagnosis remains on the differential, CT should be considered.

While more definitive evidence-based trials are warranted, it is our recommendation that younger patients, particularly younger women (younger than ages 40 to 50) should always undergo an ultrasound of the retroperitoneum, abdomen, and pelvis prior to consideration of CT scan in suspected renal colic (even new onset renal colic). Point-of-care ultrasound may allow this to be done at the bedside if appropriately trained clinicians are available. If ultrasound is non-diagnostic and symptoms are persistent or severe, CT may then be warranted.

Imaging in Trauma

Each year about 1 in 10 persons in the United States will visit an ED for a traumatic injury, with the majority male and about 70% younger than age 45.[82] From 1998 to 2007, the use of advanced imaging (CT or MRI) increased from 6% to 15%; however, the trends in prevalence of serious injuries did not match this increase, and admission rates for trauma did not change.[83] A recent study from Germany that looked retrospectively at whole body CT (sometimes called a "panscan") in "polytrauma," concluded that incorporation of this into routine care could increase survival.[84] In high-mechanism trauma, where the likelihood of injury is relatively high, the benefit of CT no doubt outweighs the risk.[85] However, because pan-scanning delivers a substantial dose of radiation (~32 mSv), often to younger patients who are more vulnerable to its carcinogenic effects, more selective use of pan-scanning has been advocated.[86,87]

An ACEP clinical policy published in 2011 on blunt abdominal trauma concluded that guidance for patients who may not require an abdominal CT included (level of evidence "C"):[88]

Patients with isolated abdominal trauma, for whom occult abdominal injury is being considered, are at low risk for adverse outcome and may not need abdominal CT scanning if the following are absent: abdominal tenderness, hypotension, altered mental status (Glasgow Coma Scale score <14), costal margin tenderness, abnormal chest radiograph, hematocrit <30% and hematuria.

The focused assessment with sonography in trauma (FAST) exam represents a rapid method to evaluate for serious injury to the thorax or abdomen in blunt or penetrating trauma without any ionizing radiation. FAST is recommended as the initial imaging modality if the patient is hemodynamically unstable.[88] If the patient is hemodynamically stable, a positive FAST should be followed with a CT scan and may expedite appropriate evaluation and therapy. In a stable patient with a negative FAST exam, further evaluation depends on suspicion for significant injury. A negative initial FAST exam does not rule out all significant traumatic injuries. However, if there is a low suspicion for significant injury, a period of observation and a repeated negative FAST 6 hours later may be a reasonable approach.[89]

While we are not aware of studies specifically targeted at imaging based on gender in trauma, many of the same principles apply as in other areas of imaging. If there is a true suspicion for serious injury to the head, chest, abdomen, pelvis, or spine, CT is likely indicated regardless of age or gender. However if suspicion for injury is low, a careful physical examination and period of observation may safely replace CT scanning, with long-term benefits to patients and society. Young males, who most commonly incur a traumatic injury, are the group in which radiation risk could be most reduced by the appropriate use of CT.

Imaging of the Head

Approximately half of all CTs performed in the ED are head CTs.[90] While risk of radiation from head CT is lower than that of other CT scans, they represent a risk based on the sheer number of studies performed and also represent a source of significant resource utilization that has relatively low diagnostic yield. Particular attention has been focused on pediatric patients due to their increased risk of cancer from radiation.[91,92] While most CTs

are for head trauma or headache, advanced imaging of the head is often used for nonspecific presentations such as dizziness or syncope.[93]

Non-contrast CT imaging of the brain is the test of choice if significant traumatic brain injury (TBI) is suspected. TBI is estimated to occur in 1.7 million patients, with about 80% of these visiting the ED and death occurring in 52,000. There is a bimodal distribution of significant TBI in the very young and elderly, but males are more likely than females to undergo significant injury at any age. While CT is certainly indicated in any situation with head trauma, if there are any persistent neurologic findings (including GCS less than 15), it is less likely to be helpful in mild traumatic brain injury (MTBI). There are two well validated and commonly used decision rules for MTBI in adults: the New Orleans and the Canadian Head CT rules.[94,95] Simply following these guidelines (regardless of gender) could reduce inappropriate imaging as often as 35% of the time.[96] For pediatrics, the Pediatric Emergency Care Applied Research Network (PECARN) has published guidelines for imaging in pediatric head trauma.[92]

Non-traumatic headache is responsible for about 2% of all ED visits in the United States, accounting for more than 2 million annual visits.[97] The prevalence of migraine headache in women is two to three times higher than in men, and women present more frequently to the ED with complaint of headache. While headache is a common ED complaint, serious etiologies that are diagnosable by CT scan (typically tumor or subarachnoid hemorrhage) are rare: 46 in 10,000 for brain tumor and 9 in 10,000 for subarachnoid hemorrhage.[98] The diagnostic yield of head CT in neurologically normal patients is less than 1%, and both ACEP and the ACR do not recommend head CT for recurrent atraumatic headache.[98,99]

Imaging in the Pregnant Patient

The general rule in pregnancy is to avoid CT scan if possible, as there is the risk of radiation to the fetus as well as the young mother. However, if a CT is necessary for the diagnosis of a significant health threat to the mother, it may still be indicated. Ultrasound is considered the first-line test for abdominal pain in pregnant women and may be able to definitively diagnose biliary colic, appendicitis, ectopic pregnancy, or significant traumatic injury. It may also identify evidence of ureteral obstruction (from kidney stone), although some hydronephrosis is physiologic in pregnancy. MRI is a safe modality in pregnancy that can often diagnose or rule out pathology if ultrasound is inconclusive.

In U.S. EDs, the incidence of ectopic pregnancy is about 8% to 12% for patients presenting with first trimester pregnancy complaints (lower abdominal/pelvic pain or vaginal bleeding). Ultrasound should thus be obtained in any patient with a first trimester complaint that could represent ectopic, regardless of beta-hCG level, as it may detect an ectopic pregnancy.[100] Bedside ultrasound may be used to rule in an intrauterine pregnancy, which in the absence of fertility agents makes coexisting ectopic or heterotopic pregnancy extremely unlikely (on the order of 1 in 4,000).[101] Bedside ultrasound may also be used to look for free intraperitoneal fluid, which if present in the right upper quadrant makes it likely that operative intervention will be required for ruptured ectopic.[102]

Appendicitis is the most common surgical emergency in pregnancy.[103] While appendicitis is no more common in pregnant patients than non-pregnant age-matched controls, the diagnosis is more often missed when pregnancy is present. If appendicitis is suspected, typically the first imaging study would be a transabdominal and transvaginal ultrasound. This may identify appendicitis or reveal an alternate cause of symptoms such as an ovarian cyst. If the ultrasound is inconclusive, MRI represents an excellent test and may be done in consultation with the surgery and obstetric specialists. While gadolinium contrast in MRI may enhance diagnostic accuracy, little is known about the risk to the fetus.[104]

Trauma in pregnancy represents a risk both to the mother and the fetus. In addition to traumatic injury to the intra-abdominal organs, patients in later pregnancy are at risk for placental abruption or even uterine rupture. A FAST exam is a typical first imaging study, which can include basic assessment of the uterus and fetus. If this is negative, typically the patient will be referred for further ultrasound evaluation of the placenta and 4-hour fetal monitoring. If suspicion for significant intra-abdominal injury is not high and the fetus is not in distress, serial examinations and repeat FAST exam may be adequate to exclude serious injury to the mother. Choice of performing CT of the abdomen and pelvis must depend on the mechanism of the trauma and level of suspicion for serious intraabdominal injury.

Pregnancy is an independent risk factor for venous thromboembolism (VTE) and PE, with risk peaking in late pregnancy and the postpartum period. While d-dimer is often used to determine if patients with a low pretest probability for PE need a CT scan, d-dimer rises during pregnancy and will typically be positive in the late pregnancy and postpartum period regardless of whether a VTE is present. However, if d-dimer is negative (particularly in early pregnancy and assuming other symptoms do not make PE highly likely), it is helpful in ruling out PE. If d-dimer is not obtained, or if PE is still suspected, most diagnostic algorithms for pregnant patients with suspected PE recommend starting with a lower extremity ultrasound. While the absence of DVT does not rule out a PE, presence of DVT with symptoms of PE can yield a presumptive diagnosis without CT. If lower extremity ultrasound is negative and PE is still suspected, either a contrast enhanced CT or a ventilation perfusion (VQ) scan may be obtained. While VQ scan used to be recommended as the preferred modality for evaluating PE in pregnant women, it has been shown that the radiation exposure is no greater from a CT scan, and CT scanning more often results in a definitive answer. Imaging may be obtained in conjunction with obstetrics consultation. MRI is safe in pregnancy and may identify proximal PE if it is present, but it has not been shown to reliably rule out more distal PEs.[105]

Conclusion

Imaging is an essential part of diagnosing and caring for ED patients. Appropriate imaging utilization is a delicate balance between not missing diagnoses that will affect outcomes while avoiding the downsides of over utilization – cost, time, and radiation that may lead to harms later in life for the individual or the population as whole. The data suggest that in the United States, we are over utilizing advanced imaging, particularly CT, in certain situations, and that there are often options that do not involve ionizing radiation. An understanding of how gender impacts prevalence of disease and risk of imaging (particularly risk of radiation from CT) may lead to better, more patient-centered care.

Case Conclusion

While pleuritic chest pain classically raises the question of whether a PE may be present, the treating clinician recognized that this 28-year-old woman meets the PE rule-out criteria (PERC), placing her risk for PE at well below 2%. Therefore, d-dimer was not obtained, as a false positive could lead to an unnecessary CT scan, with its accompanying cost, contrast exposure, time, and radiation. This patient was discharged with nonsteroidal anti-inflammatory medications for her musculoskeletal chest pain. On follow-up with her primary care physician one week later, she was doing well, with symptoms nearly resolved.

Unanswered Questions/Need for Further Research in This Area

Clinical prediction rules and decision guidelines for appropriate imaging utilization are an active area of research within emergency medicine and the larger medical community. While pediatric and pregnant patients are often treated as separate populations for imaging appropriateness guidelines, gender may be underemphasized. Development and study of gender-specific appropriateness criteria for imaging may be helpful to improve safety and long-term health outcomes.

While there is increased awareness of the risk of radiation from CT scanning, debate continues because of the lack of solid epidemiologic evidence about cancer risk from low doses of radiation (<100 mSv). Further studies are needed in this area, particularly in differentiating risk by age and gender.

References

1. NHAMCS. National Hospital Ambulatory Medical Care Survey: 2008 Emergency Department Summary Tables. *Medical Care* (2008).

2. Smith-Bindman, R. et al. Use of diagnostic imaging studies and associated radiation exposure for patients enrolled in large integrated health care systems, 1996–2010. *JAMA* **307**, 2400–9 (2013).

3. Miller, M. E. *MedPAC recommendations on imaging services. Secretary* (2005). At http://vns .aan.com/media/031705_testimonyimaging-hou .pdf.

4. Kocher, K. E., Meurer, W. J., Desmond, J. S. & Nallamothu, B. K. Effect of testing and treatment on emergency department length of stay using a national database. *Academic Emergency Medicine* **19**, 525–34 (2012).

5. Trzeciak, S. & Rivers, E. P. Emergency department overcrowding in the United States: an emergeing threat to patient safety and public health. *Emergency Medicine Journal* **20**, 402–5 (2003).

6. Volk, M. & Ubel, P. Better off not knowing. *Archives of Internal Medicine* **171**, 487–88 (2011).

7. Stone, J. H. Incidentalomas – clinical correlation and translational science required. *New England Journal of Medicine* **354**, 2748–9 (2006).

8. Center for Devices and Radiological Health, U. S. F. and D. A. Initiative to Reduce Unnecessary Radiation Exposure from Medical Imaging. *Ncrp Rep.* (2010). At www.fda.gov/downloads/Radiatio n-EmittingProducts/RadiationSafety/Radiation DoseReduction/UCM200087.pdf.

9. IMV. IMV CT Overview. At www.imvinfo.com/ index.aspx?sec=ct&sub=def.

10. Berdahl, C. T., Vermeulen, M. J., Larson, D. B. & Schull, M. J. Emergency department computed tomography utilization in the United States and Canada. *Annals of Emergency Medicine* **62**, 486–94. e3 (2013).

11. Hricak, H. et al. Managing radiation use in medical imaging: A multifaceted challenge. *Radiology* **258**, 889–905 (2011).

12. Iakovou, I. et al. Impact of gender on the incidence and outcome of contrast-induced nephropathy after percutaneous coronary intervention. *Journal of Invasive Cardiology* **15**, 18–22 (2003).

13. Lang, D. M., Alpern, M. B., Visintainer, P. F. & Smith, S. T. Gender risk for anaphylactoid reaction to radiographic contrast media. *Journal of Allergy and Clinical Immunology* **95**, 813–7 (1995).

14. Sistrom, C. L. The appropriateness of imaging: A comprehensive conceptual framework. *Radiology* **251**, 637–49 (2009).

15. U.S. Congress. Patient Protection and Affordable Care Act. (2010). At http://democrats.senate.gov/ pdfs/reform/patient-protection-affordable-care -act-as-passed.pdf.

16. Swensen, S. J. Patient-centered Imaging. *American Journal of Medicine* **125**, 115–17 (2012).

17. Pines, J. M. Trends in the rates of radiography use and important diagnoses in emergency

department patients with abdominal pain. *Medical Care* **47**, 782–6 (2009).

18. Westphalen, A. C., Hsia, R. Y., Maselli, J. H., Wang, R. & Gonzales, R. Radiological imaging of patients with suspected urinary tract stones: National trends, diagnoses, and predictors. *Academic Emergency Medicine* **18**, 699–707 (2011).

19. Gottlieb, R. H. et al. CT in detecting urinary tract calculi: Influence on patient imaging and clinical outcomes. *Radiology* **225**, 441–9 (2002).

20. Baker, L. C., Atlas, S. W. & Afendulis, C. C. Expanded use of imaging technology and the challenge of measuring value. *Health Affairs (Millwood)* **27**, 1467–78 (2008).

21. Gazelle, G. S. et al. A framework for assessing the value of diagnostic imaging in the era of comparative. *Radiology* **261**, 692–8 (2011).

22. Schuur, J. D. et al. A top-five list for emergency medicine. *JAMA Internal Medicine* (2014). doi:10.1001/jamainternmed.2013.12688

23. Lee, C. I., Haims, A. H., Monico, E. P., Brink, J. A. & Forman, H. P. Diagnostic CT scans: Assessment of patient, physician, and radiologist awareness of radiation dose and possible risks. *Radiology* **231**, 393–8 (2004).

24. Ozasa, K. et al. Studies of the mortality of atomic bomb survivors, Report 14, 1950–2003: An overview of cancer and noncancer diseases. *Radiation Research* **177**, 229–43 (2012).

25. Doss, M. Linear no-threshold model may not be appropriate for estimating cancer risk from CT. *Radiology* **270**, 307–8 (2014).

26. Boone, J. M. et al. *AAPM Report No. 204: Size-Specific Dose Estimates in Pediatric and Adult Body CT Examinations.* American Association of Physicists in Medicine 1–24 (2011).

27. *European Guidelines for Multislice Computed Tomography* Appendix 1. At www.msct.eu/PDF_FILES/Appendix MSCT Dosimetry.pdf.

28. Berrington de González, A. et al. Projected cancer risks from computed tomographic scans performed in the United States in 2007. *Archives of Internal Medicine* **169**, 2071–7 (2009).

29. Smith-Bindman, R. et al. Radiation dose associated with common computed tomography examinations and the associated lifetime attributable risk of cancer. *Archives of Internal Medicine* **169**, 2078–86 (2009).

30. National Academy of Sciences. Health Risks from Exposure to Low Levels of Ionizing Radiation: BIER VII – Phase 2 (Executive Summary). 2 (2006).

31. Pearce, M. S. et al. Radiation exposure from CT scans in childhood and subsequent risk of leukaemia and brain tumours: A retrospective cohort study. *Lancet* **6736**, 1–7 (2012).

32. American College of Radiology. *Dose Index Registry.* At www.acr.org/Quality-Safety/National-Radiology-Data-Registry/Dose-Index-Registry.

33. Lukasciewicz, A. & Moore, C. L. Radiation dose index of renal colic protocol CT studies in the United States: A report from the American College of Radiology National Radiology Data Registry. *Radiology* (2014). At http://pubs.rsna.org/doi/full/10.1148/radiol.14131601.

34. Niemann, T., Kollmann, T. & Bongartz, G. Diagnostic performance of low-dose CT for the detection of urolithiasis: A meta-analysis. *AJR. American Journal of Roentgenology* **191**, 396–401 (2008).

35. Bhuiya, F. A., Pitts, S. R. & McCaig, L. F. Emergency department visits for chest pain and abdominal pain: United States, 1999–2008. *NCHS Data Brief* 1–8 (2010). At www.ncbi.nlm.nih.gov/pubmed/20854746.

36. Redberg, R. F. Radiation minimization strategies for medical imaging. *JAMA Internal Medicine* **173**, 2014 (2013).

37. Benacerraf, B. R., McLoud, T. C., Rhea, J. T., Tritschler, V. & Libby, P. An assessment of the contribution of chest radiography in outpatients with acute chest complaints: A prospective study. *Radiology* **138**, 293–9 (1981).

38. Moore, C. L., Molina, A. & Lin, H. Ultrasonography in community emergency departments in the United States: Access to ultrasonography performed by consultants and status of emergency physician-performed ultrasonography. *Annals of Emergency Medicine* **47**, 147–53 (2006).

39. Labovitz, A. J. et al. Focused cardiac ultrasound in the emergent setting: A consensus statement of the American Society of Echocardiography and American College of Emergency Physicians. *Journal of the American Society of Echocardiography* **23**, 1225–30 (2010).

40. Taylor, R. A. et al. Point-of-care focused cardiac ultrasound for the assessment of thoracic aortic dimensions, dilation, and aneurysmal disease. *Academic Emergency Medicine* **19**, 244–7 (2012).

41. Parker, M. S. et al. Female breast radiation exposure during CT pulmonary angiography. *AJR. American Journal of Roentgenology* **185**, 1228–33 (2005).

42. Kosowsky, J. M. Approach to the ED patient with "low-risk" chest pain. *mergency Medicine Clinics of North America* **29**, 721–7, vi (2011).

43. Jones, I. D. & Slovis, C. M. Pitfalls in evaluating the low-risk chest pain patient. *Emergency Medicine Clinics of North America* **28**, 183–201, ix (2010).

44. Einstein, A. J. & York, N. Effects of radiation exposure from cardiac imaging. *Journal of Antimicrobial Chemotherapy* **59**, 553–65 (2012).

45. Einstein, A. J., Tilkemeier, P., Fazel, R., Rakotoarivelo, H. & Shaw, L. J. Radiation safety in nuclear cardiology – current knowledge and practice: Results from the 2011 American Society of Nuclear Cardiology member survey. *JAMA Internal Medicine* **173**, 2013–15 (2014).

46. Weigold, W. G. Coronary computed tomography angiography in the emergency department: The high stakes game of low risk chest pain. *Journal of the American College of Cardiology* **61**, 893–5 (2013).

47. Hausleiter, J. et al. Estimated radiation dose associated with cardiac CT angiography. *JAMA* **301**, 500–507 (2009).

48. Ayaram, D. et al. Triple Rule-out computed tomographic angiography for chest pain: A diagnostic systematic review and meta-analysis. *Academic Emergency Medicine.* **20**, 861–71 (2013).

49. Wiener, R. S., Schwartz, L. M. & Woloshin, S. Time trends in pulmonary embolism in the United States. *Archives of Internal Medicine* **171**, 831–7 (2011).

50. Kline, J. Further illumination of the test threshold approach in the care of emergency department patients with symptoms of pulmonary embolism. *Annals of Emergency Medicine* **55**, 327–30 (2010).

51. Kline, J. et al. D-dimer threshold increase with pretest probability unlikely for pulmonary embolism to decrease unnecessary computerized tomographic pulmonary angiography. *Journal of Thrombosis and Haemostasis* **10**, 572–81 (2012).

52. Wells, P. S. et al. Excluding pulmonary embolism at the bedside without diagnostic imaging. *Ann Int Med*, **135**: 98–107 (2001).

53. Kabrhel, C. et al. Factors associated with positive D-dimer results in patients evaluated for pulmonary embolism. *Academic Emergency Medicine* **17**, 589–97 (2010).

54. Venkatesh, A. et al. Evaluation of pulmonary embolism in the emergency department and consistency with a national quality measure: Quantifying the Opportunity for Improvement. *Archives of Internal Medicine* **1** (2012). doi:10.1001/archinternmed.2012.1804

55. Kline, J. *et al.* Prospective multicenter evaluation of the pulmonary embolism rule-out criteria. *Journal of Thrombosis and Haemostasis* **6**, 772–80 (2008).

56. Kocher, K. E. et al. National trends in use of computed tomography in the emergency department. *Annals of Emergency Medicine* **58**, 452–62 (2011).

57. Everhart, J. E., Khare, M., Hill, M. & Maurer, K. R. Prevalence and ethnic differences in gallbladder disease in the United States. *Gastroenterology* **117**, 632–9 (1999).

58. Privette, T. W., Carlisle, M. C. & Palma, J. K. Emergencies of the liver, gallbladder, and pancreas. *Emergency Medicine Clinics of North America* **29**, 293–317, viii–ix (2011).

59. Summers, S. M. et al. A prospective evaluation of emergency department bedside ultrasonography for the detection of acute cholecystitis. *Annals of Emergency Medicine* **56**, 114–22 (2010).

60. Jang, T. B. Bedside biliary sonography: Advancement and future horizons. *Annals of Emergency Medicine* **56**, 123–5 (2010).

61. Horn, A. E. & Ufberg, J. W. Appendicitis, diverticulitis, and colitis. *Emergency Medicine Clinics of North America* **29**, 347–68, ix (2011).

62. Parker, L. et al. Cost and radiation savings of partial substitution of ultrasound for CT in appendicitis evaluation: A national projection. *AJR. American Journal of Roentgenology* **202**, 124–35 (2014).

63. Martinez, J. P. & Mattu, A. Abdominal pain in the elderly. *Emergency Medicine Clinics of North America* **24**, 371–88, vii (2006).

64. Ernst, C. B. Current concepts: Abdominal aortic anuerysm. *New England Journal of Medicne* **328**, 1167–72 (1993).

65. Guirguis-Blake, J. M., Beil, T. L., Senger, C. A. & Whitlock, E. P. Ultrasonography screening for abdominal aortic aneurysms: A systematic evidence review for the U.S. Preventive Services Task Force. *Archives of Internal Medicine* **160**, 321–29 (2014).

66. U.S. Preventive Services Task Force. Screening for Abdominal Aortic Aneurysm. (2005). At www.uspreventiveservicestaskforce.org/uspstf/uspsaneu.htm.

67. Moore, C. L., Holliday, R. S., Hwang, J. Q. & Osborne, M. R. Screening for abdominal aortic aneurysm in asymptomatic at-risk patients using emergency ultrasound. *American Journal of Emergency Medicine* **26**, 883–7 (2008).

68. Stoker, J., VanRanden, A., Wytze, L. & Boermeester, M. A. Imaging patients with acute abdominal pain. *Radiology* **253**, 31–46 (2009).

69. Scales, C. D., Smith, A. C., Hanley, J. M. & Saigal, C. S. Prevalence of kidney stones in the United States. *European Urology* **62**, 160–5 (2012).

70. Moore, C. L., Daniels, B., Singh, D., Luty, S. & Molinaro, A. Prevalence and clinical importance of alternative causes of symptoms using a renal colic computed tomography protocol in patients with flank or back pain and absence of pyuria. *Academic Emergency Medicine* **20**, 470–8 (2013).

71. Moore, C. L. et al. Derivation and validation of a clinical prediction rule for uncomplicated ureteral stone – the STONE score: Retrospective and prospective observational cohort studies. *British Medical Journal* **348**, g2191 (2014).

72. Ghani, K. R. et al. Trends in surgery for upper urinary tract calculi in the USA using the Nationwide Inpatient Sample: 1999-2009. *BJU International* **112**, 224–30 (2013).

73. Strope, S., Wolf, J. S. & Hollenbeck, B. K. Changes in gender distribution of urinary stone disease. *Urology* **75**, 543–6, 546.e1 (2010).

74. Scales, C. D. et al. Changing gender prevalence of stone disease. *Journal of Urology* **177**, 979–82 (2007).

75. Sierzenski, P. R. et al. Applications of justification and optimization in medical imaging: Examples of clinical guidance for computed tomography use in emergency medicine. *Annals of Emergency Medicine* 1–8 (2013). doi:10.1016/j.annemergmed.2013.08.027

76. Ha, M. & MacDonald, R. D. Impact of CT scan in patients with first episode of suspected nephrolithiasis. *Journal of Emergency Medicine* **27**, 225–31 (2004).

77. Coursey, C. A. et al. ACR appropriateness criteria acute onset flank pain – suspicion of stone disease. *Ultrasound Quarterly* **28**, 227–33 (2012).

78. Moore, C. L. & Scoutt, L. Sonography first for acute flank pain? *Journal of Ultrasound Medicine* **31**, 1703–11 (2012).

79. Goertz, J. K. & Lotterman, S. Can the degree of hydronephrosis on ultrasound predict kidney stone size? *American Journal of Emergency Medicine* **28**, 813–6 (2010).

80. Jindal, G. & Ramchandani, P. Acute flank pain secondary to urolithiasis: Radiologic evaluation and alternate diagnoses. *Radiologic Clinics of North American* **45**, 395–410, vii (2007).

81. Moore, C., Meyers, A. B., Capotasto, J. & Bokhari, J. Prevalence of abnormal CT findings in patients with proven ovarian torsion and a proposed triage schema. *Emergency Radiology* **16**, 115–20 (2009).

82. National Center for Health Statistics. *Health, United States, 2012: With Special Feature on Emergency Care.* (2012). At www.cdc.gov/nchs/data/hus/hus12.pdf#087.

83. Korley, F. K., Pham, J. C. & Kirsch, T. D. Use of advanced radiology during visits. *JAMA* **304**, 1465–71 (2010).

84. Huber-Wagner, S. et al. Effect of whole-body CT during trauma resuscitation on survival: A retrospective, multicentre study. *Lancet* **373**, 1455–61 (2009).

85. Zondervan, R. L., Hahn, P. F., Sadow, C. A., Liu, B. & Lee, S. I. Body CT scanning in young adults: Examination indications, patient outcomes, and risk of radiation-induced cancer. *Radiology* **267**, 460–9 (2013).

86. Healy, D. et al. Systematic review and meta-analysis of routine total body CT compared with selective CT in trauma patients. *Emergency Medicine Journal* **31**, 101–8 (2014).

87. Gupta, M. et al. Selective use of computed tomography compared with routine whole body imaging in patients with blunt trauma. *Annals of Emergency Medicine* **58**, 407–16, e15 (2011).

88. Diercks, D. B. et al. Clinical policy: Critical issues in the evaluation of adult patients presenting to the emergency department with acute blunt abdominal trauma. *Annals of Emergency Medicine* **57**, 387–404 (2011).

89. Scalea, T. M. et al. Focused assessment with sonography for trauma (FAST): Results from an International Consensus Conference. *Journal of Trauma* **57**, 466–72 (1999).

90. Niska, R., Bhuiya, F. & Xu, J. National Hospital Ambulatory Medical Care Survey: 2007 emergency department summary. *National Health Statistics Report.* 1–31 (2010). At www.ncbi.nlm.nih.gov/pubmed/20726217.

91. Devries, A. et al. CT scan utilization patterns in pediatric patients with recurrent headache. *Pediatrics* (2013). doi:10.1542/peds.2012–3862.

92. Kuppermann, N. et al. Identification of children at very low risk of clinically-important brain injuries after head trauma: A prospective cohort study. *Lancet* **374**, 1160–70 (2009).

93. Saber Tehrani, A. S. et al. Rising annual costs of dizziness presentations to U.S. emergency departments. *Academic Emergency Medicine* **20**, 689–96 (2013).

94. Stiell, I. G. et al. The Canadian CT Head Rule for patients with minor head injury. *Lancet* **357**, 1391–6 (2001).

95. Haydel, M. J. et al. Indications for computed tomography in patients with minor head injury. *New England Journal of Medicine* **343**, 100–105 (2000).

96. Melnick, E. R. et al. CT overuse for mild traumatic brain injury. *The Joint Commission Journal on Quality and Patient Safety* **38**, 483–9 (2012).

97. Friedman, B. W. & Grosberg, B. M. Diagnosis and management of the primary headache disorders in the emergency department setting. *Emergency Medicine Clinics of North America* **27**, 71–87, viii (2009).

98. Jordan, J. E. ACR appropriateness criteria: Headache. *American Journal of Neuroradiology* **28**, 1824–6 (2007).

99. Edlow, J., Panagos, P. D., Godwin, S., Thomas, T. L. & Decker, W. W. Clinical policy: Critical issues in the evaluation and management of adult patients presenting to the emergency department with acute headache. *Annals of Emergency Medicine* **52**, 407–36 (2008).

100. Hahn, S., Lavonas, E. J., Mace, S. E., Napoli, A. M. & Fesmire, F. M. Clinical policy: Critical issues in the initial evaluation and management of patients presenting to the emergency department in early pregnancy. *Annals of Emergency Medicine* **60**, 381–90, e28 (2012).

101. Moore, C. & Promes, S. B. Ultrasound in pregnancy. *Emergency Medicine Clinics of North America* **22**, 697–722 (2004).

102. Moore, C., Todd, W. M., O'Brien, E. & Lin, H. Free fluid in Morison's pouch on bedside ultrasound predicts need for operative intervention in suspected ectopic pregnancy. *Academic Emergency Medicine* **14**, 755–8 (2007).

103. Andersen, B. & Nielsen, T. F. Appendicitis in pregnancy: Diagnosis, management and complications. *Acta Obstetricia et Gynecologica Scandinavica* **78**, 758–62 (1999).

104. Garcia-bournissen, F., Shrim, A. & Koren, G. Safety of gadolinium during pregnancy. *Canadian Family Physician* **52**, 309–11 (2006).

105. Revel, M. P. et al. Diagnostic accuracy of magnetic resonance imaging for an acute pulmonary embolism: Results of the "IRM-EP" study. *Journal of Thrombosis and Haemostasis* **10**, 743–50 (2012).

Chapter

13

Special Populations
A. Old, not Neutered: A Sex and Gender-Based Approach to the Acute Care of Elders

Elena Kapilevich and Bruce Becker

The Case of Mrs. V, Part I

Mrs. V is an 81-year-old woman who is brought to the ED by her daughter. She has fallen a number of times in the past few months according to her daughter and has some bruises on her shins from "running into the dishwasher door." Today she complains of pain in her right wrist, which is ecchymotic, swollen, and tender. She has lived alone since the death of her husband six years ago. Her daughter is "worried about her." She has lost weight in the past few months and has stopped participating in a local church charity and other community activities that she used to organize. She is responsive and conversant in the ED and states that she is just so busy getting her house fixed up and tired from her chores that she can't even think of going out. When asked specifics about the housework, she is vague about the details, makes a joke about the forgetfulness of old age, and is a bit defensive, stating "I think I'm doing pretty well for my age." She is thin but alert and oriented x 3, and, except for a tender, ecchymotic wrist, her PE is fairly unremarkable. The daughter comes out of the room to speak to you in the hallway: "She is not herself. She was always so energetic. I don't think she should be living alone anymore."

Introduction: Demographics and Variations in Longevity

On January 1, 2011, the first baby boomer turned 65, initiating a demographic upshift of epic proportions. There are more than 77 million baby boomers living in the United States, all of whom were born between 1946 and 1964. In 2010 according to the US Census Bureau, more than 40 million Americans, 13% of the population, were older than age 65. One out of every eight Americans was now "old." By 2035, one of every five will be old, and by 2050 this number will climb to almost 90 million. Among those already considered old, the proportion of people celebrating their 84th birthday is increasing at a rate three times greater than the rate of those boomers passing 64, the historical standard "retirement age" (Pleis, 2009) Demographic America is aging rapidly with substantial economic, social, and medical implications.

In most parts in the world, women live longer than men. This gender gap is most pronounced in industrialized nations such as the United States and Canada, where life expectancy rose dramatically during the twentieth century. This rise was the result of effective public health interventions, including vaccination, water and sewage treatment, and improvements in medical care, directly reducing perioperative, peri-partum, perinatal, and infant mortality. In the United States today, women outlive men by approximately 5.3 years (80.1 to 74.8 years). The younger men are succumbing to childhood diseases, traumatic injuries, homicide, and substance abuse at a higher rate than their female counterparts. Men are twice as likely as women to die from heart disease, 20% more likely to die from stroke, and more likely to perish from cirrhosis of the liver and cancer (Regan, 2013). Men have greater mortality rates than women for all the leading causes of death in the United States (Kramarow, 2007). These higher rates contribute to the changing relationship of gender to longevity for men and women. The "gender gap" is typically widest at birth and throughout young adulthood. Men have a greater infant mortality and, interestingly, are more likely to die *in utero* than women (Matthews 2010). Genetic factors seem to contribute to this disparity.

This gender gap in life expectancy narrows as men and women age. The longevity of men surviving to 65 approaches that of women; those men who reach 75 will have a lifespan equal to their female counterparts.

Currently, women make up 60% of adults older than age 65, and 70% of all those older than age 85. The remaining life expectancy of those women who survive to age 85 is an additional six years (Kramarow, 2007; Regan 2013). The life expectancy for women in many developed countries has already increased so much in the past century that most of the improvement in longevity expected in future decades will be seen in men. A number of biologic, socioeconomic, developmental, and cultural factors support women's advantage in mortality rates. Hormonal differences are primarily responsible for women's longevity, particularly the opposing effects of estrogen and testosterone on lipids and, subsequently, vasculature and vascular disease. Testosterone is known to raise LDL and lower HDL, while estrogen has the opposite effect (Pinkhasov 2010). Estrogen is also thought to protect the vascular endothelium, a benefit that persists in women for years after menopause. These differences in lipid profiles and vascular endothelial damage may account for the delayed onset of cardiovascular disease and higher median age of death from cardiovascular diseases in women, who, on average, develop cardiovascular disease 10 years later than men. Testosterone, on the other hand, may have immunosuppressant effects, leaving men more susceptible to infectious diseases and accounting for men's higher rates of death from infections (Hubbard 2011).

Smoking is a major contributor to morbidity and mortality; men are more likely than women to be current or former smokers, although this gender gap is rapidly closing. Among older men who are alive today, a greater proportion smoked at some point in their lives than older women; consequently, the likelihood of men's dying from smoking-related cancers and smoking-related cardiopulmonary disease is greater. Men and women have similar death rates from their own gender-specific malignancies such as prostate, breast, and ovarian cancer, thus supporting the theory that cancer mortality is likely unrelated to gender-specific hormonal factors or biological differences (Lasithiotakis, 2008, Underwood, 2006).

Geriatric Care in the Emergency Department

Older adults make up a large proportion of patients seeking treatment in the Emergency Department in the United States, with almost 30% of individuals older than age 75 reporting an ER visit in the past year, as compared to less than 20% of those who are younger. Furthermore, ED usage by the "old" (65–85), and the "oldest-old" (>85) is increasing. As the population of elders increases in the next few decades, the number of ED visits attributed to their demographic is expected to rise proportionately. Between 1993 and 2003, ED visits for patients ages 65–74 increased by 34% (Roberts, 2008). Between 2005 and 2010, ED visits by the old increased by 26%, and by 46% by the oldest-old. The incidence rate for ED visits by the oldest-old was twice that of the old, and they were more likely to have longer ED throughput times and greater hospital admission rates (Vilpert, 2013).

This dramatic upward trend has many implications for emergency medicine providers: Diagnosis, treatment, and dispositions for these elder patients are often vastly different from the approach that providers choose for younger patients. Geriatric patients have a higher prevalence of overlapping comorbidities, polypharmacy, adverse drug effects and drug-drug interactions, cognitive deficits, osteoporosis, and a distinctive subset of medical conditions and injury patterns. Elders come to the ED with higher acuity complaints and are more likely to be hospitalized for their complaints (LaCalle, 2010).

Adverse drug reactions were the cause of ED visits in almost 8% of patients older than age 65 in one study (Sikdar, 2010). After an ED visit, older patients are at much higher risk than younger individuals for functional decline, depression, and an overall deterioration of the quality of their lives. This is reflected in ED returns data. Patients with the highest one-year return rate (>10 visits) were most likely to be men older than age 65 (Moore, 2009). Apart from having a higher admission rate, older patients (especially men) are also more likely to have complications during their admission, to require ICU care, and to have longer hospital stays overall (Donnan, 2008; Kozal 2006). Because older women outnumber older men, they make up a larger proportion of geriatric patients living in nursing homes and assisted living facilities, seeking treatment in Emergency Departments and being admitted for inpatient care to hospitals. Thus, health care providers and facilities that provide acute care must have a broad understanding of the sex and gender issues that influence the acute medical care of these patients.

Delirium, Dementia, and Neuropsychiatric Disorders

Almost 25% of elders treated in Emergency Departments have altered mental status as a result of dementia, delirium, or both (Hustey, 2002; Jacqmin-Gadda, 2013). The incidence of dementia in these patients is directly proportional to their age, increasing from 12.7% per year in the 90- to 94-year-old age group, to 21.2% per year in the 95- to 99-year-old age group, to 40.7% per year in the 100+ age group (Corrada, 2010). Some of these elder patients who present to the ED with cognitive deficits are at their baseline level of functioning; for others, however, their altered mental status represents a subacute or acute deterioration precipitated by the emergent medical condition or injury for which they were seeking treatment. The ability of the clinician to obtain an accurate history and physical examination in the ED can often be limited. Moreover, the ED visit only represents one point in the timeline of the patient's life. Since it is difficult to ascertain the baseline, the degree of acute alteration and the exact cause for the impairment can be difficult to discern. Altered mental status in elder patients contributes to prolonged ED stays, increased use of imaging studies, and delays in diagnosis and disposition, which lead ineluctably to the increased rate of admissions that is commonly seen in this elder patient population.

It has long been suggested that women have a higher rate of dementia than men, particularly the dementia of Alzheimer's disease (AD). Since women have a longer life expectancy than men, and the risk for AD increases with age, this association does not seem to be particularly surprising. Researchers have reported that the risk for developing AD is consistently greater in women, a finding highlighted in a meta-analysis of four European population-based studies from the 1990s (Andersen, 1995; Azad 2007). Several explanations have been proposed for this observation. One focuses on anatomical differences between men's and women's brains: Women have a lower volume of gray matter, a thinner cortex, and decreased brain weight, findings that have been correlated with cognitive deficits and a greater incidence of dementia (Luders, 2002; Ikram, 2010). Another explanation focuses on the fact that men have a higher cognitive reserve than women; this reserve may support the delayed onset of dementia and cognitive decline. The cognitive reserve in men is a result of multiple socioeconomic factors: In the past, men have achieved a higher overall level of education and have worked at more cognitively challenging jobs (Stern, 2010; Letenneur, 2000). Women now surpass men in their level of education and are garnering more cognitively challenging jobs; thus, if these factors are at work, the gender gap in the prevalence of AD should close or even reverse. Other hypotheses suggest the influence of sex-specific hormones on the development of AD and gender bias in diagnostic work-ups, which may lead to a falsely increased prevalence or earlier diagnosis in women. Aside from increasing age, other risk factors for the development of dementia are sex specific. Among men, heart failure, Parkinson's disease, a family history, and mild depression were significant risk factors, while among women both mild and severe depression, increased fasting blood sugar, and a BMI <24 were significantly associated with AD (Noale, 2013).

The issue of gender and dementia remains controversial. Several recent studies, controlling for life expectancy, level of education, and cardiovascular risk factors, reported equivalent rates of AD and vascular dementia by gender. The literature also suggests that in patients with AD, male gender is associated with a greater mortality (Todd, 2013). But this too remains controversial. It may very well be that there are more women with dementia today simply because there is positive selective pressure favoring the survival of women; men die before they develop AD. A further confounding factor is that men who develop AD have a shorter lifespan than women with AD (Chene, 2014). Clearly these issues await further research.

Delirium is an acute alteration in sensorium or a change in cognition with a waxing and waning of consciousness. Delirium is a significant problem seen in patients in Emergency Departments, inpatient wards, ICUs, and nursing homes. Up to 10% of older ED patients are diagnosed with delirium. Approximately 1.5 million older patients with delirium will be evaluated in the ED each year in the United States (Han, 2009; Elie, 2000).

Delirium complicates up to 20% of hospital admissions for patients >65 and can lead to significant delays in treatment and soaring health care costs (Inouye, 2006). In the oldest-old, delirium was also associated with worsening dementia severity (OR 3.1, 95% CI, 1.5–6.3) as well as deterioration in global function score (OR 2.8, 95% CI, 1.4–5.5) (Davis, 2012). Delirium can often mask underlying medical problems and lead to difficulties in diagnosis: A delirious patient can rarely provide a useful history or participate in a meaningful physical examination. Delirium itself may be difficult to recognize, as it may fluctuate in severity over time. Delirium may be the only presenting symptom of a number of serious medical conditions such as sepsis, stroke, intracranial hemorrhage, or MI. Thus prompt recognition, diagnosis, and treatment of the underlying condition may be lifesaving. Delirium in older ED patients is an independent predictor of increased six-month mortality. Unfortunately, as many as 50% of patients presenting with delirium have a preexisting dementia, making the differentiation between the two entities problematic for emergency medical clinicians caring for these patients (Kakuma, 2003). Delirium in elders is misdiagnosed by emergency medicine practitioners in up to 75% of cases (Hustey, 2003). Many studies demonstrate the association of delirium with prolonged hospital stay, the need for institutionalization, and an overall increase in mortality in elderly patients, reinforcing the importance of early recognition and treatment. The risk factor most strongly associated with delirium is preexisting dementia, followed by medical illness, alcohol abuse, and depression (Elie, 2000). While these conditions have clear gender specificity, research focusing on the presentation and diagnosis of delirium in the ED has not focused on gender at all. This area of clinical significance has great research potential.

Gender differences have been demonstrated in postoperative delirium, a condition that is more common among elderly patients, with incidence rates as great as 55% depending on the type and duration of surgical procedure (Allen, 2012; Ansaloni, 2010). Longer and more critical surgery is associated with greater rates of delirium. In a study of orthopedic surgery patients, men were twice as likely as women to suffer from postoperative delirium after hip fracture repair (Endo, 2005). Additionally, those men were more likely to exhibit the hyperactive form of delirium with signs of aggression and over-agitation, requiring the use of antipsychotic medications with their attendant side effects and morbidity. Women with preoperative dementia were more likely to suffer postoperative delirium, while men *without* preoperative dementia had a greater incidence of delirium (Lee, 2011). Women also have the additional risk factors of greater age and lower BMI; consequently, women treated acutely for hip fractures should be evaluated for dementia; clinicians should be prepared for early diagnosis and intervention of acute postoperative delirium in women who screened positive.

Mental illness in elders is common and contributes to significant morbidity and increased risk of mortality, especially when associated with other comorbid conditions. Psychiatric illness in older adults is often unrecognized and, even when properly diagnosed, often undertreated. Inadequately treated psychiatric illness in elderly patients can lead to a lower overall quality of life, increased use of medical resources, frequent ED visits, and institutionalization (Katon, 2003; Licht-Strunk, 2009). The patient's family, the primary care provider, or the patient him- or herself may mistake the early, subtle signs and symptoms of psychiatric illness in elders for normal aging or dementia. The provider must remember that even though elders often experience an increase in the frequency and severity of chronic and acute illness, a decrease in functional status, and the premature loss of loved ones and friends, the development of depression or other mental illness is never a "normal" or acceptable consequence of these events.

The three most common major psychiatric disorders encountered in elderly patients are depression, bipolar disorder, and schizophrenia. Late onset depression is the most common geripsychiatric disorder. This diagnosis includes those patients who have had a past (even distant) history of depression who now present with a depressive episode, and others who develop their first depressive episode after the age of 65. Clinically significant depressive symptoms affect between 8% and 20% of elders (65+) and are associated with increased morbidity (Barry, 2008). In a study by Luppa, 38.2% of patients older than age 75 reported symptoms on a commonly used instrument (the CES_D) consistent with depression. Depressive symptoms in these patients were significantly associated with divorced or widowed marital status, low educational level, poor self-rated health status, functional impairment, mild cognitive impairment, stressful life events, and poor social network (Luppa, 2012).

Depression in elders (as in their younger peers) is more common in women. Elder women who are not depressed are more likely than men to become depressed and are more likely to remain depressed; depressed women are less likely to receive aggressive pharmacologic treatment but are also less likely to die while depressed (Barry, 2008). More than 7% of women older than age 65 have clinically significant major depression (McGuire, 2006) and up to 12% have symptomatic depressive disorders (Luppa, 2012). This high prevalence has important medical implications, as depression in this demographic group is correlated with an increased frequency of falls, a greater probability of an unhealthy BMI, a greater overall likelihood of ED and outpatient visits, and a higher incidence of fractures.

Several factors may account for this gender discrepancy. Men are less commonly diagnosed with depression than women. Elder men present differently, often coming to medical attention because of anger, agitation, anhedonia, withdrawal, or apathy. Men are less likely to acknowledge or admit feelings of sadness. Men with nondysphoric depression showed overall poorer long-term outcomes and an increased risk of

death at 13-year follow-up than women (Marcus 2005; Crossett, 2004). Men were also less likely to seek help for their symptoms from a physician or mental health professional and had higher successful suicide rates than women (Callanan, 2012). While adults >65 make up 13% of the total population, they account for 24% of completed suicides in the United States. White men older than age 85 have the highest rate of successful suicides with an incidence of 55 per 100,000. Most were in their first episode of depression at the time of successful suicide (Yeates, 2002).

Bipolar disorder and schizophrenia account for a significant proportion of mentally ill older adults. Unlike younger bipolar patients, whose prevalence is roughly equal among men and women, geriatric patients with bipolar disorder tend to be mostly female – approximately 69% according to an epidemiologic review of 17 studies (Depp, 2004). Similarly, women account for the majority of patients presenting with late onset schizophrenia and schizophrenia-like psychosis, with a ratio of approximately 3:2 women to men. This finding is vastly different from that of younger cohorts, in which men with new onset schizophrenia predominate at a ratio of 1.4:1 (Howard, 2000; Haffner, 2003)). One interpretation is that women are more predisposed to psychiatric illness later in life; however, the ratio of women to men increases with age. It could simply be that female longevity accounts for this age discrepancy. Regardless, it is important to suspect, identify, and diagnose psychiatric illness in elderly patients and make appropriate referrals for evaluation to facilitate prompt effective treatment, ameliorating or avoiding adverse outcomes including the increased morbidity and mortality often associated with these disorders.

The Case of Mrs. V, Part II

Mrs. V has some concerning symptoms including avoidance of social activities (isolation), disinterest in leaving her home (anhedonia), "forgetfulness," a jocularity about her forgetfulness, weight loss (poor nutrition, vitamin and mineral deficiency, osteoporosis, occult malignancy), minor trauma (leaving the dishwasher door open), and falls. She has social risk factors: She is widowed, lives alone, and is female. In the ED, she should be screened for minimal cognitive impairment

(MCI), or early dementia, and depression. She screened positive on the CES-D for depression and a basic MSE revealed some deficits in recall and drawing tasks. Additional labs were obtained including a B12 and folate, thyroid stimulating hormone, and VDRL. The ED MD should inform her PCP that Mrs. V would benefit from an outpatient evaluation for depression. Her positive screen for MCI suggests that she is at higher risk for postoperative delirium should her wrist require operative intervention.

Traumatic Injuries

Trauma remains a major cause of morbidity and mortality among older adults. Patients older than age 65 account for almost 25% of all trauma patients; in fact, trauma has become the fifth leading cause of death within this population after cardiovascular, neoplastic, cerebrovascular, and pulmonary diseases. The elderly account for 5.9% of all injury-related ED visits. Their rate of injury increases rapidly after age 75; the prevalence of fractures and open wounds is up to five times greater for patients older than age 85 as compared to those between 65 and 75. Treating the injured elderly in the ED costs twice as much as treating younger patients. Elders are also twice as likely to require EMS transport and are five times more likely to require hospital and intensive care admission (Schwartz, 2005).

Every year, more than a third of all elderly sustain falls. Falls account for two-thirds of elders' accidental deaths, followed by motor vehicle accidents. Polypharmacy is a leading risk factor for elder falls, but only if the patient is taking one of the established fall risk-increasing drugs (diuretics, quinine and derivatives, or psychotropics) (Ziere, 2006). Additionally, the distinct anatomy and physiology of elder patients increase their susceptibility to trauma and predispose them to specific types of injury patterns. While both men and women are predisposed to fall injuries and subsequent hospitalizations, older women are more likely to fall than older men and account for approximately two-thirds of falls (Stevens, 2005). Falls increase dramatically with age; they are four to five times more likely to occur in elders older than age 85 as compared to those between the ages of 65 and 85. Women older than age 65

who fall are much more likely to be injured than those who are younger. Women were more likely than men to inform others of their fall. Not surprisingly, these women were more likely than men to seek treatment in an Emergency Department. They were also more likely to need hospitalization for their traumatic injuries. Nevertheless, if men required hospitalization, their length of stay for acute care and rehabilitation exceeded that of women, and they were less likely to return to their homes and independent living (Close, 2012). The types of sustained injuries, responses to treatment, and overall outcomes also differ between elderly men and women. For example, elder men were 43% less likely than women to have any kind of fracture and less than half as likely to have a hip fracture (Schwartz, 2005). They were also less likely to have a contusion but significantly more likely to have an open wound.

The reasons for elder women's increased rates of significant injury, ED use, and hospitalization from falls have not been fully elucidated and are difficult to explain, especially in light of women's decrease in physical activity with advancing age. Women are more likely to limit their physical activity as they age compared to men, probably in part due to their age-related greater fear of falling, often in the setting of osteoporosis. Older men (similar to younger men) tend to engage in higher risk behavior that is not in keeping with their actual physical and balancing skills (Etman, 2012). It has been well established that elders who live alone are more likely to sustain falls, and women who live alone were more likely to sustain falls than men living alone, women living with men, or women living with other women. The positive effect of social support is seen in elders of Hispanic ethnicity who have a reduced risk of fatal falls across all age and gender subgroups, likely reflecting the cultural values of *familia* (Landy, 2012). As women have historically outlived men, more older women are living, and living alone, who are at a greater risk for falls. Women's propensity to seek medical attention after a fall may also lead to a greater number of recorded injuries among women (Painter, 2009). From a preventive health perspective, both elder men and women who were treated in an ED for fall-related injuries had a higher likelihood of one or more previous ED visits in the prior year.

Furthermore, women with a history of Colles wrist fracture had a lifetime hip fracture risk of 13%. Those with spinal fracture had a risk of 15% as compared to the general population of elderly women, who had a rate of 9% (Haentjens, 2004). Thus, ED treatment for non-hip fracture injuries or illness can provide opportunities for identifying patients at risk for falls, implementing screening, and initiating falls prevention intervention programs to help prevent further serious or fatal injury.

Hip fractures, with an annual incidence of more than 200,000 cases and a cost of more than $10 billion, are the most expensive, morbid, and prevalent fractures among the elderly (Gerson, 2004; Braithwaite, 2003). A majority of elders sustaining these fractures lose significant function; six-month mortality approaches 20% and almost a quarter will require skilled nursing facility placement (Hawkes, 2006). The lifetime risk of hip fracture is about 14% for postmenopausal women and 6% for men (Kanis, 2008). Fracture rates are highest for white women and lowest for black men in all age groups more than age 70 (Trombetti, 2002).

The higher rates of fracture among women can be attributed to more frequent falls, longer life span, and lower bone mass and bone density. The higher prevalence of osteoporosis in elderly women contributes significantly to the greater incidence of injuries in women who do fall. Bone mass for both men and women peaks at age 30 and declines at a rate of approximately 0.5% per year for men and 1% per year for women (Schuit, 2004). The decline of estrogen during menopause further contributes to the rapid progression of osteopenia in this population, making them much more susceptible to fractures (Ensrud, 2007). Women who suffer hip fractures have lower body weight and are taller than those who do not and tend to have less soft tissue covering the hip; the average BMI for these women is <27 (Kanis, 2008).

Although women are almost twice as likely to sustain hip fractures than men, men with hip fractures have a higher mortality rate than women (15% at one month vs. 10%) and are twice as likely to die within the first year after sustaining this injury (Gerson, 2004; Trombetti, 2002). Male gender also seems to be an independent risk factor for postoperative complications such as pneumonia and heart failure in patients with hip fractures

(Roche, 2005). At the time of fracture, men tend to be older than women, suffer from more comorbid conditions, have diminished capacity for completing activities of daily living, and are more likely to live in a nursing home and to suffer from depression (Moore, 2009); these factors probably are responsible for the increased mortality. Although moderate drinking has not been demonstrated to increase the risk of hip fracture, heavy alcohol use has been associated with a higher incidence of hip fracture among men.

Depression, more prevalent in elderly women, is strongly associated with hip fractures. In a five-year study of all fractures among 7,518 older women, depressed women had a rate of hip fracture 40% higher than women who were not depressed (Forsen, 1999). This relationship has been attributed to the diminished bone density associated with depression from a decreased propensity to exercise, poor nutrition, alcohol and tobacco use, and the correlation of SSRI use with osteoporosis (Diem, 2007). Insomnia and anxiety can cause sleep deprivation, and pharmacologic treatment with anxiolytics, antidepressants, psychotropics, and sleep medications can result in difficulty concentrating, ignoring environmental hazards, impaired gait and reaction time, and balance disturbance, predisposing the patient to falls. Hormone replacement and calcium supplementation seem to lower the risk of hip fracture among depressed older women (Greenspan, 2003; Hlatky, 2002).

For survivors of hip fracture, disability remains a serious concern (Roche, 2005). Gender may be associated with outcome, as women are more likely to experience moderate disability and men to experience severe disability and increased mortality (Endo, 2005; Holt, 2008). Depression has been associated with delayed recovery and with lasting disability after hip fracture for both men and women. A prospective survey of 374 hip fracture patients hospitalized over a six-month period identified strong correlations between anxiety or depression and severe disability for both sexes (Bertram, 2011).

The Case of Mrs. V, Part III

While her trauma evaluation revealed only a Colles fracture, Mrs. V revealed that she has been having frequent falls. Elders are at increased risk for subdural hematomas, which can affect mental status mimicking MCI, anorexia leading to inadequate nutrition and weakness, and impaired balance resulting in additional falls. A CT brain scan was performed; it demonstrated cortical atrophy and no bleed. Mrs. V is at high risk for a hip fracture in the future; therefore, a falls prevention program with a home inspection for hazards would be helpful. Mrs. V should get be getting regular bone scans to assess bone density and osteoporosis especially in light of her weight loss and decreased physical activity. She should receive appropriate treatment if necessary as well as a nutritional assessment and dietary counseling with her daughter (who is the caregiver in this case).

A case manager evaluated Mrs. V in the ED to address her home living situation. During that conversation, Mrs. V revealed that her falls have been occurring at night while making her way to the bathroom. She reported, when asked, that she often had to get out of bed three to four times a night to urinate and that she went repeatedly during the day, with frequency, urgency, a constant sense of bladder discomfort, and occasional incontinence necessitating adult diapers, which were a source of great embarrassment to her. The case manager reported this to the physician who sent a urinalysis and culture and performed a post-void bladder scan to check residual volume, which was 175 cc.

Urinary Tract Symptoms: Retention, Incontinence, and Infection

While acute urinary retention is 10 times less common in women than men, chronic urinary retention and incomplete emptying, with post-void residual volumes exceeding 100 cc, can be found in more than a third of elderly women. In contra distinction to acute retention, which causes immediate and obvious morbidity, chronic retention may be asymptomatic and lead to recurrent UTI or urinary incontinence (Malik, 2014). Chronic urinary retention in women is associated with uterine prolapse, diabetes mellitus, polypharmacy, and frailty. Symptoms may begin subtly and progress slowly, unreported by patients who have decreased bladder sensation, cognitive

impairment or shame about their condition and go undiagnosed by health care providers. Retention often comes to medical attention when the elder presents with recurrent urinary tract infections or stress urinary incontinence (Mody, 2014). Women without any urinary symptoms who have two clean catch urine samples that grow out $< 10^5$ CFU/mL of the same bacteria are presumed to have asymptomatic bacteriuria and are "colonized." They are not infected and do not need antibiotic treatment (Nicolle, 2009).

Asymptomatic bacteriuria is present in 3.5% of women across all demographic groups and in up to 50% in women older than age 70 (Monane, 1995). Asymptomatic bacteriuria is considered to be benign in these women and can wax and wane. Thirty percent of these patients' urine samples obtained at six-month intervals demonstrated resolving bacteriuria and 30% of those whose cultures had been negative turned positive. Regardless of culture results, a significant percentage reported GU symptoms: urgency, incontinence, dysuria, and general symptoms including anorexia, fatigue, malaise, and weakness.

Elder women with physical disabilities who are chronically incontinent have a high prevalence of bacteriuria (43%) and pyuria (45%) (Lekan-Rutledge 2004). These women meet the laboratory criteria for UTI but often remain asymptomatic (Nicolle, 2006). In frail older adults who are institutionalized, there was significant association between laboratory-confirmed UTI and acute dysuria, change in character of urine, and change in mental status. Because subclinical bacteriuria and pyuria are common in elder women, using urine dipstick testing, UA, and urine culture to guide treatment is challenging.

Sensitivity and specificity for urinary dipstick testing to evaluate for leukocyte esterase, nitrites, or both vary in older adults by the age of study participants, clinical suspicion of UTI, and the chosen laboratory definition for UTI (i.e., bacteriuria alone, level of bacteriuria [>102–105CFU/mL], or bacteriuria plus pyuria). The sensitivity and specificity for a positive dipstick test in older patients with symptoms were 82% and 71%, respectively (Devillé, 2004). Other studies of elderly patients showed that the negative predictive value for dipstick testing ranges from 92% to 100% (Ducharme, 2007).

New dysuria is the most discriminating clinical finding in patients with symptomatic UTI. The practitioner should note the timing, severity, and location of symptoms; however, worsening frequency and urgency can occur in both UTI and urinary incontinence without infection. To make matters even more confusing, several randomized controlled trials found that 25% to 50% of women presenting with UTI symptoms will have recovered in one week without using antibiotics (Christiaens, 2002; Ferry, 2007).

Urinalysis and culture should not be routinely ordered for a patient with chronic nocturia or incontinence. These studies should be done for patients with fever, acute dysuria, new or worsening urinary urgency, frequency, new urinary incontinence, gross hematuria, and suprapubic or costovertebral angle pain or tenderness. In a cognitively impaired patient, persistent change in mental status and change in character of the urine not responsive to other interventions (i.e., hydration) suggests the need for urine studies (Mody, 2014).

Local resistance rates, adverse side-effect profile, patient comorbidities, and urinary pathogens, if known, will guide therapy. Among community-dwelling elderly women, *E. coli* is the predominant pathogen, followed by *Klebsiella pneumoniae*, *Proteus mirabilis*, and *Enterococcus faecalis* (Linhares, 2013).

Fluoroquinolone resistance is most common in women ≥65 (Zhanel, 2005). Between 2005 and 2009, the incidence of *E. coli* isolates resistant to fluoroquinolone and fluoroquinolones plus trimethoprim-sulfamethoxazole more than doubled in women ≥80 (Swami, 2012). Extended-spectrum β-lactamase-producing gram-negative pathogens highly resistant to penicillin-clavulanate, ciprofloxacin, and trimethoprim-sulfamethoxazole have been cultured from urine in community-dwelling and institutionalized elderly women with acute UTI. Nitrofurantoin and fosfomycin remain effective against these bacteria (Meier, 2011). Nitrofurantoin is a safe choice in patients with creatinine clearance ≥40 mL/min. This antibiotic is primarily concentrated and excreted in the urine with low plasma concentrations, low rates of antibiotic resistance, and excellent cost effectiveness; it is a great choice for cystitis in elderly women who retained normal kidney function (Bains, 2009;

Oplinger, 2013; McKinnell, 2011). Pulmonary toxicity has been reported for nitrofurantoin; thus women taking this medication with new onset pulmonary complaints need careful evaluation. Fosfomycin should be considered in elderly women who fail nitrofurantoin therapy or in those whose culture results suggest resistance.

The most effective duration of antibiotic administration for elderly women remains controversial. A review of 15 studies involving 1,644 women showed no difference in UTI treatment failure rates between a short course (3–6 days) and a longer course (7–14 days) of oral antibiotic therapy. While patients preferred single dose therapy, persistent infection rates were significant (Lutters, 2008). Repeating urine cultures after treatment to document the successful eradication of infection is not recommended as asymptomatic recurrent and self-limited bacteriuria are common in elderly women. These women should be reevaluated for termination or persistence of urinary symptoms as the basis of determining clinical success (Mody, 2014).

Clinicians treating elderly women who present with urinary symptoms must ask about recent sexual intercourse and new partners. Sexual intercourse in these women has been associated with a higher incidence of symptomatic UTIs. It is important to remember that "honeymoon" cystitis is not limited by age of the patient and should not bias the practitioner. Sexually transmitted infections can also cause urinary symptoms in the absence of UTI, and testing should be performed where appropriate. Older baby boomers, no longer fertile and spurning the use of condoms, are a new and growing demographic for STIs (Moore, 2008). Multiple preventive interventions for these sexually active elderly women have been proposed but remain to be studied for effectiveness, including early postcoital voiding, liberalized fluid intake during the daytime hours, and postcoital antibiotic prophylaxis (Albert, 2004).

Several prophylactic approaches have been proposed in elderly women who are not taking medications promoting urinary retention and who do not have other GU pathology such as renal calculi, pelvic floor prolapse, or other structural bladder, intestinal, or reproductive organ pathology. Ingestion of cranberry juice or its active ingredients may be useful in elderly women with risk factors for UTI or a history of recurrent UTIs (Wang, 2012). Vaginal estrogen cream has been demonstrated to reduce the incidence of UTIs in elderly, postmenopausal women; however, oral estrogen was not effective (Perrotta, 2008).

The Case of Mrs. V, Conclusion

A clean catch was sent and revealed positive leukocyte esterase, positive nitrites, nine WBCs, squamous cells, and some bacteria. A culture was sent, no antibiotics were given, and Mrs. V was referred to her PCP for follow up in two to three days. A culture grew out mixed flora with 104 CFUs of *E. Coli*. She was told to drink two glasses of cranberry juice a day. Her PCP was informed of her elevated postvoid residual and urinary retention. She was subsequently referred to a urologist for urodynamic testing and further evaluation. She denied recent sexual activity and, in fact, seemed slightly embarrassed but made a joke about it. STI testing was not performed. An orthopedist was able to reduce and cast the fracture. She was given a sling, a Carter Pillow, and a follow-up appointment. She was discharged to the care of her daughter with the understanding that she would stay at her daughter's house until follow-up evaluations were performed including a home safety inspection.

Take Home Points

1) The population of elders is growing geometrically and women comprise the majority of ED and in-hospital patients.
2) Presentations for acute illness or injury often represent the tip of the iceberg or leading edge of a bevy of physical, psychological, social, and cognitive problems in the life of the geriatric patient.
3) Delirium is present in 50% of elderly ED patients and may be masked by the presence of dementia. It portends a worse prognosis and leads to an increase in admissions and longer hospital stays.
4) Chronic urinary retention, often asymptomatic and presenting itself with symptoms of urinary incontinence, significantly predisposes elderly women to recurrent urinary tract infections. However, asymptomatic bacteriuria and pyuria are common in older women, and routine urine testing is not indicated until development of *new* urinary symptoms.
5) Nitrofurantoin and fosfomycin are excellent antibiotic choices for treatment of symptomatic UTI in elderly women due to high rates of resistance and treatment failure with ciprofloxacin and trimethoprim-sulfamethoxazole.
6) The astute emergency medicine or acute care clinician must understand these issues, screen and test for the problems surrounding the chief complaint, arrange appropriate follow-ups, involve case managers, and negotiate with families to provide the most effective, safe care and disposition for their patients.

Areas for Future Research

1) Development of point-of-care approaches for differentiating urinary symptoms of incontinence and bladder retention from infection requiring antibiotic treatment in elderly women.
2) Point-of-care approaches to evaluating future fall risk: social, musculoskeletal, neurologic, domestic, and effective and acceptable approaches to falls prevention.
3) Causes of delirium and differences in outcomes between men and women who suffer from delirium in the hospital.
4) Usefulness of antibiotics for UTI prophylaxis in high-risk elderly women with frequent and resistant infections.
5) Trends in incidence of Alzheimer's disease and other types of dementia in men and women over the next 10 to 20 years.
6) Approach for bedside depression screening in elderly adults in the ER, and early psychiatric consults and interventions in suspected cases.

References

Albert X, Huertas I, Pereiro I, Sanfélix J, Gosalbes V, Perrotta. 2004. Antibiotics for preventing recurrent urinary tract infection in non-pregnant women (Review) *The Cochrane Library* 2004, Issue 3 http://www.thecochranelibrary.com.

Allen SR, Frankel HL. 2012. Postoperative complications: delirium. *Surg Clin North Am* **92**(2): 409–431.

Ansaloni L, Catena F, Chattat R, et al. 2010. Risk factors and incidence of postoperative delirium in elderly patients after elective and emergency surgery. *Brit J Surg* **97**(2): 273–280.

Azad NA, Bugami MA, Loy-English I. 2007. Gender differences in dementia risk factors. *Gender Med* **4**(2): 120–129.

Bains A, Buna D, and Hoag N. 2009. A Retrospective Review Assessing the Efficacy and Safety of Nitrofurantoin in Renal Impairment. *Can Pharm J / Revue des Pharmaciens du Canada* **142**(5): 248–252.

Bertram M, Norman R, Kemp L, Vos T. 2011. Review of the long-term disability associated with hip fractures. *Inj Prev* **17**: 365–370.

Braithwaite RS, Col NF, Wong JB. 2003. Estimating hip fracture morbidity, mortality and costs. *Am Geriatr Soc* **51**(3): 364–370.

Callanan VJ, Davis MS. 2012. Gender differences in suicide methods. *Soc Psych Psych Epid* **47**(6): 857–869.

Chene G, Beiser A, Au R, Preis SR, Wolf PA, Dufouil C, Seshadri S. 2013. Gender and incidence of dementia in the Framingham Heart Study from mid-adult life. *Alzheimer's Demen*: 1–11.

Close JC, Lord SR, Antonova EJ, et al. 2012. Older people presenting to the emergency department after a fall: a population with substantial recurrent healthcare use. *Emerg Med J* **29**(9):742–747.

Corrada MM, Brookmeyer R, Paganini-Hill A, Berlau D, Kawas CH. 2010. Dementia incidence continues to increase with age in the oldest old: the 90+ study. *Annals of Neurology* **67**(1):114–121.

Crossett JH. 2004. The best is yet to be: preventing, detecting, and treating depression in older women. *J Am Med Womens Assoc* **59**:210.

Depp CA, Jeste DV. 2004. Bipolar disorder in older adults: a critical review. *Bipolar Disord* **6**:343–367.

Deville WLJM, Yzermans JC, van Duijn NP, et al. 2004. The urine dipstick test useful to rule out infections. A meta-analysis of the accuracy. *BMC Urol* **4**:4.

Diem SJ, Blackwell TL, Stone KL et al. 2007. Use of antidepressants and rates of hip bone loss in older women: the study of osteoporotic fractures. *Arch Intern Med*. **167**(12):1240–1245.

Donnan PT, Dorward DW, Mutch B, Morris AD. Development and validation of a model for predicting emergency admissions over the next year (PEONY): a UK historical cohort study. *Arch Intern Med* **168**(13):1416–1422.

Ducharme J, Neilson S, and Ginn JL. 2007. Can urine cultures and reagent test strips be used to tract infection in elderly emergency department patients without focal urinary symptoms? *CJEM* **9**(02): 87–92.

Elie M, Rousseau F, Cole M, Primeau F, McCusker J, Bellavance F. 2000. Prevalence and detection of delirium in elderly emergency department patients; *CMAJ* **163**(8):977–981.

Endo, Yoshimi, et al. Gender differences in patients with hip fracture: a greater risk of morbidity and mortality in men. *J Orthop Trauma* **19**(1):29–35.

Ensrud KE, Ewing S, Taylor BC, et al. 2007. Frailty and risk of falls, fracture, and mortality in older women. the study of osteoporotic fractures. *J Gerontol A Biol Sci Med Sci* **62**(7):744–751.

Etman A, Wijlhuizen GJ, van Heuvelen MJ, Chorus A, Hopman-Rock M. 2012. Falls incidence underestimates the risk of fall-related injuries in older age groups: a comparison with the FARE (Falls risk by Exposure). *Age Ageing* **41**(2):190–195.

Gerson LW, Emond JA, Camargo CA, Jr. 2004. US emergency department visits for hip fracture, 1992–2000. *Eur Emerg Med* **11**(6):323–328.

Greenspan SL, Resnick NM, Parker RD. 2003. Combination therapy with hormone replacement and alendronate for prevention of bone loss in elderlywomen: a randomized controlled trial *JAMA* **289**(19):2525–2533.

Haentjens P, Johnell O, Kanis JA, et al. 2004. Evidence from data searches and life-table analyses for gender-related differences in absolute risk of hip fracture after Colles' or spine fracture: Colles' fracture as an early and sensitive marker of skeletal fragility in white men. *J Bone Miner Res* **19**(12):1933–1944.

Hafner H. 2003. Gender differences in schizophrenia. *Psychoneuroendocrino* **28**, Supplement 2:17–54.

Han JH, Zimmerman EE, Cutler N. 2009. Delirium in older emergency department patients: recognition, risk factors, and psychomotor subtypes. *Acad Emerg Med* 1069–6563 1553–2712 **16**(3):193–200.

Hawkes WG, Wehren L, Orwig D, et al. 2006. Gender differences in functioning after hip fracture. *J Gerontol Biol Sciences and Medical Sci* **61**(5):495–499.

Hlatky MA, Boothroyd D, Vittinghoff E. 2002. Quality-of-life and depressive symptoms in postmenopausal women after receiving hormone therapy: results from the Heart and Estrogen/Progestin Replacement Study (HERS) trial. *JAMA*. **287**(5):591–597.

Holt G, Smith R, Duncan K, et al. 2008. Gender differences in epidemiology and outcome after hip fracture: Evidence from the Scottish Hip Fracture Audit. *J Bone Joint Surg Br* **90**-B(4):480–483.

Howard R, Rabins PV, Seeman MV, Jeste DV 2000. Late-onset schizophrenia and very-late-onset schizophrenia-like psychosis: an international consensus. *Am J Psychiat*; **157**(2):172–178.

Hubbard RE, Rockwood K. 2011. Frailty in older women. *Maturitas 0378–5122 1873–4111* **69**(3):203–207.

Hustey FM, Meldon SW. 2002. The prevalence and documentation of impaired mental status in elderly emergency department patients. *Ann Emerg Med* 39:248–253.

Ikram MA, Vrooman HA, Vernooij MW, Heijer TD, Hofman A, Niessen WJ, et al. 2010. Brain tissue volumes in relation to cognitive function and risk of dementia. *Neurobiol Aging* 31:378–386.

Inouye SK. 2006. Delirium in older persons. *N Engl J Med* 354:1157–1165.

Jacqmin-Gadda H, Alperovitch A, Montlahuc C, et al. 20-Year prevalence projections for dementia and impact of preventive policy about risk factors. *Eur J Epidemiol* **28**(6):493–502.

Kakuma R, du Fort GG, Arsenault L, et al. 2003. Delirium in older emergency department patients discharged home: effect on survival. *J Am Geriatr Soc* **51**:443–450.

Kamalesh M, Shen J. Diabetes and peripheral arterial disease in men: trends in prevalence, mortality, and effect of concomitant coronary disease. *Clin Cardiol* **32**(8):442–446.

Kanis JA, Johnell O, Oden A, et al. 2008, FRAX™ and the assessment of fracture probability in men and women from the UK. *Osteoporosis Int* **19** (4):385–397.

Katon WJ, Lin E, Russo J, Unutzer J. 2003. Increased medical costs of a population-based sample of depressed elderly patients. *Arch Gen Psychiat* **60**:897.

Kozak LJ, DeFrances CJ, Hall MJ. 2006. National hospital discharge survey: 2004 annual summary with detailed diagnosis and procedure data. *Vital Health stat* 13 0083–2006 2333–0856 (162) pp. 1–209.

Kramarow E, Lubitz J, Lentzer H, Gorina Y. 2007. Trends in the health of older Americans. *Health Affairs* 26.5 1417–1425.

LaCalle E, Rabin E. 2010. Frequent users of emergency departments: the myths, the data, and the policy implications. *Ann Emerg Med* **56**(1):42–48.

Landy DC, Mintzer MJ, Silva AK, Dearwater SR, Schulman CI. 2012. Hispanic ethnicity and fatal fall risk: do age, gender, and community modify the relationship? *J Surg Res.* **175**(1):113–117.

Lasithiotakis K, Leiter U, Meier F 2008. Age and gender are significant independent predictors of survival in primary cutaneous melanoma. *Cancer 0008–543X 1045–7410* **112**(8):1795–1804.

Lekan-Rutledge D. 2004. Urinary incontinence strategies for frail elderly women. *Urologic Nursing* **24**(4)281–301.

Letenneur L, Launer LJ, Andersen K, Dewey ME, Ott A, Copeland JR, et al. 2000. Education and the risk for Alzheimer's disease: sex makes a difference. EURODEM Pooled Analyses. *Am J Epidemiol*; **151**(11):1064–1071.

Licht-Strunk E, Van Marwijk HW, Hoekstra T, et al. 2009. Outcome of depression in later life in primary care: longitudinal cohort study with three years' follow-up. *BMJ*; 338:a3079.

Luders E, Steinmetz H, Jancke L. 2002. Brain size and grey matter volume in the healthy human brain. *Neuro Report* 13:2371–2374.

Luppa M, Sikorski C, Luck T, et al. 2012. Prevalence and risk factors of depressive symptoms in latest life–results of the Leipzig Longitudinal Study of the Aged (LEILA 75+). *Int J Geriatr Psychiatry.* **27**(3):286–295.

Luppa M, Sikorski C, Luck T, et al. 2012. Age- and gender-specific prevalence of depression in latest-life–systematic review and meta-analysis. *J Affect Disord* **136**(3):212–221.

Lutters M, Vogt-Ferrier NB. 2008. Antibiotic duration for treating uncomplicated, symptomatic lower urinary tract infections in elderly women (Review); Cochrane review, prepared and maintained by The Cochrane Collaboration and published in *The Cochrane Library* 2008, Issue 3.

Marcus SM, Young EA, Kerber KB, et al. 2005. Gender differences in depression: Findings from the STAR*D study. *Affect Disorders* **87**(2–3):141–150.

Malik RD, Cohn JA, Bales GT. 2014. Urinary retention in elderly women: diagnosis & management, *lower urinary tract symptoms & voiding dysfunction. Curr Urol Rep* 15:454.

Mathews TJ, MacDorman MF. 2010. Infant mortality statistics from the 2006 period linked birth/infant death data set. *Nat Vital Statistics Rep* **58**(17).

McGuire LC, Strine TW, Vachirasudlekha S, Mokdad AH, Anderson LA. 2008. The prevalence of depression in older U.S. women: 2006 behavioral risk factor surveillance system. *J Womens Health (Larchmt)***17** (4):501–507.

McKinnell JA, Stollenwerk NS, Jung CW, and Miller LG. 2011. Nitrofurantoin compares favorably to recommended agents as empirical treatment of uncomplicated urinary tract Infections in a decision and cost analysis. *Mayo Clin Proc*, **86**(6): 480–488.

Moore EE, Hawes SE, Scholes D, et al. 2008. Sexual intercourse and risk of symptomatic urinary infection in post-menopausal women *J Gen Intern Med* **23**(5):595–599.

Mody L and Juthani-Mehta M. 2014. Urinary tract infections in older women: a clinical review. *JAMA* **311** (8):844–854.

Moore L, Deehan A, Seed P, Jones R. 2009. Characteristics of frequent attenders in an emergency department: analysis of 1-year attendance data. *Emerg Med J* **26**(4):263–267.

Nicolle LE. 2006. Asymptomatic bacteriuria: review and discussion of the IDSA guidelines. *Int Antimicrob Ag* **28**, Supplement 1:42–48.

Nicolle LE. 2009. Urinary tract infections in the elderly. *Clin Geriatr Med* **25**(3): 423–36.

Noale M, Limongi F, Zambon S, Crepaldi G, Maggi S. 2013. Incidence of dementia: evidence for an effect modification by gender. The ILSA Study. *Int Psychogeriatr* **25**(11):1867–1876.

Oplinger M, Andrews CO. 2013. Contraindication in patients with a creatinine clearance below 60 mL/min: looking for the evidence. *Ann Pharmacother* **47**(1) 106–111.

Painter JA, Elliott SJ, Hudson S. 2009. Falls in community-dwelling adults aged 50 years and older: prevalence and contributing factors. *J Allied Health* **38** (4):201–207.

Perrotta C, Aznar M, Mejia R, et al. 2008. Oestrogens for preventing recurrent urinary tract infection in postmenopausal women Editorial Group: Cochrane Kidney and Transplant Group Published Online: 23 April 2008.

Pinkhasov RM, Shteynshlyugen A, Hakimian P. 2010. Are men shortchanged on health? Perspective on life expectancy, morbidity, and mortality in men and women in the United States. *Int j Clin* **64**(4): 465–474.

Pleis JR, Lucas JW, Ward BW. 2009. Summary health statistics for U.S. adults: *National Health Interview Survey, 2008. Vital Health Stat. Series 10*, **242**:1–157.

Regan JC and Partridge L. 2013. Gender and longevity: Why do men die earlier than women? Comparative and experimental evidence. *Endocrinol Aging Male* **27**(4): 467–479.

Roberts DC, McKay MP, Shaffer A. 2008. Increasing rates of emergency department visits for elderly patients in the United States, 1993 to 2003. *Ann Emerg Med* 51:769–774.

Roche JJ, Wenn RT, Sahota O, Moran CG. 2005. Effect of comorbidities and postoperative complications on mortality after hip fracture in elderly people: prospective observational cohort study. *BMJ* 331:1374.

Schuit SCE, van der Klift M, Weel AEAM, et al. 2004. Fracture incidence and association with bone mineral density in elderly men and women: the Rotterdam Study. *Bone* **34**(1): 195–202.

Schwartz SW, Rosenberg DM, Wang CP, Sanchez-Anguiano A, Ahmed S. Demographic differences in injuries among the elderly: an analysis of emergency department visits. *J Trauma* **58**(2):346–352.

Sikdar KC, Alaghehbandan R, MacDonald D, et al. Adverse drug events in adult patients leading to emergency department visits. *Ann Pharmacother* **44** (4):641–649.

Stern Y. 2012. Cognitive reserve in ageing and Alzheimer's disease. *Lancet Neurol* 11:1006–12.

Stevens JA, E D Sogolow ED. 2005. Gender differences for non-fatal unintentional fall related injuries among older adults. *Injury Prevention* 11:115–119.

Swantek SS and Goldstein MZ. 2000. Practical geriatrics: age and gender differences of patients with hip fracture and depression. *Psychiatr Serv* **51** (12):1501–1503.

Todd S, Barr S, Roberts M, Passmore AP. Survival in dementia and predictors of mortality: a review. *Int J Geriatr Psychiatry* **28**(11):1109–1124.

Trombetti A, Herrmann P, Hoffmeyer MA, et al. 2002. Survival and potential years of life lost after hip fracture in men and age-matched women. *Osteoporosis Int* **13** (9): 731–737.

Underwood W, Dunn RL, Williams C. 2006. gender and geographic influence on the racial disparity in bladder cancer mortality in the US. *j Am Coll Surgeons 1072-7515 1879-1190* **202**(2): 284–290.

Vilpert S, Ruedin HJ, Trueb L, Monod-Zorzi S, Yersin B, Bula C. 2013. Emergency department use by oldest-old patients from 2005 to 2010 in a

Swiss university hospital. *BMC Health Serv Res* 13:344.

Wang CH, Fang CC, Chen NC, et al. 2012. Cranberry-containing products for prevention of urinary tract infections in susceptible populations: systematic review and meta-analysis of randomized controlled trials. *Arch Intern Med*; **172**(13):988–996.

Yeates C, Duberstein PR, and Caine ED. 2002. Risk Factors for Suicide Later in Life. *Biol Psychiat* **52**(3): 193–204.

Ziere G, Dieleman JP, Hofman A, Pols HA, van der Cammen TJ, Stricker BH. 2006. Polypharmacy and falls in the middle age and elderly population. *Br J Clin Pharmacol.* **61**(2):218–223.

Special Populations

B. Girls and Boys: Sex and Gender in Pediatrics

Therese L. Canares, Marleny Franco and George M. Lazarus

Introduction

There are many physiologic differences between boys and girls during childhood development. In this chapter, we present four cases that illustrate acute pediatric conditions in which sex affects pathophysiology, differential diagnosis, evaluation, or management. Although these cases do not delineate all of the sex differences impacting the clinical practice of pediatricians, they illustrate scenarios wherein sex and gender should be considered when planning the management of children who are acutely ill. It is essential that the practitioner understands these cases and develops an effective approach to diagnosis and treatment.

Case 1: Fever in an infant

An 11-month-old female presented with fever for 3 days to 39.1°C. Review of systems was positive only for rhinorrhea. Vital Signs: heart rate 130 beats per minute, respiratory rate 30 breaths per minute, blood pressure 100/70, O_2 saturation 99%, and rectal temperature 39.5°C. The infant cried but was consolable; the remainder of the exam was unremarkable.

Introduction

Fever without a source (FWS) is a common pediatric complaint in the acute care setting. FWS is defined as a fever that is not associated with signs or symptoms uncovered in the history or seen during the physical examination, indicating a diagnosis (e.g., viral upper respiratory infection, acute otitis media, gastroenteritis) (Baraff, 2008). Infants with FWS are at risk for serious bacterial illness, including urinary tract infection (UTI), bacteremia, pneumonia, or meningitis. As opposed to the other serious bacterial illnesses, risk factors for infants with UTI are affected by the sex of the patient. Therefore, an understanding of the influence of sex on UTI should

guide the clinician in the workup of the febrile infant. The following discussion will be applicable to febrile infants 3–24 months of age. Alternative guidelines apply for febrile infants less than 3 months of age and are not discussed here.

Prevalence and Risk Factors of UTI

Epidemiologic data highlight the difference in the prevalence of UTI by sex. The prevalence of UTI in all febrile infants with no source of fever is 5% (Baraff, 2008). However, the prevalence in girls is almost twice that seen in boys (6.5% vs. 3.3%), with a relative risk of 2.27 (Baraff, 2008; Subcommittee on Urinary Tract Infection et al., 2011).

Girls

Demographic and historical factors affect girls' risk for UTI. While developing clinical decision rules, one group of investigators found that the most sensitive predictors of UTI in febrile girls <24 months old were white race, age <12 months, fever >39°C, fever >2 days, and absence of other source of fever (Gorelick and Shaw, 2000). These risk factors have been validated as a screening tool and adapted by the American Academy of Pediatrics (AAP) (Subcommittee on Urinary Tract Infection et al., 2011).

Behavioral factors such as bathroom habits and hygiene also influence girls' risk for UTIs. A study of girls ages 5–17 identified independent risk factors for recurrent UTIs, including abnormal voiding frequency, voiding postponement, functional stool retention, normal to large bladder capacity, poor fluid intake, and residual urine (Rudaitis et al., 2009).

Boys

Age and circumcision status affect boys' risk of UTI. A study of all children <2 years presenting with their first UTI found that boys with their first UTIs are significantly younger than girls (mean ages: boys 6 months vs. girls 10 months, p<0.001) (Hansson et al., 1999). In children of all ages, uncircumcised, febrile males <3 months of age had the highest prevalence of UTIs of any group, male or female. The increased prevalence of UTI <3 months is supported by other epidemiologic studies that document that the highest rates of UTI occur in the first month of life (Shaikh et al., 2008).

Some of the anatomical differences that decrease the risk of UTIs in boys (and men) are the increased distance between the anus and the urethral meatus, the drier environment surrounding the male urethra, the increased length of the urethra, and the antibacterial activity of prostatic fluid (Lipsky, 1989).

Circumcision lowers the risk of UTI in boys (Craig et al., 1996; Singh-Grewal et al., 2005; Subcommittee on Urinary Tract Infection et al., 2011). A meta-analysis of boys with UTI found the prevalence in uncircumcised versus circumcised male infants <3 months was 20.1% versus 2.4% (Shaikh et al., 2008). Circumcision also reduces relative risk of admission for UTI in boys <12 months (To et al., 1998).

Reflux

Vesicoureteral reflux (VUR) is an important risk factor for UTIs, although VUR often is not detected until the patient develops her or his first UTI. Vesicoureteral reflux is more prevalent in infant girls than boys with first UTI (36% vs. 24%, respectively) (Hansson et al., 1999). This difference extends beyond infancy. A study of children ages 0–21 with first UTI found that girls were nearly twice as likely as boys to have VUR (OR 1.88) (Chand et al., 2003).

Posterior urethral valves (PUV) are a common cause of VUR in boys, and also a risk factor for development of UTI. Boys with PUV who are circumcised are eight times less likely to develop a UTI (Mukherjee et al., 2009). With or without PUV, boys with VUR who are circumcised have reduced rates of recurrent UTI (Singh-Grewal et al., 2005).

Diagnosis of UTI

In febrile infants of either sex, the risk of UTI is high, and the clinician must decide which patients require urinary testing as part of a complete work-

Table 13B.1 Guidelines for Diagnostic Testing of Infants With Fever without a Source (FWS) (Adapted from Baraff, 2008)

Infants >3 Months of Age, FWS >39°C, Received HIB & PCV-7 Vaccines
Obtain urinalysis (or "urine dip") and urine culture for: • all females and uncircumcised males <24 months • circumcised males <6 months • all infants with history of prior UTI

up. Guidelines followed by most pediatricians when faced with infants >3 months with fever without a source are listed in Table 13B.1.

Further recommendations are elaborated in the AAP clinical practice guidelines for febrile infants with UTI (Subcommittee on Urinary Tract Infection et al., 2011). The AAP found that the quality of evidence for obtaining a sterile urine culture by catheterization or suprapubic aspiration prior to starting antibiotics in both girls and boys with FWS was robust, and that urine cultures obtained from urine that had been collected using a bag had an unacceptably high false positive rate. These guidelines also recommend that if the clinician determines that a child is well appearing and antibiotics are withheld, well-defined risk factors can help predict the probability of a UTI (Table 13B.2). This probability can then guide the clinician's decisions about whether to obtain a sterile urine culture, to obtain a urinalysis bag specimen followed by sterile urine culture if urinalysis is abnormal, or to utilize clinical follow-up monitoring without testing. To diagnose a UTI, urinalysis should demonstrate pyuria and/or bacteriuria and the urine culture should grow at least 50,000 single species bacterial colony-forming units per milliliter (cfu/mL).

The most common pathogens causing UTIs in children are *E. coli*, *Proteus*, *Klebsiella*, *Enterobacter*, *Pseudomonas*, and *Enterococcus*. A multi-institutional study found that in children <18 years, the prevalence of *E. coli* is higher in girls (83%) than in boys (50%), p<0.001. All of the other pathogens causing UTIs had higher prevalence in boys than in girls (Edlin et al., 2013).

A number of virulence factors of *E. coli* strains in UTI have been identified with a clear sex predilection. P-fimbriated strains (mediators of

Table 13B.2 Probability of UTI in Infants with FWS (Adapted from Subcommittee on Urinary Tract Infection et al., 2011)

Risk Factor	Probability of UTI	Number of Factors Present	
Girls		≤1	
• white race	≤1%		
• age <12 mo			
• fever ≥39°C	≤2%	≤2	
• fever ≥2 days			
• absence of other source of infection			
Boys		Uncircumcised	Circumcised
• nonblack race	≤1%	Probability >1% with 0 risk factors	≤2
• fever ≥39°C			
• fever ≥24 hours	≤2%	0	≤3
• absence of other source of infection			

uroepithelial cell adherence) are more common in boys with pyelonephritis and VUR than in girls. The aerobactin system in *E. coli* strains is seen more often in pyelonephritis, cystitis, or bacteremia in girls than boys. The aerobactin system is thought to promote bacterial growth and potential for antibiotic resistance. Certain capsular polysaccharides associated with UTIs in girls have an increased virulence because they shield bacteria from phagocytosis or the alternative complement pathway. These virulence factors may contribute in part to the increased prevalence of *E. coli* in girls (Johnson, 1991; Westerlund et al., 1988).

Management of UTI

The decision to use enteral or parenteral antibiotics depends on clinical judgment. Initial antibiotic selection should be based on local antimicrobial sensitivity. The AAP recommends a 7–14 day course of treatment, which has been proven to be more efficacious than single dose treatment (Subcommittee on Urinary Tract Infection et al., 2011; Fitzgerald et al., 2012). Current evidence supports a uniform approach to treating UTI for both girls and boys.

Complications and Post-Emergency Department (ED) Care of UTI

The rate of complications of UTIs and the post-ED management do not differ with the sex of the patient. The acute care clinician should emphasize the importance of following-up with the primary care provider (PCP) to obtain a renal and bladder ultrasound after the first UTI. In the acute setting, untreated UTI may progress to pyelonephritis, perinephric abscess, bacteremia, or urosepsis. The major cause of long-term morbidity associated with untreated first UTI is renal scarring, thus highlighting the importance of proper diagnosis and treatment of pediatric UTIs (Wennerstrom et al., 2000; Shaikh et al., 2010).

Conclusion

The preceding section reviews the risk factors that contribute to the differences in prevalence of UTI by sex in infants. These risk factors include race, age, fever, and anatomic differences. The AAP guidelines presented will help the acute care clinician decide which febrile infants need further diagnostic testing for UTI after the acute intervention.

Case Conclusion

The 11-month-old girl underwent urethral catheterization based on increased risk of UTI (see Table 13B.2). Urinalysis revealed 0 nitrites, 2+ leukocyte esterase, 150 white blood cells, and 20 red blood cells per high-powered field, few squamous cells and many bacteria.

She was initially treated for presumptive UTI with cephalexin, based on local antimicrobial sensitivity profiles. At follow-up with her pediatrician, her urine culture grew >50,000 cfu/mL of *E. coli*, sensitive to cephalosporins. She had a normal renal and bladder ultrasound.

Gaps in Knowledge/Research Questions

Areas of potential research include continued surveillance of how sex affects antimicrobial resistance patterns. The prevalence of bacteria that are resistant to multiple antibiotics is increasing and the relationship, if any, between sex and multidrug-resistant bacteria has not been well studied. Currently, investigators are evaluating point-of-care testing on transcriptional signatures from blood tests that identify bacterial infection in febrile infants and developing biomarkers to improve early diagnosis of pyelonephritis. As technology progresses, comprehensive blood tests will allow clinicians to forgo invasive procedures such as urinary tract catheterization, replacing them with point-of-care accurate and sensitive blood and urine testing.

Case 2: Infant not feeding well and more sleepy

A two-week-old full-term boy presented with three days of worsening emesis and decreased feeding and one day of increased sleeping. His review of systems was notable for decreased urine output and failure to regain birth weight. Vital Signs: heart rate 175 beats per minute, respiratory rate 40 breaths per minute, blood pressure 60/30, O_2 saturation 96% on room air, and rectal temperature 36.9°C. On physical examination, he appeared listless, the anterior fontanelle was sunken, and lips and mucous membranes were dry. Genitourinary examination revealed a circumcised male with normal external genitalia. Skin was ashen. Extremities were cool with four-second capillary refill. The remainder of the cardiac, pulmonary, and abdominal examination was unremarkable. Shock was not reversed despite 60 mL/kg of 0.9% normal saline, prostaglandins, and dopamine infusion.

Introduction

It is imperative that clinicians recognize the signs of compensated shock in a neonate: tachycardia,

mild tachypnea, slight delayed capillary refill, orthostatic changes, and mild irritability (Fleisher and Ludwig, 2010). The causes of neonatal shock include septic shock, cardiogenic shock resulting from closure of the patent ductus arteriosus in patients with ductal-dependent congenital heart disease, and genetic disorders such as inborn errors of metabolism or congenital adrenal hyperplasia (CAH). Clinicians treating a neonate with fluid and catecholamine-refractory shock must consider a diagnosis of adrenal insufficiency. Adrenal insufficiency in neonates may be caused by CAH. The following section will elaborate on the varying presentations of CAH by sex.

Pathophysiology of CAH

Congenital adrenal hyperplasia (CAH) is caused by enzymatic deficiencies of the adrenal cortisol biosynthesis pathway (Figure 13B.1). CAH, which is inherited in an autosomal recessive manner, is seen in 1 in 15,000 live births. The prevalence of CAH in developed nations is the same in both sexes. Reports from developing nations note increased prevalence in girls, although this may reflect missed cases in boys who may die before receiving a proper diagnosis (Speiser et al., 2010).

The most common enzyme deficiency found in children with CAH is 21-hydroxylase deficiency (21OHD), accounting for approximately 95% of cases (Speiser et al., 2010). These patients have varying levels of deficiency in mineralocorticoids (aldosterone) and glucocorticoids (cortisol) and an excess of androgens. Cortisol deficiency leads to stimulation of adrenocorticotropic hormone (ACTH) and results in hyperplasia of the adrenal gland (Sharma and Seth, 2013). Since 21OHD is the most common cause of CAH, the remainder of this discussion will focus on this enzyme deficiency.

Clinical Manifestations of CAH

The clinical manifestations of CAH are the result of adrenal insufficiency, accumulated precursors proximal to the enzymatic block, and androgen excess. CAH can be divided into classic and nonclassic forms based on symptoms and the degree of enzyme activity. Classic CAH can then be subdivided into salt-wasting (SW) and non-salt-wasting (NSW) types.

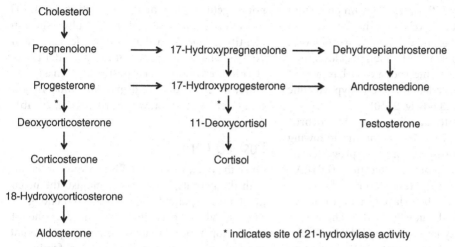

Figure 13B.1 The cortisol biosynthesis pathway affected by 21OH deficiency in CAH

Salt-wasting CAH comprises 75% of classic CAH cases and is characterized by the complete absence of 21OH, which results in a deficiency of cortisol and aldosterone production and excess testosterone production. Lack of aldosterone leads to renal sodium loss, hypovolemia, and hyperkalemia. Clinically, patients usually present in the second week of life with nonspecific and insidious symptoms such as poor feeding, poor weight gain, emesis, and irritability (Fleisher and Ludwig, 2010). Symptoms may progress to adrenal crisis and potentially fatal hypovolemic shock, as with the infant in the vignette. Girls with SW-CAH may be diagnosed at an earlier age, due to ambiguous genitalia. These girls are virilized in utero resulting in phenotypes ranging from clitoral hypertrophy and partial labioscrotal fusion to completely phenotypically male genitalia. An apparently male neonate with no palpable testes warrants careful scrutiny. Ambiguous genitalia should prompt urgent genetic and gonadal sex determination. Boys with SW-CAH may have more subtle effects of androgen and ACTH excess, such as mild phallic enlargement or hyperpigmentation (due to stimulation of melanocyte-stimulating hormone along with ACTH) (Sharma and Seth, 2013). The subtle changes in male genitalia can lead to delayed diagnosis until the infant presents in shock.

The remaining 25% of classic cases are non-salt-wasting CAH. In these patients, 1% to 2% of enzyme activity remains, resulting in mild virilization, sparing of aldosterone, and no salt wasting. Girls may have ambiguous genitalia; however, diagnosis is often delayed until puberty. Boys may present with precocious puberty (Sharma and Seth, 2013).

In non-classic CAH, remaining 21OH activity is 20% to 50%. Most patients are asymptomatic or exhibit mild symptoms such as precocious pubarche or signs of androgen excess in female adolescence, such as acne, hirsutism, and menstrual irregularities (Sharma and Seth, 2013). The following discussion focuses on classic congenital adrenal hyperplasia.

Diagnosis of CAH

Although CAH screening is included in the newborn screening program in all 50 states in the United States and at least 40 other countries, the ED clinician should note that these results might not be available for three to four weeks (Antal and Zhou, 2009; Fleisher and Ludwig, 2010; Merke, 2014a). The diagnosis of CAH in the ED is based on clinical suspicion, physical examination including vital signs and a genitourinary exam, and laboratory abnormalities.

The most urgent blood tests to obtain are serum electrolytes and blood glucose. The first clue to an underlying diagnosis of CAH in a boy with normal appearing genitalia is often the combination of hyperkalemia and hyponatremia. It is important to note that expected elevation in serum potassium seen in CAH may be obscured by ongoing GI losses caused by the acute salt-wasting crisis leading to an initial normal serum potassium level. Blood glucose levels may be low due to decreased oral intake and decreased cortisol levels, or they may be normal. Metabolic acidosis, evidenced by low pH and bicarbonate level, is present in patients in moderate to severe hypovolemic shock (Fleisher and Ludwig, 2010).

Ideally, prior to administering hydrocortisone, blood should be drawn for the following laboratory tests: cortisol, 17-hydroxyprogesterone (17OHP), dehydroepiandrosterone (DHEA), androstenedione, and testosterone; however, treatment should not be delayed in a critically ill infant (Fleisher and Ludwig, 2010). The serum level of 17-hydroxyprogesterone (17OHP) is elevated in CAH (usually greater than 100 ng/mL in the classic form) (Sharma and Seth, 2013).

Management of CAH

The infant in hypovolemic shock from a salt-wasting crisis requires aggressive intravenous (IV) fluid resuscitation. A time-sensitive and goal-directed algorithm for pediatric shock includes 60 mL/kg normal saline bolus in the first 15 minutes, followed by catecholamines if there is no response to fluids. In neonates of both sexes, with fluid and catecholamine-refractory shock, the clinician should administer hydrocortisone, as there is a high risk of adrenal insufficiency caused by CAH.

Maintenance fluids for CAH patients should include 5% dextrose at 1.5 to 2 times maintenance rates for adrenal crisis (Sharma and Seth, 2013). Hydrocortisone should be administered as 50–100 mg/m^2 IV bolus (typically 25 mg for a neonate) followed by 50–100 mg/m^2 of hydrocortisone per day divided every 6 hours. Mineralocorticoid replacement is unnecessary in the acute setting due to the mineralocorticoid effects of hydrocortisone at high doses. CAH-induced hyperkalemia usually requires only fluid resuscitation. In the setting of a hyperkalemia-induced arrhythmia, 10% calcium gluconate should be administered to stabilize the cardiac membranes. Hypoglycemia can be treated with glucose 0.25 g/kg and subsequent inclusion of 10% dextrose in IV fluids.

Once the patient is stabilized in the ED, the patient should be admitted to a pediatric intensive care unit (PICU) for further management and

non-urgent aspects of the evaluation for CAH, including karyotype and pelvic ultrasound to identify gonadal structures. The female infant (46XX) who is diagnosed in the neonatal period after in utero androgen exposure is given a Prader score, which grades the degree of genital virilization (Fleisher and Ludwig, 2010; Merke, 2014b).

Post-ED Care

Once the diagnosis of CAH is made, a conference with the parents, the endocrinologist, the urologist (and the patient if the child is old enough to understand and participate) may include the following topics: growth and hormone replacement, gender assignment, sexual orientation, feminizing surgery, and fertility.

Both girls and boys with CAH display rapid growth during the neonatal period, due to androgen excess. Boys with undetected CAH may have brisk increase in height with precocious puberty; however, they may also have early fusion of physes leading to short stature as adults. Preservation of full adult height requires close follow-up by an endocrinologist (Sharma and Seth, 2013).

Development of gender identity depends on the degree of in utero androgen exposure and a host of other factors during childhood, including gender assignment (Jordan-Young, 2012). Gender assignment in the female child (46XX) with highly virilized genitalia is an issue that requires sensitivity and the expertise of a multidisciplinary team. A study of 12 46XX people who were assigned male gender at birth (based on high Prader scores) and diagnosed with CAH after age 3 found that most subjects maintained male gender identity with sexual attraction to females. Two of these subjects were reassigned to female gender in childhood but subsequently reassigned themselves to male. Those patients with ambiguous gender who did the poorest with regard to self-esteem, body image, masculinity, and social adjustment had less familial and social support (Lee et al., 2010). Consultation with a mental health specialist may be helpful for patients with CAH (Speiser et al., 2010). These reports underscore the significance of psychosocial support for children with CAH.

In utero androgen exposure affects sexual orientation. Females (46XX) with CAH recalled more "male-typical" play during childhood, had reduced satisfaction with identifying as female gender, reduced heterosexual interest, and increased rates of bisexual and homosexual orientation when compared to controls. Males with CAH did not differ from unaffected males in these respects (Hines et al., 2004). Moreover, homosexual and bisexual identity among a cohort of females (46XX) with CAH was correlated with the degree of prenatal androgenization as well as global measures of masculinization of nonsexual behavior (Meyer-Bahlburg et al., 2008). These findings are explained by the brain organization theory, which suggests that in utero androgen exposure affects brain development and consequently sexual orientation, gender identity, and nonsexual behavior (such as aggression or play activity levels in children) (Meyer-Bahlburg, 2011; Jordan-Young, 2012; Pasterski et al., 2007).

Females (46XX) with virilized genitalia may require feminizing surgery. Current literature suggests that the effects of feminizing surgery on sexual function are not satisfactory. Clitoral sensitivity after clitoroplasty has been shown to be impaired and is associated with anorgasmia (Crouch et al., 2008; Nordenstrom, 2011). Vaginal reconstruction carries the risk of stricture formation, vaginal penetration difficulties, dyspareunia, stenosis, and lower urinary tract problems (Gastaud et al., 2007; Crouch et al., 2008; Lee et al., 2012; van der Zwan et al., 2013). Current trends and guidelines favor postponing feminizing surgery unless patients have moderate or severe signs of virilization (Nordenstrom, 2011).

Subfertility is common in both female and male CAH patients. In females, the subfertility depends on the severity of virilization, combined with psychosocial and psychosexual issues related to gender identity (Gastaud et al., 2007; van der Zwan et al., 2013). Subfertility in males is related to aberrant adrenal tissue that can cause testicular adrenal rest tumors and abnormal sperm quality (Falhammar et al., 2012).

Although growth, gender identity, sexual orientation, and fertility are not strictly pediatric or acute care issues, these problems can be predicted at the onset of illness and highlight the importance of early pediatric endocrinology and urology consultation (Otten et al., 2005).

Conclusion

Clinicians treating infants in fluid and catecholamine-refractory shock should consider congenital adrenal hyperplasia in the differential diagnosis and administer corticosteroids early. Because of the variations in the severity of CAH, girls may present with ambiguous genitalia, while boys may have hyperpigmented genitalia or phallic enlargement, although most affected male infants have normal appearing genitalia.

Case Conclusion

The boy received IV hydrocortisone, which immediately improved his vital signs and perfusion. His response strongly suggested that he was in adrenal crisis, likely secondary to CAH. Pediatric endocrinology, urology, and the PICU were notified, and the patient was admitted for ongoing management of adrenal crisis and a workup for CAH.

Gaps in Knowledge

There are too few prospective long-term studies on the psychological and functional effects of early feminizing surgery compared to delayed (postpubertal) feminizing surgery (Braga and Pippi Salle, 2009). Additionally, more neuroanatomic research studies are needed to clarify the effects of in utero androgen exposure on brain development and gender identity (Meyer-Bahlburg, 2011). More complete evidence would provide families with the knowledge necessary to make life-altering decisions for their female children with CAH. Furthermore, as surgical expertise increases, more effective feminizing surgery techniques that yield more satisfactory results for sexual function will improve quality of life for female patients with CAH.

Case 3: Lower abdominal pain in an adolescent

A 14-year-old female presented with two days of severe right lower quadrant abdominal pain. Review of systems was positive for two episodes of non-bilious, non-bloody emesis and was otherwise negative. Vital Signs: heart rate 110 beats per minute, respiratory rate 20 breaths per minute, blood pressure 110/80, O_2 saturation 99%, and oral temperature 36.7°C Exam: She was in moderate discomfort from pain, her abdomen was soft with moderate tenderness in the right lower quadrant, and involuntary guarding without rebound tenderness.

Introduction

The differential diagnosis of lower abdominal pain in adolescents is broad and varies depending on the sex of the patient. Illnesses that cause lower abdominal pain in both sexes range in severity from mild conditions to surgical emergencies, including appendicitis, nephrolithiasis, and constipation.

In girls, lower abdominal pain can be gynecologic in origin and encompass entities such as pelvic inflammatory disease (PID), ovarian pathology, and ectopic pregnancy. A surgical emergency that can cause similar, nonspecific symptoms in boys is testicular torsion. Significant components of the adolescent history that the clinician must obtain are the date of the most recent menses in girls, sexual history, and high-risk behaviors. When interviewing the adolescent, the clinician should consider local consent laws and confidentiality issues (Kruszka and Kruszka, 2010). Work-up always includes a pregnancy test in all menstruating females, even if the history and exam seem conclusive (Balachandran et al., 2013). The following discussion reviews sex differences in each of these conditions.

Appendicitis

Clinical Presentation of Appendicitis

While appendicitis is more common in boys (and men), the clinical presentation of appendicitis is similar in children and adults and there is no difference in boys' and girls' presentation. Symptoms and diagnostic findings may include periumbilical pain that migrates to the right lower quadrant, anorexia, nausea, vomiting, leukocytosis with left shift, and fever. The incidence of appendicitis in children peaks in the second decade of life, with median age of 10–11. The male to female ratio is approximately 1.4:1 (Pepper et al., 2012; Shah, 2013).

Diagnosis of Appendicitis

The most well-studied clinical prediction rules for appendicitis in children include the modified Alvarado score and the Pediatric Appendicitis Score (PAS) (Kulik et al., 2013). Both scores were more accurate in boys than in girls, which was consistent with studies of the Alvarado score in adults of both sexes (Mandeville et al., 2011).

Efforts to reduce ionizing radiation exposure in children have led to the use of ultrasound (US) as the preferred first-line imaging modality for appendicitis in children and young women (Shademan and Tappouni, 2013). The approach of US followed by computed tomography (CT) or magnetic resonance imaging (MRI) when US is non-diagnostic has shown increased cost effectiveness and high accuracy when compared to CT alone for both sexes (Wan et al., 2009; Aspelund et al., 2014). US was more successful for diagnosis of appendicitis in children than adults and in boys as compared to girls (Yu et al., 2005b). In a multi-institutional study comparing US to CT for diagnosis of appendicitis, all children younger than age 5 and girls older than age 10 had a higher negative appendectomy rate (NAR) when using US alone for diagnosis. NAR is defined as a normal appendix on histopathology. US is more challenging in younger children and in pubescent females (Bachur et al., 2012). This is consistent with other reports that NAR was independently associated with younger age and female sex (Oyetunji et al., 2012). The larger number of abdominal conditions that mimic appendicitis may have contributed to US's decreased accuracy diagnosing appendicitis in girls. Pelvic MRI may be an alternative to CT scan for difficult cases (Shademan and Tappouni, 2013).

Pubertal females are diagnostically challenging because they are more likely to present with non-classical symptoms of appendicitis, and they may have gynecologic conditions that mimic appendicitis. Pelvic examination was not found to delay the diagnosis of appendicitis in women; therefore, this examination should be performed if clinically indicated and feasible (McGann Donlan and Mycyk, 2009). Obesity in children can obscure physical examination findings. Obese girls with appendectomies have significantly higher NAR than obese boys (24.6% vs. 17.4%, p<0.05) (Kutasy and Puri, 2013).

The clinician may consider observation rather than immediate CT in adolescent girls with mild lower abdominal pain. A study of adolescents and adults in whom US found normal pelvic structures but did not visualize the appendix determined that these patients were at significantly lower risk for appendicitis. These results suggest that if the appendix is not visualized on US, the clinician may follow a staged approach, with clinical observation rather than immediate CT; the CT can then be obtained for persistent or worsening abdominal pain (Stewart et al., 2012).

Management of Appendicitis

The primary management of uncomplicated appendicitis is appendectomy, either laparoscopic appendectomy (LA) or open appendectomy (OA). LA has additional benefits in girls and women of reproductive age because it allows direct visualization of the abdominal and pelvic contents, an improved cosmetic outcome, and less risk of postoperative adhesions that can increase the risk of infertility (Markar et al., 2012; Sauerland et al., 2010; Tzovaras et al., 2007). The benefit of LA is reduced in prepubescent females who are less likely to have abdominal pain caused by gynecologic pathology (Markar et al., 2012). LA is as safe as OA in boys but has not proved to provide any clear benefit (Tzovaras et al., 2007). Retrospective reviews note that boys were more likely to have open appendectomy, whereas girls had higher rates of laparoscopic appendectomy (Markar et al., 2012; Oyetunji et al., 2011).

Complications of Appendicitis

Perforation of the appendix is a potential complication of appendicitis. In studies combining children and adults, men had an earlier and greater rate of perforation than women; this complication was more common in elderly patients than in children (Augustin et al., 2011; Barreto et al., 2010; Sulu et al., 2010).

Nephrolithiasis

Clinical Presentation of Nephrolithiasis

Children with nephrolithiasis present to Emergency Departments with abdominal or flank pain, hematuria, fever, or dysuria (Alpay et al., 2013). In contrast to stones formed by adults, pediatric kidney stones are more often caused by genetic or metabolic conditions. In recent decades, the overall prevalence of pediatric kidney stones has been increasing in both sexes (Matlaga et al., 2010; Novak et al., 2009). Boys have a predilection for kidney stones in the first decade of life due to genetic and metabolic conditions diagnosed in infancy, and girls in the second decade of life (Sas, 2011; Sas et al., 2010; Wood et al., 2013; Matlaga et al., 2010; Novak et al., 2009; Habbig et al., 2011).

One theory explaining young boys' increased risk of stone formation is that boys are more likely to have anatomical malformations resulting in urinary obstruction and stasis. Another theory associates puberty in girls with kidney stone formation, suggesting that estrogen has a lithogenic effect; this theory has its basis in studies of postmenopausal women on hormone replacement therapy (Matlaga et al., 2010; Novak et al., 2009). Estrogen may also affect stone formation in pubertal girls by stimulating adiposity and enhanced bone mineralization. These theories are not well studied and remain an area of exploration for future research.

Diagnosis of Nephrolithiasis

Pediatric kidney stones are often found incidentally, presenting only with nonspecific symptoms (Habbig et al., 2011). Initial assessment of a child with symptoms of renal colic may include urinalysis for microscopic hematuria and urine calcium/creatinine ratio. Imaging may include abdominal ultrasound, X-ray, or CT scan, based on clinical presentation (Kalorin et al., 2009). Efforts to limit radiation in children are encouraged.

Management of Nephrolithiasis

Management of pediatric kidney stones is the same for either sex. Prevention is the primary approach to management of pediatric kidney stones. Hydration, which decreases solute concentration in the urine, dietary modifications, and certain medications are important aspects of prevention (Habbig et al., 2011). Pain control is accomplished with oral therapy or parenteral analgesia if oral medication is not tolerated. Overall stone passage rate has been reported at 34% for children younger than age 10 and 29% for children older than age 10, with no apparent differences by sex (Kalorin et al., 2009).

Invasive management of kidney stones may be pursued for obstruction, infection, or depressed renal function. These interventions include ureteroscopy, shock wave lithotripsy, and percutaneous nephrolithotomy, with similar approaches in both sexes (Kalorin et al., 2009).

Complications of Nephrolithiasis

Complications of kidney stones include upper urinary tract infection; ureteral obstruction; hydronephrosis; and, if chronic and untreated obstruction is present, renal failure (Alexander et al., 2012; Alpay et al., 2013; Habbig et al., 2011). One study noted that kidney stones were a common cause of acute renal failure in older children and that acute renal failure was more common in boys than girls, for unclear reasons (Jamal and Ramzan, 2004).

Constipation

Clinical Presentation of Constipation

Constipation presents with abdominal pain and infrequent stooling. The passage of infrequent, large-caliber stools is highly suggestive of functional constipation (Biggs and Dery, 2006). During the toilet training period, straining at defecation and infrequent stooling were reported significantly more often for girls, whereas fecal soiling of underclothes and passage of large bowel movements were reported more often in boys (Wald et al., 2009; de Lorijn et al., 2004). Encopresis in children with constipation is more common in boys (Biggs and Dery, 2006; Nurko and Scott, 2011; de Lorijn et al., 2004).

Clinicians have identified an association between bowel and bladder dysfunction, which is termed "dysfunctional elimination syndrome." Different types of dysfunctional elimination were described in each sex. Constipation and dysfunctional voiding were more common in girls, whereas boys had more encopresis and idiopathic detrusor overactivity disorder (Combs et al., 2013).

Diagnosis of Constipation

The diagnosis of constipation does not differ by sex. Diagnosis of functional constipation is usually based on bowel hygiene history and physical examination. The clinician should perform a digital rectal exam and visual inspection of the anus. The presence of impacted stool or anal fissures suggests functional constipation (Biggs and Dery, 2006). A thorough history and review of systems is important to rule out organic causes of constipation such as Hirschsprung's disease, spinal cord abnormality, hypothyroidism, cystic fibrosis, gluten enteropathy, congenital anorectal malformations, or sexual abuse (Biggs and Dery, 2006). The clinician may use radiography when the diagnosis of constipation is uncertain, but there is insufficient evidence to support routine imaging (Berger et al., 2012; Reuchlin-Vroklage et al., 2005). Treatment and complications of functional constipation are similar for both boys and girls and are beyond the scope of this discussion.

Pelvic Inflammatory Disease

Clinical Presentation of PID

Pelvic inflammatory disease (PID) is an ascending infection that spreads from the lower to the upper genital tract. The mechanism of infection begins with attachment of infectious agents to columnar epithelium of the cervix (Banikarim and Chacko, 2005). PID is common among sexually active women, with an increased prevalence in adolescents in part due to high-risk behaviors (Abu Raya et al., 2013; Datta et al., 2012).

Microbiology of PID includes *Neisseria gonorrhea*, *Chlamydia trachomatis*, and other aerobic and anaerobic microorganisms (Banikarim and Chacko, 2005; Abu Raya et al., 2013). In the United States, Chlamydia infections are more common in women than in men ages 14 to 39 (2.2% vs. 1.1%, respectively). There was a declining prevalence of Chlamydia infections in both sexes from 1999 to 2008, with a more notable decline in men and adolescents of both sexes (Datta et al., 2012).

PID presents with nonspecific symptoms including lower abdominal or pelvic pain, cramping, vaginal bleeding or discharge, urinary symptoms, fever, or dyspareunia (Abu Raya et al., 2013).

Gonorrhea and Chlamydia infections in men often present as urethritis but may also cause epididymitis or prostatitis. Urethritis from either organism may present with urethral discharge or dysuria, or may be asymptomatic. Asymptomatic urethritis occurs more commonly with Chlamydia than with Gonorrhea and is more common in women than in men (Cecil et al., 2001; Detels et al., 2011; Sherrard and Barlow, 1996).

Diagnosis of PID

PID is a clinical diagnosis based on either uterine/adnexal tenderness or cervical motion tenderness. Additional diagnostic criteria may include fever >38.3°C, abnormal cervical discharge, white blood cells on wet mount of cervical discharge, elevated erythrocyte sedimentation rate or C-reactive protein, or identification of *N. gonorrhea* or *C. trachomatis* in cervical discharge (Banikarim and Chacko, 2005).

N. gonorrhea or *C. trachomatis* can be diagnosed with the gold standard test of cervical culture, but the test most frequently utilized is the highly sensitive and specific nucleic acid amplification test (NAAT) (Abu Raya et al., 2013). NAAT can be performed on urine or on material obtained from vaginal swabs that the patient can self-administer.

Management of PID

The CDC recommends parenteral and oral regimens for PID (Table 13B.3) (Banikarim and Chacko, 2005; Abu Raya et al., 2013). Hospitalization for parenteral treatment is indicated for failed outpatient therapy, inability to tolerate oral intake, or clinical signs of peritoneal inflammation and should be considered in patients who are at high risk for noncompliance (Banikarim and Chacko, 2005).

The US Preventative Services Task Force (USPSTF) recommends screening all sexually active women age 25 and younger, and screening all high-risk women older than age 25 (Abu Raya

Table 13B.3 CDC Recommendations for Treatment of PID (2010)

Parenteral Regimens
Option A
• Cefotetan 2g IV every 12 hours OR Cefoxitin 2g IV every 6 hours
PLUS
• Doxycycline 100 mg orally or IV every 12 hours
Option B
• Clindamycin 900 mg IV every 8 hours
PLUS
• Gentamicin loading dose IV or IM (2 mg/kg), followed by a maintenance dose (1.5 mg/kg) every 8 hours. Single daily dosing (3–5 mg/kg) may be substituted.
Oral Regimens
Option A
• Ceftriaxone 250 mg IM in a single dose
PLUS
• Doxycycline 100 mg orally twice a day for 14 days
WITH OR WITHOUT
• Metronidazole 500 mg orally twice a day for 14 days
Option B
• Cefoxitin 2g IM in a single dose and Probenecid, 1g orally administered concurrently in a single dose
PLUS
• Doxycycline 100 mg orally twice a day for 14 days
WITH OR WITHOUT
• Metronidazole 500 mg orally twice a day for 14 days
Option C
• Other parenteral third-generation cephalosporin (e.g., ceftizoxime or cefotaxime)
PLUS
• Doxycycline 100 mg orally twice a day for 14 days
WITH OR WITHOUT
• Metronidazole 500 mg orally twice a day for 14 days

et al., 2013). Outpatient screening of women at risk, coupled with appropriate treatment, has been shown to reduce hospitalized PID, ectopic pregnancies, and ED-diagnosed Gonorrhea and

Chlamydia (Anschuetz et al., 2012; Gray-Swain and Peipert, 2006).

Complications of PID

PID can lead to significant morbidity, including infertility, ectopic pregnancy, chronic pelvic pain, recurrent infections, tubo-ovarian abscess, and possibly ovarian cancer (Abu Raya et al., 2013; Banikarim and Chacko, 2005).

Tubo-ovarian abscess occurs when bacteria and inflammatory material collect in the fallopian tubes, forming an abscess. Pathogens include aerobes and anaerobes, including those causing PID. The clinician should suspect this diagnosis in patients with moderate to severe pain who are ill appearing. Often, however, these patients' presentations are similar to those of women who have PID. Pelvic ultrasound can identify the abscess. Treatment includes hospitalization for parenteral triple antibiotic therapy, with broad spectrum agents including clindamycin, ampicillin, and gentamicin, and serial ultrasounds to monitor response to therapy (Banikarim and Chacko, 2005). Surgical drainage must be considered if medical therapies fail.

Ovarian Cysts

Clinical Presentation of Ovarian Cysts

Follicular cysts result when follicles fail to regress after completion of the menstrual cycle. Large ovarian cysts may rupture, causing an abrupt onset of pain, or may become the lead point for ovarian torsion (Ackerman et al., 2013). Hemorrhagic cysts are uncommon in early adolescence but have the potential to cause massive hemoperitoneum or hypotension (Ackerman et al., 2013; Kayaba et al., 1996).

Ovarian cysts may occur in prepubertal girls, but their diameter is usually less than 2 cm. These are usually asymptomatic, are found incidentally, and regress spontaneously. Occasionally, recurrent bleeding is due to hormonally active cysts and may suggest a genetic disorder, such as McCune-Albright syndrome. McCune-Albright syndrome has a variable presentation, including precocious puberty, café-au-lait spots, and polyostotic fibrous dysplasia. Ovarian cysts are one of several manifestations of this condition (Pienkowski et al., 2012).

Diagnosis of Ovarian Cysts

Ultrasound is the imaging modality of choice to visualize the adnexa and uterus. Pelvic US that is performed in the ED requires advanced imaging skills and experience and should be performed by experienced sonographers rather than the bedside clinician (Leeson and Leeson, 2013). Follicular cysts appear as simple, unilocular, or minimally complicated cysts with thin walls, sharply marginated borders, internal fluid, and no internal vascularity. Hemorrhagic cysts have variable appearance depending on the age of the blood products, including a complex cystic appearance with internal echoes, thickened walls, or fluid levels (Ackerman et al., 2013).

Management of Ovarian Cysts

Simple cysts <3 cm in diameter are considered physiologic. Cysts 3–5 cm are usually benign and do not require follow up. Cysts 5–7 cm should be reimaged annually and cysts that are >7 cm should be further evaluated by MRI or a surgical consultant (Ackerman et al., 2013). Cystectomy is indicated for cysts that are growing, persistent, symptomatic, or appear suspicious for malignancy (Tofteland et al., 2010). Non-ruptured hemorrhagic cysts generally resolve in 8 weeks, but if they are >5 cm, they should be reimaged to ensure resolution (Ackerman et al., 2013). Cystectomy and oophorectomy can be done laparascopically in children (Akkoyun and Gulen, 2012; Savasi et al., 2009).

Ovarian Torsion

Clinical Presentation of Ovarian Torsion

Adnexal torsion (AT) is the cause of approximately 3% of episodes of acute abdominal pain in girls (Appelbaum et al., 2013). AT involves the rotation of the ovary, fallopian tube, or both, on its vascular pedicle. In children, intermittent or non-radiating abdominal or pelvic pain has been significantly associated with AT (Appelbaum et al., 2013). Pain from AT has a predilection for the right ovary and thus is more often right sided (Spinelli et al., 2013). Additional findings may include nausea and vomiting; occasionally a mass can be palpated on physical examination (Breech and Hillard, 2005; Ackerman et al., 2013).

Diagnosis

Torsion is often associated with increased adnexal size, an ovarian cyst, or mass (Appelbaum et al., 2013; Spinelli et al., 2013; Ackerman et al., 2013). The most common lesions found in torsed ovaries of adolescents are follicular or corpus luteal cysts, often >5 cm (Ackerman et al., 2013). Ultrasound with Doppler is the test of choice to evaluate the pelvic organs in females. In AT, US may identify adnexal masses or enlargement, and Doppler may identify absence of venous or arterial flow. The most frequent finding is a decrease or absence of venous flow (Ackerman et al., 2013). However, presence of blood flow seen with Doppler does not always exclude torsion, because the patient may be having intermittent torsion or have developed collateral blood flow (Breech and Hillard, 2005; Cass, 2005). At times, CT scan may be necessary to rule out alternative causes of nonspecific abdominal pain (Ackerman et al., 2013).

Clinicians must maintain a high index of suspicion for AT in girls with atypical abdominal pain (Breech and Hillard, 2005). Delayed diagnosis is more common in ovarian torsion than in testicular torsion. This disparity is in part the result of the anatomy of male genitalia; the testes and scrotum are more easily palpated and examined by the clinician. Furthermore, abdominal pain in girls generates a broader differential than abdominal or scrotal pain in boys. Girls with gonadal torsion present later after the onset of pain, wait 2.5 times longer for diagnostic imaging, wait 2.7 times longer to go to the operating room for definitive treatment, and have a gonadal salvage rate that is less than half that of boys (Piper et al., 2012). More liberal use of diagnostic laparoscopy in girls, when imaging is non-diagnostic, would improve ovary salvage rate (Piper et al., 2012).

Management of Ovarian Torsion

Laparoscopic detorsion has become the preferred approach in children with AT, with consideration of oophoropexy at the time of surgery (Ackerman et al., 2013; Cass, 2005; Breech and Hillard, 2005). Cystectomy is performed if needed and efforts to limit oophorectomy are encouraged to preserve reproductive function as well as sexual development in prepubertal children (Breech and Hillard, 2005). A number of studies report viability of the ovary despite a necrotic appearance; most experts recommend leaving the ovary in situ regardless of duration of symptoms or gross appearance (Spinelli et al., 2013; Piper et al., 2012).

Ectopic Pregnancy

Clinical Presentation of Ectopic Pregnancy

Ectopic pregnancies may present with crampy abdominal or pelvic pain that is often unilateral; sometimes vaginal bleeding occurs. Cervical motion tenderness, adnexal mass, and adnexal tenderness increase the likelihood of ectopic pregnancy (Crochet et al., 2013). A ruptured ectopic pregnancy is a surgical emergency and can present with hypotension, tachycardia, or shock (Barnhart, 2009).

Diagnosis of Ectopic Pregnancy

Unruptured ectopic pregnancy is diagnosed by pelvic ultrasound in conjunction with βhCG (Barnhart, 2009). A study of ED physicians performing ultrasound for possible ectopic pregnancy demonstrated a sensitivity of 99.3% and a negative predictive value of 99.96%, suggesting that visualization of intrauterine pregnancy by emergency physicians was sufficient to rule out ectopic pregnancy (Stein et al., 2010). A single βhCG value does not identify the location of a pregnancy, but trending values may be used to estimate gestational age and determine viability of a pregnancy (Barnhart, 2009).

Management of Ectopic Pregnancy

Medical or surgical management of an ectopic pregnancy must be determined by an obstetrician. Medical management includes administration of systemic methotrexate if there are no signs of rupture, the βhCG is <5,000 IU/L, routine lab tests are normal, and the patient is reliable to follow-up. Surgical management includes saplingetcomy or salpingostomy. Surgery is indicated for patients with signs of rupture, βhCG >5,000 IU/L, need for laparoscopic diagnosis, or suspicion for a concurrent viable intrauterine pregnancy (known as a heterotopic pregnancy). Expectant management may be considered when a reliable patient has no evidence of rupture and has a βhCG <1,500 IU/L that decreases within 48 hours (Farquhar, 2005; Lozeau and Potter, 2005).

Testicular Torsion

Clinical Presentation of Testicular Torsion

Testicular torsion typically presents with testicular or abdominal pain, often unilateral, with nausea and vomiting (Gunther and Rubben, 2012). Physical examination may show the testis in a horizontal lie, scrotal induration, swelling or discoloration, and an absent cremasteric reflex. Intermittent torsion may present with repeated, severely painful episodes with spontaneous resolution (Eaton et al., 2005).

Diagnosis of Testicular Torsion

Significant ischemic damage is estimated to occur after four to eight hours (Gunther and Rubben, 2012). Urinalysis with evidence of pyuria may suggest an alternative diagnosis of epididymitis or orchitis, although this may be present in torsion as well. The diagnostic study of choice is US with color Doppler, which identifies a torsed testis with absent blood flow (Gunther and Rubben, 2012). Presence of blood flow, however, does not definitively rule out torsion, and a high clinical suspicion warrants surgical consultation regardless of Doppler results (Mellick, 2012). Studies of emergency physicians performing ultrasound of the testes are ongoing (Leeson and Leeson, 2013).

Management of Testicular Torsion

Surgical detorsion should be performed without delay when torsion is identified or highly suspected. Bilateral orchiopexy is performed at the time of surgery to reduce the likelihood of torsion of the contralateral testis. Orchiectomy may be indicated for a nonviable testis (Gunther and Rubben, 2012).

Conclusion

The differential diagnosis of lower abdominal pain in the adolescent includes several life-threatening or fertility-threatening diagnoses that the clinician must not miss. It is essential to consider the anatomical differences between sexes, as well as high-risk behaviors common in adolescents when evaluating teenagers with abdominal pain. Building rapport with a young patient to obtain a thorough history and a complete examination of reproductive organs is important.

Case Conclusion

This patient had persistent pain despite the administration of morphine and had a normal white blood cell count. The pelvic US with Doppler identified an enlarged right ovary with absent venous or arterial flow, consistent with ovarian torsion. She was transferred to the operating room for laparoscopic detorsion.

Gaps in Knowledge/Research Questions

Boys with gonadal torsion are diagnosed earlier and have a higher gonad salvage rate than girls (Piper et al., 2012). The reproductive consequences of a nonviable gonad after torsion are substantial. Future research should explore ways to reduce delay in diagnosis of ovarian torsion. Early laparoscopic intervention to evaluate nonspecific abdominal pain in girls needs study.

Case 4: Knee pain

A 13-year-old boy presented with right-sided knee pain for one week. There was no preceding trauma, although the patient played soccer daily before the pain began. Pain was worse with ambulation, mildly improved with rest or ibuprofen. Review of systems was notable for a cold the previous week and was negative for fever or other complaints. Vital Signs: heart rate 110 beats per minute, respiratory rate 20 breaths per minute, blood pressure 110/80, O_2 saturation 99%, and oral temperature 36.7°C Exam: Antalgic gait involving the right leg, no point tenderness at the knee, decreased range of motion of the right hip and knee due to pain; the right lower extremity was neurovascularly intact. There was no tenderness with varus or valgus stress at the knee joint, and no excess laxity on anterior and posterior drawer testing; the Lachman test was negative.

Introduction

Knee pain in children can be caused by several orthopedic conditions, some of which are more likely depending on the sex of the patient. The differential diagnosis for knee pain in children includes slipped capital femoral epiphysis (SCFE), Osgood-Schlatter disease, and anterior cruciate ligament (ACL) injury. The following discussion highlights the differences in each of these conditions by sex.

Slipped Capital Femoral Epiphysis (SCFE)

Prevalence and Risk Factors of SCFE

Slipped capital femoral epiphysis (SCFE) is anterior-superior displacement of the femoral metaphysis while the epiphysis remains in the acetabulum (Peck and Herrera-Soto, 2014). The incidence in the United States is 10.8 per 100,000 children, with an increased incidence in adolescent boys (average age of onset is 12 years), African Americans or Hispanics, and obese patients (Lehmann et al., 2006; Benson et al., 2008). Several studies report an increasing incidence of SCFE in girls and an increasing incidence in children overall. These authors suggest that this change may be due to increasing childhood obesity (Murray and Wilson, 2008; Witbreuk et al., 2013).

The etiology of SCFE is believed to be multifactorial; contributing factors include obesity, growth spurts, or endocrine disorders (e.g., hypothyroidism, hypogonadism, or panhypopituitarism). More than half of children with SCFE exceed the 90th percentile in body weight (Peck, 2010; Peck and Herrera-Soto, 2014).

Clinical Presentation of SCFE

SCFE presents similarly in both sexes. The classic presentation of SCFE includes hip or groin pain, a waddling gait, and a preference for holding the affected leg externally rotated and abducted. Referred pain along the obturator nerve may cause approximately 15% of patients with SCFE

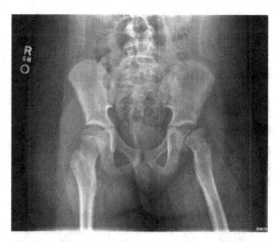

Figure 13B.2 X-ray with AP view of a left hip with SCFE (Peck, 2010)

to complain of pain only at the thigh or knee (Peck, 2010). For this reason, children with knee pain should always have a thorough hip examination (Adirim and Cheng, 2003). SCFE presents bilaterally in 18% to 50% of patients and sequentially (e.g., hips are affected within 18 months of each other) in a significant subgroup of these patients.

Diagnosis of SCFE

Diagnostic X-rays should include anteroposterior (AP) and frog-leg views of the hips, as well as AP and lateral views of the knee, when knee pain is present (Figure 13B.2). The degree of displacement of the epiphysis demonstrates the severity of the condition (Peck, 2010). The diagnostic approach to SCFE is the same for both sexes; however, clinicians should remember to obtain a pregnancy test in reproductive-age females prior to obtaining X-rays.

Management and Complications of SCFE

The management and complications of SCFE are the same for both sexes. The patient should not bear weight on the affected extremity, using crutches or a wheelchair, and should be referred to an orthopedic surgeon. Treatment is surgical fixation with a single screw, which prevents progression of the slip. Avascular necrosis and chondrolysis (loss of articular cartilage) are complications of severe displacement (Peck, 2010).

Osgood-Schlatter Disease

Prevalence and Risk Factors of Osgood-Schlatter Disease

Osgood-Schlatter is an inflammatory condition that causes knee pain in children and adolescents. Most affected children are ages 10 to 14. Osgood-Schlatter occurs in approximately 20% of adolescents involved in sports, compared to 5% who are non-athletes. Up to 30% of patients can have bilateral knee involvement. It is caused by repetitive traction on the apophysis of the tibial tubercle, at the site of patella tendon insertion (Atanda et al., 2011; Kujala et al., 1985). Sports with cutting and jumping movements predispose to Osgood-Schlatter disease and include soccer, basketball, gymnastics, and volleyball (Cassas and Cassettari-Wayhs, 2006).

Historically this condition was reported more frequently in boys; however, the current literature reports an equal prevalence in boys and girls. This change is likely the result of girls' increased participation in sports. Osgood-Schlatter generally presents one to two years earlier in girls than in boys, consistent with girls' earlier pubertal growth spurt. The occurrence of Osgood-Schlatter primarily during puberty reflects the accelerated bone growth that occurs in response to increased hormone activity in puberty (de Lucena et al., 2011; Duri et al., 2002; Kienstra, 2014).

Diagnosis and Management of Osgood-Schlatter Disease

Osgood-Schlatter's disease is diagnosed and managed similarly in both sexes. Diagnosis is made clinically, by finding tenderness with direct pressure on the tibial apophysis, tenderness with resisted knee extension, and reported pain with jumping and physical activities (de Lucena et al., 2011). Radiography may be considered to rule out fracture, tumor, or osteomyelitis. X-rays may detect soft tissue swelling and fragmentation of the tibial tubercle. The natural history is self-limited. Symptomatic treatment includes pain relief with nonsteroidal anti-inflammatory drugs,

stretching, and physical therapy (Atanda et al., 2011).

Anterior Cruciate Ligament Injury

Prevalence and Risk Factors for ACL Injury

There is a significant sex discrepancy in anterior cruciate ligament (ACL) injuries in high school and collegiate athletes. Girls are 2 to 10 times more likely to sustain ACL injuries than boys (Brophy et al., 2010b; Barber-Westin et al., 2009; Boles and Ferguson, 2010). Risk factors that predispose girls to injure their ACLs include biomechanic, neuromuscular, anatomic, hormonal, and environmental factors (Barber-Westin et al., 2009).

Sex differences in biomechanics are apparent in studies of athletes. The ACL is under increased stress during faulty landing techniques, deceleration, pivoting, or cutting movements with anterior shear forces (Brophy et al., 2010a). Girls' biomechanics and neuromuscular activation differ from those of boys during landing and cutting movements. Girls demonstrate increased knee and hip extension, increased quadriceps muscle activation, and increased knee valgus angles, thus placing a greater load on the ACL (Powers and Fisher, 2010; Brophy et al., 2010b; Yu et al., 2005a; Elliot et al., 2010). The tendency for girls to land with increased knee extension becomes evident after age 12 and is more pronounced through adolescence (Yu et al., 2005a). Another biomechanical cause of ACL injury in girls participating in sports occurs during deceleration of a planted foot with an internally rotated hip and a valgus knee (Elliot et al., 2010). An additional risk factor for ACL injury is the presence of leg dominance, more common in females, which affects their balance, strength, and flexibility. Girls tend to injure the ACL of their supporting leg, while boys more often injure their kicking leg (Boles and Ferguson, 2010; Brophy et al., 2010a).

Anatomic characteristics of the ACL and the knee contribute to the sex differences. The ACL is smaller in girls, has less linear stiffness, and tolerates lower load and energy absorption before failure. Physiologic studies found that the female knee has less resistance to translation and rotation in sagittal, frontal, and transverse planes (Brophy et al., 2010b). These sex differences contribute to girls' increased risk of ACL injury. Hormonal influences may impact ACL integrity as well. Prepubescent boys and girls demonstrate similar rates of ACL injury. During puberty, the pelvic width–femoral length ratio becomes greater in girls than in boys, which increases the quadriceps-femoris angle, thereby affecting limb alignment and forces on the ACL. Receptors for estrogen and testosterone have been identified on ACL fibroblasts. Increased estrogen levels during puberty may reduce collagen production, causing joint laxity (Elliot et al., 2010; Brophy et al., 2010b; Giugliano and Solomon, 2007; Renstrom et al., 2008; Boles and Ferguson, 2010).

Certain environmental and behavioral factors that can affect athletic performance, including nutritional deficiencies and eating disorders, are more common in girls than in boys (Elliot et al., 2010). Nutritional concerns including calcium or vitamin D deficiencies may contribute to ACL injury by weakening supporting structures in the knee.

Diagnosis and Management of ACL Injury

The principles of diagnosis and management of ACL injures are not sex specific. Diagnosis is suggested by a history of pivoting and rapid deceleration movements during athletics, followed by a "popping" sensation and immediate swelling and pain. Physical exam demonstrates joint laxity on the anterior drawer or Lachman tests. X-rays of the knee are performed to rule out fracture. MRI is the test of choice to diagnose ACL injury, but it has decreased sensitivity and specificity in children younger than age 12 (Al-Hadithy et al., 2013). Thus, the clinician must conduct a thorough history and physical exam and use imaging as an adjunct for diagnosis.

Acute care of a suspected or confirmed ACL injury includes pain control, ice, and elevation to reduce swelling, non-weight-bearing with crutches or a wheelchair, and a knee immobilizer. Specialist consultation from an orthopedist who is familiar with arthroscopic ACL reconstruction and pediatric injuries should be obtained. The approach to surgery in a child with open growth plates is controversial. The risks of secondary meniscal injury from non-operative or delayed surgical treatment must be weighed against the risks of iatrogenic injury to the physes with immediate surgical treatment (Al-Hadithy et al., 2013; Renstrom et al., 2008).

Post-ED Care of ACL Injury

ACL injuries have a significant impact on an athlete's quality of life. Immediately, a torn ACL limits sports participation and long term there is a high risk of osteoarthritis of the knee (Boles and Ferguson, 2010). The clinician should stress appropriate rest and supportive care until the patient has surgical intervention or follow-up. Neuromuscular retraining programs have been developed to help athletes incorporate safer movement patterns to prevent ACL injury (Barber-Westin et al., 2009; Brophy et al., 2010a; Powers and Fisher, 2010).

Conclusion

Pediatric conditions with discrepancies by sex that present with knee pain in the child or adolescent were discussed. Biomechanics of the musculoskeletal system and hormonal factors predispose boys and girls to orthopedic conditions. SCFE has a predilection for obese boys; Osgood-Schlatter has equal incidence by sex in recent reports; and ACL injury is more common in adolescent girls. Although SCFE is a condition affecting the hip, the clinician should be aware that pathology in the hip might cause referred pain to the knee. Thus the clinician should perform a thorough lower extremity examination, including range of motion, gait, and neurovascular status in any patient presenting with pain and injury of the lower extremity.

Case Conclusion

The patient had an X-ray that was consistent with SCFE. Orthopedics consultation was obtained from the ED. The patient received IV morphine for pain control and was admitted for surgical intervention the next day.

Gaps in Knowledge/Research Questions

The incidence of Osgood-Schlatter in boys and girls appears to be changing, with an increasing incidence in young women. Further studies may show whether this trend is solely the result of girls' increasing participation in sports or whether there are other causes.

Programs have recently been developed focusing on injury prevention training by improving the biomechanics of athletes. The principles and practices of these neuromuscular retraining programs have not yet been generally accepted, nor have they pervaded the training of coaches and physical education instructors who are responsible for young athletes. Researchers have not yet carried out long-term prospective studies to determine whether these programs have lasting protective effects, improving athletes' movements and preventing sports-related musculoskeletal injuries.

References

Abu Raya, B., Bamberger, E., Kerem, N. C., Kessel, A. & Srugo, I. 2013. Beyond "safe sex"– can we fight adolescent pelvic inflammatory disease? *European Journal of Pediatrics*, 172, 581–90.

Ackerman, S., Irshad, A., Lewis, M. & Anis, M. 2013. Ovarian cystic lesions: A current approach to diagnosis and management. *Radiologic Clinics of North America*, 51, 1067–85.

Adirim, T. A. & Cheng, T. L. 2003. Overview of injuries in the young athlete. *Sports Medicine*, 33, 75–81.

Akkoyun, I. & Gulen, S. 2012. Laparoscopic cystectomy for the treatment of benign ovarian cysts in children: An analysis of 21 cases. *Journal of Pediatric & Adolescent Gynecology*, 25, 364–6.

Al-Hadithy, N., Dodds, A. L., Akhtar, K. S. & Gupte, C. M. 2013. Current concepts of the management of anterior cruciate ligament injuries in children. *Bone Joint Journal*, 95-B, 1562–9.

Alexander, R. T., Hemmelgarn, B. R., Wiebe, N., Bello, A., Morgan, C., Samuel, S., Klarenbach, S. W., Curhan, G. C. & Tonelli, M. 2012. Kidney stones and kidney function loss: A cohort study. *British Medical Journal*, 345, e5287.

Alpay, H., Gokce, I., Ozen, A. & Biyikli, N. 2013. Urinary stone disease in the first year of life: Is it dangerous? *Pediatric Surgery International*, 29, 311–6.

Anschuetz, G. L., Asbel, L., Spain, C. V., Salmon, M., Lewis, F., Newbern, E. C., Goldberg, M. & Johnson, C. C. 2012. Association between enhanced screening for Chlamydia trachomatis and Neisseria gonorrhoeae and reductions in sequelae among women. *Journal of Adolescent Health*, 51, 80–5.

Antal, Z. & Zhou, P. 2009. Congenital adrenal hyperplasia: Diagnosis, evaluation, and management. *Pediatrics Review*, 30, e49–57.

Appelbaum, H., Abraham, C., Choi-Rosen, J. & Ackerman, M. 2013. Key clinical predictors in the early diagnosis of adnexal torsion in children. *Journal of Pediatric & Adolescent Gynecology*, 26, 167–70.

Aspelund, G., Fingeret, A., Gross, E., Kessler, D., Keung, C., Thirumoorthi, A., Oh, P. S., Behr, G., Chen, S., Lampl, B., Middlesworth, W., Kandel, J. & Ruzal-Shapiro, C. 2014. Ultrasonography/MRI versus CT for diagnosing appendicitis. *Pediatrics*, 133, 586–93.

Atanda, A., Jr., Shah, S. A. & O'Brien, K. 2011. Osteochondrosis: Common causes of pain in growing bones. *American Family Physician*, 83, 285–91.

Augustin, T., Cagir, B. & Vandermeer, T. J. 2011. Characteristics of perforated appendicitis: Effect of delay is confounded by age and gender. *Journal of Gastrointestinal Surgery*, 15, 1223–31.

Bachur, R. G., Hennelly, K., Callahan, M. J., Chen, C. & Monuteaux, M. C. 2012. Diagnostic imaging and negative appendectomy rates in children: Effects of age and gender. *Pediatrics*, 129, 877–84.

Balachandran, B., Singhi, S. & Lal, S. 2013. Emergency management of acute abdomen in children. *Indian Journal of Pediatrics*, 80, 226–34.

Banikarim, C. & Chacko, M. R. 2005. Pelvic inflammatory disease in adolescents. *Seminars in Pediatric Infectious Diseases*, 16, 175–80.

Baraff, L. J. 2008. Management of infants and young children with fever without source. *Pediatric Annals*, 37, 673–9.

Barber-Westin, S. D., Noyes, F. R., Smith, S. T. & Campbell, T. M. 2009. Reducing the risk of noncontact anterior cruciate ligament injuries in the female athlete. *The Physician and Sportsmedicine*, 37, 49–61.

Barnhart, K. T. 2009. Clinical practice. Ectopic pregnancy. *New England Journal of Medicine*, 361, 379–87.

Barreto, S. G., Travers, E., Thomas, T., Mackillop, C., Tiong, L., Lorimer, M. & Williams, R. 2010. Acute perforated appendicitis: An analysis of risk factors to guide surgical decision making. *Indian Journal of Medical Sciences*, 64, 58–65.

Benson, E. C., Miller, M., Bosch, P. & Szalay, E. A. 2008. A new look at the incidence of slipped capital femoral epiphysis in New Mexico. *Journal of Pediatric Orthopaedics*, 28, 529–33.

Berger, M. Y., Tabbers, M. M., Kurver, M. J., Boluyt, N. & Benninga, M. A. 2012. Value of abdominal radiography, colonic transit time, and rectal ultrasound scanning in the diagnosis of idiopathic constipation in children: A systematic review. *Journal of Pediatrics*, 161, 44–50.e1–2.

Biggs, W. S. & Dery, W. H. 2006. Evaluation and treatment of constipation in infants and children. *American Family Physician*, **73**, 469–77.

Boles, C. A. & Ferguson, C. 2010. The female athlete. *Radiologic Clinics of North America*, **48**, 1249–66.

Braga, L. H. & Pippi Salle, J. L. 2009. Congenital adrenal hyperplasia: A critical appraisal of the evolution of feminizing genitoplasty and the controversies surrounding gender reassignment. *European Journal of Pediatric Surgery*, **19**, 203–10.

Breech, L. L. & Hillard, P. J. 2005. Adnexal torsion in pediatric and adolescent girls. *Current Opinion in Obstetrics and Gynecology*, **17**, 483–9.

Brierley, J., Carcillo, J. A., Choong, K., Cornell, T., Decaen, A., Deymann, A., Doctor, A., Davis, A., Duff, J., Dugas, M. A., Duncan, A., Evans, B., Feldman, J., Felmet, K., Fisher, G., Frankel, L., Jeffries, H., Greenwald, B., Gutierrez, J., Hall, M., Han, Y. Y., Hanson, J., Hazelzet, J., Hernan, L., Kiff, J., Kissoon, N., Kon, A., Irazuzta, J., Lin, J., Lorts, A., Mariscalco, M., Mehta, R., Nadel, S., Nguyen, T., Nicholson, C., Peters, M., Okhuysen-Cawley, R., Poulton, T., Relves, M., Rodriguez, A., Rozenfeld, R., Schnitzler, E., Shanley, T., Kache, S., Skippen, P., Torres, A., Von Dessauer, B., Weingarten, J., Yeh, T., Zaritsky, A., Stojadinovic, B., Zimmerman, J. & Zuckerberg, A. 2009. Clinical practice parameters for hemodynamic support of pediatric and neonatal septic shock: 2007 update from the American College of Critical Care Medicine. *Critical Care Medicine*, **37**, 666–88.

Brophy, R., Silvers, H. J., Gonzales, T. & Mandelbaum, B. R. 2010a. Gender influences: The role of leg dominance in ACL injury among soccer players. *British Journal of Sports Medicine*, **44**, 694–7.

Brophy, R. H., Silvers, H. J. & Mandelbaum, B. R. 2010b. Anterior cruciate ligament injuries: Etiology and prevention. *Sports Medicine and Arthroscopy Review*, **18**, 2–11.

CDC. 2010. Pelvic Inflammatory Disease Treatment. *Sexually Transmitted Diseases Treatment Guidelines* [Online]. Available: www.cdc.gov/std/treatment/2010/pid.htm.

Cass, D. L. 2005. Ovarian torsion. *Seminars in Pediatric Surgery*, **14**, 86–92.

Cassas, K. J. & Cassettari-Wayhs, A. 2006. Childhood and adolescent sports-related overuse injuries. *American Family Physician*, **73**, 1014–22.

Cecil, J. A., Howell, M. R., Tawes, J. J., Gaydos, J. C., Mckee, K. T., Jr., Quinn, T. C. & Gaydos, C. A. 2001. Features of Chlamydia trachomatis and Neisseria gonorrhoeae infection in male Army recruits. *Journal of Infectious Diseases*, **184**, 1216–9.

Chand, D. H., Rhoades, T., Poe, S. A., Kraus, S. & Strife, C. F. 2003. Incidence and severity of vesicoureteral reflux in children related to age, gender, race and diagnosis. *Journal of Urology*, **170**, 1548–50.

Combs, A. J., Van Batavia, J. P., Chan, J. & Glassberg, K. I. 2013. Dysfunctional elimination syndromes – how closely linked are constipation and encopresis with specific lower urinary tract conditions? *Journal of Urology*, **190**, 1015–20.

Craig, J. C., Knight, J. F., Sureshkumar, P., Mantz, E. & Roy, L. P. 1996. Effect of circumcision on incidence of urinary tract infection in preschool boys. *Journal of Pediatrics*, **128**, 23–7.

Crochet, J. R., Bastian, L. A. & Chireau, M. V. 2013. Does this woman have an ectopic pregnancy?: The rational clinical examination systematic review. *JAMA*, **309**, 1722–9.

Crouch, N. S., Liao, L. M., Woodhouse, C. R., Conway, G. S. & Creighton, S. M. 2008. Sexual function and genital sensitivity following feminizing genitoplasty for congenital adrenal hyperplasia. *Journal of Urology*, **179**, 634–8.

Datta, S. D., Torrone, E., Kruszon-Moran, D., Berman, S., Johnson, R., Satterwhite, C. L., Papp, J. & Weinstock, H. 2012. Chlamydia trachomatis trends in the United States among persons 14 to 39 years of age, 1999–2008. *Sexually Transmitted Diseases*, **39**, 92–6.

De Lorijn, F., Van Wijk, M. P., Reitsma, J. B., Van Ginkel, R., Taminiau, J. A. & Benninga, M. A. 2004. Prognosis of constipation: Clinical factors and colonic transit time. *Archives of Disease in Childhood*, **89**, 723–7.

De Lucena, G. L., Dos Santos Gomes, C. & Guerra, R. O. 2011. Prevalence and associated factors of Osgood-Schlatter syndrome in a population-based sample of Brazilian adolescents. *American Journal of Sports Medicine*, **39**, 415–20.

Detels, R., Green, A. M., Klausner, J. D., Katzenstein, D., Gaydos, C., Handsfield, H., Pequegnat, W., Mayer, K., Hartwell, T. D. & Quinn, T. C. 2011. The incidence and correlates of symptomatic and asymptomatic Chlamydia trachomatis and Neisseria gonorrhoeae infections in selected populations in five countries. *Sexually Transmitted Diseases*, **38**, 503–9.

Duri, Z. A., Patel, D. V. & Aichroth, P. M. 2002. The immature athlete. *Clinics in Sports Medicine*, **21**, 461–82, ix.

Eaton, S. H., Cendron, M. A., Estrada, C. R., Bauer, S. B., Borer, J. G., Cilento, B. G., Diamond, D. A., Retik, A. B. & Peters, C. A. 2005. Intermittent testicular torsion: Diagnostic features and management outcomes. *Journal of Urology*, **174**, 1532–5; discussion 1535.

Edlin, R. S., Shapiro, D. J., Hersh, A. L. & Copp, H. L. 2013. Antibiotic resistance patterns of outpatient pediatric urinary tract infections. *Journal of Urology*, **190**, 222–7.

Elliot, D. L., Goldberg, L. & Kuehl, K. S. 2010. Young women's anterior cruciate ligament injuries: An expanded model and prevention paradigm. *Sports Medicine*, **40**, 367–76.

Falhammar, H., Nystrom, H. F., Ekstrom, U., Granberg, S., Wedell, A. & Thoren, M. 2012. Fertility, sexuality and testicular adrenal rest tumors in adult males with congenital adrenal hyperplasia. *European Journal of Endocrinology*, **166**, 441–9.

Farquhar, C. M. 2005. Ectopic pregnancy. *Lancet*, **366**, 583–91.

Fitzgerald, A., Mori, R., Lakhanpaul, M. & Tullus, K. 2012. Antibiotics for treating lower urinary tract infection in children. *Cochrane Database Systematic Reviews*, **8**, CD006857.

Fleisher, G. R. & Ludwig, S. 2010. *Textbook of Pediatric Emergency Medicine*. Philadelphia: Wolters Kluwer/ Lippincott Williams & Wilkins Health.

Gastaud, F., Bouvattier, C., Duranteau, L., Brauner, R., Thibaud, E., Kutten, F. & Bougneres, P. 2007. Impaired sexual and reproductive outcomes in women with classical forms of congenital adrenal hyperplasia. *Journal of Clinical Endocrinology & Metabolism*, **92**, 1391–6.

Giugliano, D. N. & Solomon, J. L. 2007. ACL tears in female athletes. *Physical Medicine and Rehabilitation Clinics of North America*, **18**, 417–38, viii.

Gorelick, M. H. & Shaw, K. N. 2000. Clinical decision rule to identify febrile young girls at risk for urinary tract infection. *Archives of Pediatrics and Adolescent Medicine*, **154**, 386–90.

Gray-Swain, M. R. & Peipert, J. F. 2006. Pelvic inflammatory disease in adolescents. *Current Opinion in Obstetrics and Gynecology*, **18**, 503–10.

Gunther, P. & Rubben, I. 2012. The acute scrotum in childhood and adolescence. *Deutsches Arzteblatt International*, **109**, 449–57; quiz 458.

Habbig, S., Beck, B. B. & Hoppe, B. 2011. Nephrocalcinosis and urolithiasis in children. *Kidney International*, **80**, 1278–91.

Hansson, S., Bollgren, I., Esbjorner, E., Jakobsson, B. & Marild, S. 1999. Urinary tract infections in children below two years of age: A quality assurance project in Sweden. The Swedish Pediatric Nephrology Association. *Acta Paediatrica*, **88**, 270–4.

Hines, M., Brook, C. & Conway, G. S. 2004. Androgen and psychosexual development: Core gender identity, sexual orientation and recalled childhood gender role behavior in women and men with congenital adrenal hyperplasia (CAH). *The Journal of Sex Research*, **41**, 75–81.

Jamal, A. & Ramzan, A. 2004. Renal and post-renal causes of acute renal failure in children. *Journal of the College of Physicians and Surgeons Pakistan*, **14**, 411–5.

Johnson, J. R. 1991. Virulence factors in Escherichia coli urinary tract infection. *Clinical Microbiology Reviews*, **4**, 80–128.

Jordan-Young, R. M. 2012. Hormones, context, and "brain gender": A review of evidence from congenital adrenal hyperplasia. *Social Science & Medicine*, **74**, 1738–44.

Kalorin, C. M., Zabinski, A., Okpareke, I., White, M. & Kogan, B. A. 2009. Pediatric urinary stone disease–does age matter? *Journal of Urology*, **181**, 2267–71; discussion 2271.

Kayaba, H., Tamura, H., Shirayama, K., Murata, J. & Fujiwara, Y. 1996. Hemorrhagic ovarian cyst in childhood: A case report. *Journal of Pediatric Surgery*, **31**, 978–9.

Kienstra, A. J. M., Charles G 2014. *Osgood-Schlatter disease (tibial tuberosity avulsion)*, UpToDate. Topic 6289, Version 11.0.

Kruszka, P. S. & Kruszka, S. J. 2010. Evaluation of acute pelvic pain in women. *American Family Physician*, **82**, 141–7.

Kujala, U. M., Kvist, M. & Heinonen, O. 1985. Osgood-Schlatter's disease in adolescent athletes. Retrospective study of incidence and duration. *American Journal of Sports Medicine*, **13**, 236–41.

Kulik, D. M., Uleryk, E. M. & Maguire, J. L. 2013. Does this child have appendicitis? A systematic review of clinical prediction rules for children with acute abdominal pain. *Journal of Clinical Epidemiology*, **66**, 95–104.

Kutasy, B. & Puri, P. 2013. Appendicitis in obese children. *Pediatric Surgery International*, **29**, 537–44.

Lee, P., Schober, J., Nordenstrom, A., Hoebeke, P., Houk, C., Looijenga, L., Manzoni, G., Reiner, W. & Woodhouse, C. 2012. Review of recent outcome data of disorders of sex development (DSD): Emphasis on surgical and sexual outcomes. *Journal of Pediatric Urology*, **8**, 611–5.

Lee, P. A., Houk, C. P. & Husmann, D. A. 2010. Should male gender assignment be considered in the markedly virilized patient with 46, XX and congenital adrenal hyperplasia? *Journal of Urology*, **184**, 1786–92.

Leeson, K. & Leeson, B. 2013. Pediatric ultrasound: Applications in the emergency department. *Emergency Medicine Clinics of North America*, **31**, 809–29.

Lehmann, C. L., Arons, R. R., Loder, R. T. & Vitale, M. G. 2006. The epidemiology of slipped capital femoral epiphysis: An update. *Journal of Pediatric Orthopaedics*, **26**, 286–90.

Lipsky, B. A. 1989. Urinary tract infections in men. Epidemiology, pathophysiology, diagnosis, and treatment. *Annals of Internal Medicine*, **110**, 138–50.

Lozeau, A. M. & Potter, B. 2005. Diagnosis and management of ectopic pregnancy. *American Family Physician*, **72**, 1707–14.

Mandeville, K., Pottker, T., Bulloch, B. & Liu, J. 2011. Using appendicitis scores in the pediatric ED. *American Journal of Emergency Medicine*, **29**, 972–7.

Markar, S. R., Blackburn, S., Cobb, R., Karthikesalingam, A., Evans, J., Kinross, J. & Faiz, O. 2012. Laparoscopic versus open appendectomy for complicated and uncomplicated appendicitis in children. *Journal of Gastrointestinal Surgery*, **16**, 1993–2004.

Matlaga, B. R., Schaeffer, A. J., Novak, T. E. & Trock, B. J. 2010. Epidemiologic insights into pediatric kidney stone disease. *Urological Research*, **38**, 453–7.

Mcgann Donlan, S. & Mycyk, M. B. 2009. Is female sex associated with ED delays to diagnosis of appendicitis in the computed tomography era? *American Journal of Emergency Medicine*, **27**, 856–8.

Mellick, L. B. 2012. Torsion of the testicle: It is time to stop tossing the dice. *Pediatric Emergency Care*, **28**, 80–6.

Merke, D. P. 2014a. *Diagnosis of classic congenital adrenal hyperplasia due to 21-hydroxylase deficiency*, UpToDate.

Merke, D. P. 2014b. *Treatment of classic congenital adrenal hyperplasia due to 21-hydroxylase deficiency in infants and children*, UpToDate.

Meyer-Bahlburg, H. F. 2011. Brain development and cognitive, psychosocial, and psychiatric functioning in classical 21-hydroxylase deficiency. *Endocrine Development*, **20**, 88–95.

Meyer-Bahlburg, H. F., Dolezal, C., Baker, S. W. & New, M. I. 2008. Sexual orientation in women with classical or non-classical congenital adrenal hyperplasia as a function of degree of prenatal androgen excess. *Archives of Sexual Behavior*, **37**, 85–99.

Mukherjee, S., Joshi, A., Carroll, D., Chandran, H., Parashar, K. & Mccarthy, L. 2009. What is the effect of circumcision on risk of urinary tract infection in boys with posterior urethral valves? *Journal of Pediatric Surgery*, **44**, 417–21.

Murray, A. W. & Wilson, N. I. 2008. Changing incidence of slipped capital femoral epiphysis: A relationship with obesity? *The Journal of Bone & Joint Surgery*, **90**, 92–4.

Nordenstrom, A. 2011. Adult women with 21-hydroxylase deficient congenital adrenal hyperplasia, surgical and psychological aspects. *Current Opinion in Pediatrics*, **23**, 436–42.

Novak, T. E., Lakshmanan, Y., Trock, B. J., Gearhart, J. P. & Matlaga, B. R. 2009. Sex prevalence of pediatric kidney stone disease in the United States: An epidemiologic investigation. *Urology*, **74**, 104–7.

Nurko, S. & Scott, S. M. 2011. Coexistence of constipation and incontinence in children and adults. *Best Practice & Research: Clinical Gastroenterology*, **25**, 29–41.

Otten, B. J., Stikkelbroeck, M. M., Claahsen-Van Der Grinten, H. L. & Hermus, A. R. 2005. Puberty and fertility in congenital adrenal hyperplasia. *Endocrine Devopment*, **8**, 54–66.

Oyetunji, T. A., Nwomeh, B. C., Ong'Uti, S. K., Gonzalez, D. O., Cornwell, E. E., 3rd & Fullum, T. M. 2011. Laparoscopic appendectomy in children with complicated appendicitis: Ethnic disparity amid changing trend. *Journal of Surgical Research*, **170**, e99–103.

Oyetunji, T. A., Ong'Uti, S. K., Bolorunduro, O. B., Cornwell, E. E., 3rd & Nwomeh, B. C. 2012. Pediatric negative appendectomy rate: Trend, predictors, and differentials. *Journal of Surgical Research*, **173**, 16–20.

Pasterski, V., Hindmarsh, P., Geffner, M., Brook, C., Brain, C. & Hines, M. 2007. Increased aggression and activity level in 3- to 11-year-old girls with congenital adrenal hyperplasia (CAH). *Hormones and Behavior*, **52**, 368–74.

Peck, D. 2010. Slipped capital femoral epiphysis: Diagnosis and management. *American Family Physician*, **82**, 258–62.

Peck, K. & Herrera-Soto, J. 2014. Slipped capital femoral epiphysis: what's new? *Orthopedic Clinics of North America*, **45**, 77–86.

Pepper, V. K., Stanfill, A. B. & Pearl, R. H. 2012. Diagnosis and management of pediatric appendicitis, intussusception, and Meckel diverticulum. *Surgical Clinics of North America*, **92**, 505–26, vii.

Pienkowski, C., Cartault, A., Carfagna, L., Ernoult, P., Vial, J., Lemasson, F., Le Mandat, A., Galinier, P. & Tauber, M. 2012. Ovarian cysts in prepubertal girls. *Endocrine Development*, **22**, 101–11.

Piper, H. G., Oltmann, S. C., Xu, L., Adusumilli, S. & Fischer, A. C. 2012. Ovarian torsion: Diagnosis of inclusion mandates earlier intervention. *Journal of Pediatric Surgery*, **47**, 2071–6.

Powers, C. M. & Fisher, B. 2010. Mechanisms underlying ACL injury-prevention training: the brain-behavior relationship. *Journal of Athletic Training*, **45**, 513–5.

Renstrom, P., Ljungqvist, A., Arendt, E., Beynnon, B., Fukubayashi, T., Garrett, W., Georgoulis, T., Hewett, T. E., Johnson, R., Krosshaug, T., Mandelbaum, B., Micheli, L., Myklebust, G., Roos, E., Roos, H.,

Schamasch, P., Shultz, S., Werner, S., Wojtys, E. & Engebretsen, L. 2008. Non-contact ACL injuries in female athletes: An International Olympic Committee current concepts statement. *British Journal of Sports Medicine*, **42**, 394–412.

Reuchlin-Vroklage, L. M., Bierma-Zeinstra, S., Benninga, M. A. & Berger, M. Y. 2005. Diagnostic value of abdominal radiography in constipated children: A systematic review. *Archives of Pediatrics and Adolescent Medicine*, **159**, 671–8.

Rudaitis, S., Pundziene, B., Jievaltas, M., Uktveris, R. & Kevelaitis, E. 2009. Recurrent urinary tract infection in girls: Do urodynamic, behavioral and functional abnormalities play a role? *Journal of Nephrology*, **22**, 766–73.

Sas, D. J. 2011. An update on the changing epidemiology and metabolic risk factors in pediatric kidney stone disease. *Clinical Journal of the American Society of Nephrology*, **6**, 2062–8.

Sas, D. J., Hulsey, T. C., Shatat, I. F. & Orak, J. K. 2010. Increasing incidence of kidney stones in children evaluated in the emergency department. *Journal of Pediatrics*, **157**, 132–7.

Sauerland, S., Jaschinski, T. & Neugebauer, E. A. 2010. Laparoscopic versus open surgery for suspected appendicitis. *Cochrane Database Systematic Reviews*, CD001546.

Savasi, I., Lacy, J. A., Gerstle, J. T., Stephens, D., Kives, S. & Allen, L. 2009. Management of ovarian dermoid cysts in the pediatric and adolescent population. *Journal of Pediatric & Adolescent Gynecology*, **22**, 360–4.

Shademan, A. & Tappouni, R. F. 2013. Pitfalls in CT diagnosis of appendicitis: Pictorial essay. *Journal of Medical Imaging and Radiation Oncology*, **57**, 329–36.

Shah, S. 2013. An update on common gastrointestinal emergencies. *Emergency Medicine Clinics of North America*, **31**, 775–93.

Shaikh, N., Ewing, A. L., Bhatnagar, S. & Hoberman, A. 2010. Risk of renal scarring in children with a first urinary tract infection: A systematic review. *Pediatrics*, **126**, 1084–91.

Shaikh, N., Morone, N. E., Bost, J. E. & Farrell, M. H. 2008. Prevalence of urinary tract infection in childhood: A meta-analysis. *The Pediatric Infectious Disease Journal*, **27**, 302–8.

Sharma, R. & Seth, A. 2013. Congenital adrenal hyperplasia: Issues in diagnosis and treatment in children. *The Indian Journal of Pediatrics*. November, 1–8.

Sherrard, J. & Barlow, D. 1996. Gonorrhoea in men: Clinical and diagnostic aspects. *Genitourinary Medicne*, **72**, 422–6.

Singh-Grewal, D., Macdessi, J. & Craig, J. 2005. Circumcision for the prevention of urinary tract infection in boys: A systematic review of randomised trials and observational studies. *Archives of Disease in Childhood*, **90**, 853–8.

Speiser, P. W., Azziz, R., Baskin, L. S., Ghizzoni, L., Hensle, T. W., Merke, D. P., Meyer-Bahlburg, H. F., Miller, W. L., Montori, V. M., Oberfield, S. E., Ritzen, M. & White, P. C. 2010. Congenital adrenal hyperplasia due to steroid 21-hydroxylase deficiency: An Endocrine Society clinical practice guideline. *Journal of Clinical Endocrinology & Metabolism*, **95**, 4133–60.

Spinelli, C., Buti, I., Pucci, V., Liserre, J., Alberti, E., Nencini, L., Alessandra, M., Lo Piccolo, R. & Messineo, A. 2013. Adnexal torsion in children and adolescents: New trends to conservative surgical approach – our experience and review of literature. *Gynecological Endocrinology*, **29**, 54–8.

Stein, J. C., Wang, R., Adler, N., Boscardin, J., Jacoby, V. L., Won, G., Goldstein, R. & Kohn, M. A. 2010. Emergency physician ultrasonography for evaluating patients at risk for ectopic pregnancy: A meta-analysis. *Annals of Emergency Medicine*, **56**, 674–83.

Stewart, J. K., Olcott, E. W. & Jeffrey, B. R. 2012. Sonography for appendicitis: Nonvisualization of the appendix is an indication for active clinical observation rather than direct referral for computed tomography. *Journal of Clinical Ultrasound*, **40**, 455–61.

Subcommittee on Urinary Tract Infection, S. C. O. Q. I., Management & Roberts, K. B. 2011. Urinary tract infection: Clinical practice guideline for the diagnosis and management of the initial UTI in febrile infants and children 2 to 24 months. *Pediatrics*, **128**, 595–610.

Sulu, B., Gunerhan, Y., Palanci, Y., Isler, B. & Caglayan, K. 2010. Epidemiological and demographic features of appendicitis and influences of several environmental factors. *Ulus Travma Acil Cerrahi Derg*, **16**, 38–42.

To, T., Agha, M., Dick, P. T. & Feldman, W. 1998. Cohort study on circumcision of newborn boys and subsequent risk of urinary-tract infection. *Lancet*, **352**, 1813–6.

Tofteland, N. D., Stuart-Hilgenfeld, M., Hunt, R., Tamma, P., Canares, T. L., Yao-Cohen, M. & Nazif, J. 2010. Index of suspicion, case 1: hemoptysis, dyspnea, and hematuria, case 2: rash and headache in a wrestler, case 3: abdominal distention in a teenage girl. *Pediatrics Review*, **31**, 477–82.

Tzovaras, G., Liakou, P., Baloyiannis, I., Spyridakis, M., Mantzos, F., Tepetes, K., Athanassiou, E. & Hatzitheofilou, C. 2007. Laparoscopic appendectomy: Differences between male and female patients with suspected acute appendicitis. *World Journal of Surgery*, **31**, 409–13.

Van Der Zwan, Y. G., Janssen, E. H., Callens, N., Wolffenbuttel, K. P., Cohen-Kettenis, P. T., Van Den

Berg, M., Drop, S. L., Dessens, A. B. & Beerendonk, C. 2013. Severity of virilization is associated with cosmetic appearance and sexual function in women with congenital adrenal hyperplasia: A cross-sectional study. *Journal of Sexual Medicine*, **10**, 866–75.

Wald, E. R., Di Lorenzo, C., Cipriani, L., Colborn, D. K., Burgers, R. & Wald, A. 2009. Bowel habits and toilet training in a diverse population of children. *Journal of Pediatric Gastroenterology and Nutrition*, **48**, 294–8.

Wan, M. J., Krahn, M., Ungar, W. J., Caku, E., Sung, L., Medina, L. S. & Doria, A. S. 2009. Acute appendicitis in young children: Cost-effectiveness of US versus CT in diagnosis – a Markov decision analytic model. *Radiology*, **250**, 378–86.

Wennerstrom, M., Hansson, S., Jodal, U. & Stokland, E. 2000. Primary and acquired renal scarring in boys and girls with urinary tract infection. *Journal of Pediatrics*, **136**, 30–4.

Westerlund, B., Siitonen, A., Elo, J., Williams, P. H., Korhonen, T. K. & Makela, P. H. 1988. Properties of Escherichia coli isolates from urinary tract infections in boys. *Journal of Infectious Diseases*, **158**, 996–1002.

Witbreuk, M. M., Van Royen, B. J., Van Kemenade, F. J., Witte, B. I. & Van Der Sluijs, J. A. 2013. Incidence and gender differences of slipped capital femoral epiphysis in the Netherlands from 1998–2010 combined with a review of the literature on the epidemiology of SCFE. *Journal of Children's Orthopaedics*, **7**, 99–105.

Wood, K. D., Stanasel, I. S., Koslov, D. S., Mufarrij, P. W., Mclorie, G. A. & Assimos, D. G. 2013. Changing stone composition profile of children with nephrolithiasis. *Urology*, **82**, 210–3.

Yu, B., Mcclure, S. B., Onate, J. A., Guskiewicz, K. M., Kirkendall, D. T. & Garrett, W. E. 2005a. Age and gender effects on lower extremity kinematics of youth soccer players in a stop-jump task. *American Journal of Sports Medicine*, **33**, 1356–64.

Yu, S. H., Kim, C. B., Park, J. W., Kim, M. S. & Radosevich, D. M. 2005b. Ultrasonography in the diagnosis of appendicitis: Evaluation by meta-analysis. *Korean Journal of Radiology*, **6**, 267–77.

Chapter 13

Special Populations
C. Acute Medical Care for the Transgender Patient

Elizabeth Samuels and Michelle Forcier

Case, Part 1

A 32-year-old presents with shortness of breath. The patient is listed as male in the electronic medical record (EMR), but the patient appears to be female, with long hair, makeup, and a long skirt. The physician first thinks this is the wrong room and says, "Is this John Jones's room?" The patient states it is the right room, and the physician asks, "Has he stepped out?" Between labored breaths, the patient clarifies, "I am John Jones." She is somewhat withdrawn, makes poor eye contact during the interview, appears to be in mild respiratory distress, and tells you she is having chest pain and difficulty breathing.

Introduction

"Transgender" is a broad umbrella term used to describe individuals whose gender identity or gender expression differs from the gender they were assigned at birth (see Figure 13C.1 and Glossary of Terms).

Glossary of Terms*

Transgender or trans: Literally "across gender"; sometimes interpreted as "beyond gender"; an

---

* Definitions adapted from the National Center for Transgender Equality. *Transgender Terminology.* January 2014, accessed at transequality.org/Resources/TransTerminology_2014.pdf.; UCSF Center of Excellence for Transgender Health. "Transgender Terminology" in *Primary Care Protocol for Transgender Patient Care,* Center of Excellence for Transgender Health, University of California, San Francisco, Department of Family and Community Medicine, April 2011; Bauer et al. Reported Emergency Department Avoidance, Use and Experiences of Transgender Persons in Ontario, Canada. *Annals of Emergency Medicine,* October 2013: 1–10.

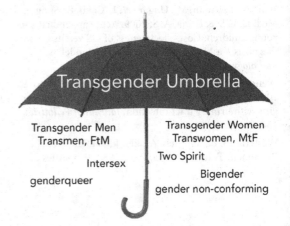

Figure 13C.1 Transgender is an umbrella term (adj.) for people whose gender identity and/or gender expression differs from the sex they were assigned at birth

umbrella, community-based term that describes a wide variety of cross-gender behaviors and identities. Transgender is not a diagnostic term; it does not imply a medical or psychological condition. Avoid using this term as a noun: a person is not "a transgender" or, as a verb, "transgendered"; they may be a transgender person.

Transsexual: An older more specific, clinical term applied to individuals who seek hormonal (and often, but not always) surgical treatment to modify their bodies so they may live full time as members of the sex category opposite to their birth-assigned sex (including legal status). Some transsexuals may simply identify as transgender or trans. This term is generally falling out of favor. Avoid using this term as a noun: a person is not "a transsexual"; they may be a transsexual person.

Transgender man, female to male (FtM) or transman: A transgender person assigned female at birth who identifies as male or masculine.

Transgender woman, male to female (MtF) or transwoman: A transgender person assigned male at birth who identifies as female or feminine.

Cisgender: Nontransgender; refers to those whose gender identity is aligned with their assigned gender at birth.

Gender identity: An individual's sense of being male, female, or something else; a person's innate and expressed masculinity, femininity, or something else.

Gender expression: How a person represents or expresses gender identity, often through behavior, clothing, hairstyles, voice, or body characteristics.

Cross-dresser: A term for people who dress in clothing traditionally or stereotypically worn by the other sex but who generally have no intent to live full time as the other gender. The older term "transvestite" is considered derogatory by many in the United States.

Queer: A term used to refer to lesbian, gay, bisexual, and often also transgender people. Some use "queer" as an alternative to "gay" in an effort to be more inclusive. Depending on the user, the term has either a derogatory or an affirming connotation, as many have sought to reclaim the term that was once widely used in a negative way.

Genderqueer: A term used by individuals who identify as neither entirely male nor entirely female.

Gender nonconforming: A term for individuals whose gender expression is different from societal expectations related to gender; prepubertal children are sometimes described as gender nonconforming as their gender identity is sometimes still fluid and for many, their gender trajectory unclear.

Gender fluid: A gender identity on a spectrum between male and female, perhaps changing over time.

Bigender: A gender identity that combines coexisting male and female gender identities.

Two-spirit: A term used by North American Native peoples to describe those who identify with both male and female gender roles and expressions.

Gender confirmation or affirmation surgery: Surgical procedures that change one's body to better reflect a person's gender identity. Previous terminology that is considered perjorative at present includes: sex reassignment or sex change operation. This may include different procedures, including those sometimes also referred to as "top surgery" (breast augmentation or removal); "bottom surgery" (altering genitals); or facial feminization surgery (altering the facial structures to appear more feminine). Contrary to popular belief, there is not one surgery; in fact, there are many different surgeries. These surgeries are medically necessary for some people; however, not all people want, need, or can have surgery as part of their transition. "Sex change surgery" is considered a derogatory term by many.

Sexual orientation: A term describing a person's attraction to members of the same sex and/or a different sex, and identification with commonly defined sexual identification as lesbian, gay, bisexual, heterosexual, or asexual.

Transition: The time and process when a person begins to live as the gender with which they identify rather than the gender they were assigned at birth. Transitioning may or may not also include medical and legal aspects, including taking hormones, having surgery, or changing identity documents (e.g., driver's license, Social Security record) to reflect one's gender identity. Some people use this term to describe their medical condition with regard to their gender until they have completed the medical procedures that are relevant for them.

Intersex: A term used for people who are born with a reproductive or sexual anatomy and/or chromosome pattern that does not seem to fit typical definitions of male or female. Intersex conditions are also known as differences of sex development (DSD).

Drag queen or king: Used to refer to male or female performers who dress as women or men for the purpose of entertaining others at bars, clubs, or other events. It is also sometimes used in a derogatory manner to refer to transgender women.

Transgender, also known as trans, individuals continue to be among the most marginalized in the lesbian, gay, bisexual, transgender, and queer (LGBTQ) community, despite some gains in LGBTQ civil rights. Trans patients have unique medical and mental health needs, facing significant barriers to care, primarily because of discrimination and insurance coverage.[1] Trans people of color experience some of the highest rates of unemployment, poverty, harassment, discrimination, and health inequalities.[2] Transwomen and transgender people of color are at especially high risk for HIV.[3] Gender nonconforming or gender queer youth are frequently targets of harassment, assault, or sexual violence in home, school, and community settings.[4] Historically, the transgender community has generally been disproportionately affected by psychiatric disorders,[5] assault,[6] cigarette smoking, and drug and alcohol use[7] and is much more likely to attempt suicide compared to the general population (41% vs. 1.6%).[8] These disparities are intimately linked to the chronic stress of societal stigma; discrimination and violence; socioeconomic status; denial of rights; and internalized, self-directed shame.[9]

As social discourse progresses regarding the health and human rights of all genders and sexualities, trans individuals are presenting to medical and mental health providers in increased numbers. Some medical schools have recognised the need to improve efforts training future clinicians in trans health,[10] however most medical students and residents at present will receive little or no training in medical school or residency about caring for the transgender patient.[11] Emergency medicine (EM) providers are critical front line ambassadors to improving the transgender person's experience and willingness to engage with health care that can reduce health disparities and negative health outcomes EM providers can more competently care for all patients, including transgender patients, using a developmental approach to gender that incorporates modern gender paradigms and ensures health access and equity to a broad range of gender diverse patients.

[1] Grant, J.M., Mottet L.A., Tanis J. et al. (2011). *Injustice at Every Turn: A Report of the National Transgender Discrimination Survey*. Washington: National Center for Transgender Equality and National Gay and Lesbian Task Force.

[2] Ibid.

[3] Clements-Nolle, K., Mark, R., Guzman, R., and Katz, M. (2001). HIV prevalence, risk behaviors, health care use, and mental health status of transgender persons: Implications for public health intervention. *American Journal of Public Health*, **91**(6), 915–21; Grant et al., *Injustice at Every Turn*, 2; United Nations Programme on HIV/AIDS (UNAIDS) and World Health Organization (WHO). (2007). 2007 AIDS Epidemic Update. *Accessed at* http://data.unaids.org/pub/EPISli des/2007/2007_epiupdate_en.pdf.

[4] Grant et al., *Injustice at Every Turn*, 3.

[5] McLaughlin, K.A., Hatzenbuehler, M.L., and Keyes K.M. (2010). Responses to discrimination and psychiatric disorders among black, Hispanic, female, and lesbian, gay, and bisexual individuals. *American Journal of Public Health*, **100**(8), 1477–84.

[6] Roberts, A.L., Austin, S.B., Corliss, H.L. et al. (2010). Pervasive trauma exposure among US sexual orientation minority adults and risk of posttraumatic stress disorder. *American Journal of Public Health*, **100**(12), 2433–2441.

[7] Remafedi, G., French, S., Story, M. et al. (1998). The relationship between suicide risk and sexual orientation: Results of a population-based study. *American Journal of Public Health*, **88**(1), 57–60.

[8] Grant et al., *Injustice at Every Turn*, 2.

[9] This idea is known as a minority stress model. Institute of Medicine. (2011). *The Health of Lesbian, Gay, Bisexual, and Transgender People: Building a Foundation for Better Understanding*. Washington,

DC: The National Academies Press; Herek, G.M. (2009). Sexual stigma and sexual prejudice in the United States: A conceptual framework. In *Contemporary Perspectives on Lesbian, Gay, and Bisexual Identities*, edited by D. A. Hope. New York: Springer Science 1 Business Media, 65–111; Nemoto, T., Iwamoto, M., and Operario, D. (2003). HIV risk behaviors among Asian and Pacific Islander male-to-female transgenders. *The Community Psychologist*, **36**, 31–35.

[10] De Vries, A.L. and Cohen-Kettenis, P.T. (2012). Clinical management of gender dysphoria in children and adolescents: The Dutch approach. *Journal of Homosexuality*, **59**, 301–20; Wood, H., Sasaki, S., Bradley, S.J. et al. (2013). Patterns of referral to a gender identity service for children and adolescents (1976–2011): Age, sex ratio, and sexual orientation. *Journal of Sex and Marital Therapy*, **39**, 1–6; Zucker, K.J., Bradley, S.J., Owen-Anderson, A. et al. (2008). Is gender identity disorder in adolescents coming out of the closet? *Journal of Sex and Marital Therapy*, **34**(4), 287–290; Pleak, R.R. (2011). Gender-variant children and transgender adolescents. *Child and Adolescent Clinics of North America*, **20**(4), xv–xx.

[11] Moll, J., Krieger, P., Moreno-Walton, L. et al. (2014). The prevalence of lesbian, gay, bisexual, and transgender health education and training in emergency medicine residency programs: What do we know? *Academic Emergency Medicine*, **21**, 608–11; Obedin-Maliver, J., Goldsmith, E.S., Stewart, L. et al. (2011). Lesbian, gay, bisexual, and transgender-related content in undergraduate medical education. *JAMA*, **306**(9), 971–7.

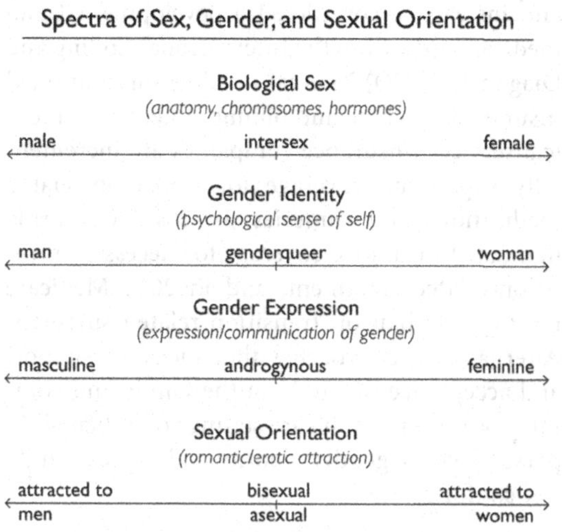

Spectra of Sex, Gender, and Sexual Orientation

Biological Sex
(anatomy, chromosomes, hormones)

male   intersex   female

Gender Identity
(psychological sense of self)

man   genderqueer   woman

Gender Expression
(expression/communication of gender)

masculine   androgynous   feminine

Sexual Orientation
(romantic/erotic attraction)

attracted to men   bisexual asexual   attracted to women

Figure 13C.2 Figurative representation of the spectrums of sex, gender, and sexual orientation

Background

Most trans patients present to the ED for problems unrelated to their gender identity, such as sprained ankles, upper respiratory tract infections, or motor vehicle accidents. They may also present with concerns related to their gender: pain, depression and suicidality, injury from abuse or assault, or complications from either supervised or unsupervised medical or surgical gender transition adjuncts. The foundation for clinical competence and comfort providing care to transgender people for any presenting concern is understanding that there may be a range of gender identity and expression among individuals, and that the gender spectrum is an aspect of both biodiversity and human development (Figure 13C.2).

Differentiating between gender, our sense of male or female self, and sexuality, who we are attracted to and the sexual behaviors we engage in, is an important developmental concept that informs care for all patients.

Gender relies on the interplay of biological, psychosocial, and cultural factors imbued with specific expectations and norms. Everyone experiences gender and individuals' understanding of their own gender identity and role is a necessary and normal component of child and adolescent development. Both identities and expression may fall in a wide spectrum and can range from constant to fluid and may change throughout a person's lifespan (see Figure 13C.2). Gender is usually assigned at birth as male or female typically based on the appearance of external genitalia. Chromosomes, gonads, hormones, and observable secondary gender sexual characteristics are typically used to determine or assign gender. Historically, intersex infants born with "ambiguous" genitalia would have surgery shortly after birth to make their genitalia less ambiguous and according to the best potential cosmetic outcome as determined by the surgical team. The results of this practice have been varied and, for many, have created significant distress when they were assigned a gender incongruent with their gender identity. More recently, intersex infants have not been assigned a definitive gender at birth but allowed to grow and mature to see how their unique gender evolves. Understanding biologically intersex persons has helped inform our understanding that the primary source of gender is more dependent on neurodevelopment than gonads and secondary gender sex characteristics. Most patients identifying as transgender will not be biologically intersex but fall elsewhere under the trans umbrella.

Epidemiological studies' population estimates of people who identify as transgender vary wildly and are often methodologically flawed. Thse estimates generally reflect counts of individuals presenting to gender speciality clinics, who have sought medical or surgical transition, thus likely underrepresentative. The fluidity and wide spectrum of identity, in addition to widespread external transphobia, too often internalized by transgender persons, make accurate studies difficult to obtain and result in underreporting. Current estimates based on population surveys show 0.6% of individuals born assigned male and 0.2% of individuals born assigned female would like to pursue hormones or surgery for gender transition. The process by which one actualizes gender identity is called transitioning. Some may transition through entirely reversible measures such as binding their breasts, attire, and hair styling, which require no medical interventions, while others may opt for partially reversible medical or hormonal therapies or irreversible surgical interventions to help match their gender presentation with their gender identity. While hormones and surgeries can be essential elements of gender transitioning, careful planning for disclosure, safety, and other social support is just as important to successful transition.

As our understanding of gender has evolved over the years, the American Psychiatric Association in 2013 appropriately removed Gender Identity Disorder from the *Diagnostic and Statistical Manual of Mental Disorders* (DSM-V). Instead of pathologizing gender nonconformity, the APA appropriately shifted the diagnostic focus to gender dysphoria, distress or discomfort caused by "a marked incongruence between one's experienced/expressed gender and assigned gender."[12] Universally, medical and mental health societies, including the American Medical Association, the American Psychiatric Association, the American Psychological Association, and the American Academy of Pediatrics, reject reparative therapies that attempt to convert a transgender individual to cisgender (or a gay individual to heterosexual), as these are regarded as illegitimate, ineffective, and harmful.[13]

Many believe gender dysphoria should be removed from the psychiatric coding altogether and instead be considered a developmental and medical need within the International Coding and Diagnostic (ICD) Manual to allow for continued insurance coverage and billing of necessary medical services. Insurance companies are incrementally expanding coverage for transition-related medications and surgeries. In 2013, California mandated insurance coverage for necessary transition-related treatment, and in 2014 Medicare removed its ban on transition-related surgeries. Alternatively, approaches that focus on support and acceptance within both the family and community and in health care settings offer benefit to persons whose gender identity and expression do not conform.

Caring for the Transgender Patient

Trans patients may have had prior difficult or stigmatizing experiences in other health settings.[14] Fear of stigma and discrimination may prevent patients from sharing important information about hormone use, recent surgeries, illicit substances, or suicidality. Respect, courtesy, and a patient-centered approach are universally desirable to all patients. It is best to avoid assumptions and directly ask each patient the preferred name or title, gender, and pronouns. This information should be noted and shared with the entire clinical team so as to use it consistently and coherently during the course of treatment. Using any patient's correct name and pronoun conveys respect, builds trust, and enhances rapport that may help a patient more easily share sensitive health information.

Many transgender individuals seek medical attention before name and gender marker are changed on their identification or insurance to reflect their authentic gender identity. It is common to take care of patients before their name and gender have been legally changed on their identification and health insurance. EMRs are generally limited to two gender options and do not have an option for a preferred name or space to indicate a patient's preferred pronoun. Not knowing this information can lead to confusing, awkward, and alienating initial interactions. The Institute of Medicine, World Professional Association for Transgender Health, and the Gay and Lesbian

[12] American Psychiatric Association. (2013). *Diagnostic and Statistical Manual of Mental Disorders* (5th ed.). Arlington, VA: American Psychiatric Publishing.

[13] American Medical Association. H-160.991 Health Care Needs of the Homosexual Population. Accessed February 10, 2014 at www.ama-assn.org/ama/pub/about-ama/our-people/member-groups-sections/glbt-advisory-committee/ama-policy-regarding-sexual-orientation; American Psychiatric Association. (2000). Position Statement on Therapies Focused on Attempts to Change Sexual Orientation (Reparative or Conversion Therapies). March 2000. Accessed February 10, 2014 at www.psychiatry.org/file%20library/advocacy%20and%20newsroom/position%20statements/ps2000_ reparativetherapy.pdf; APA Task Force on Appropriate Therapeutic Responses to Sexual Orientation. (2009). *Report of the Task Force on Appropriate Therapeutic Responses to Sexual Orientation.* Washington, DC: American Psychological Association; American Academy of Pediatrics. (1993). Homosexuality and adolescence. *Pediatrics*, **92**, 631; National Association of Social Workers. (2000). Position Statement: "Reparative" and "Conversion" Therapies for Lesbians and Gay Men. Accessed February 10, 2014 at www.naswdc.org/diversity/lgb/reparative.asp.

[14] Grant et al. *Injustice at Every Turn.*

Table 13C.1 Suggested Gender Identity, Sex, and Pronoun Data Collection Fields

Step 1: Current Gender Identity	Sex Assigned at Birth	Pronoun
Male	Male	Masculine pronouns
Female	Female	Feminine pronouns
Transmale/transman/FTM	Other	Neutral pronouns
Transfemale/transwoman/MTF		No pronouns
Genderqueer/gender-nonconforming		Something else (please specify)
Different Identity: Please state_____		

Medical Association recognize the need to adapt EMRs to collect information about a patient's gender identity, sexual orientation, and preferred name and pronoun. This information is important not only for patient care but also for epidemiological surveillance of quality metrics and health inequalities. A summary of suggested EMR entries appears in Table 13C.1, but for more information see the citations in the accompanying note.[15]

Differentiating between gender and sexuality allows ED clinicians to build trust with their patients and take a more thorough and detailed medical history, when relevant to a patient's visit. Understanding medical and surgical methods of transitioning, in addition to knowing the well-documented poorer health outcomes in the transgender community, provides a solid foundation for providing culturally competent care. Gratuitous curiosity about the transgender experience is not professional and has no place in patient care. As with their cisgender counterparts, clinicians should take a detailed history regarding medications, surgeries, and social practices and health-risk behaviors if relevant to

their chief complaint. Your history may give you details vital to the correct diagnosis, especially when an individual presents with abdominal pain, fever, genitourinary concerns, chest pain, or shortness of breath. When clinically appropriate, screen patients for depression, suicidality, substance use and abuse, and interpersonal violence. When asking about sexual partners, ask about specific sexual behaviors rather than the gender of their partners so you can glean necessary information for risks of pregnancy, infection, sexually transmitted diseases, and HIV transmission.

Prior or concurrent hormone use or surgeries may alter your differential diagnosis. Many transgender individuals have not had surgery because of disinterest, lack of access, or cost. Those who have should be asked specifically what structures were removed or created, and whether these procedures were done in medical settings. Clinical scenarios where hormone use or surgeries are especially relevant are in cases of abdominal pain, genitourinary concerns, sepsis, or chest pain. For example, a transwoman who has not had an orchiectomy with lower abdominal pain may have testicular torsion. Similarly, a transman presenting with suprapubic pain who has not had a hysterectomy may be pregnant, may have pelvic inflammatory disease, or perhaps ovarian torsion. Postoperative bleeding and infection should always be suspected for any recent procedure. You may need to alter the malignancies in your differential to include organ or hormone specific malignancies, such as prostate cancer in transwomen or cervical, ovarian, or breast cancer in transmen.

Physical exams can be uncomfortable and psychologically difficult for many patients, including

[15] Deutsch, M.B., Green, J., Keatley, J. et al. (2013). Electronic medical records and the transgender patient: Recommendations from the World Professional Association for Transgender Health EMR Working Group. *Journal of the American Medical Information Association*, 20, 700–703; Institute of Medicine, *The Health of Lesbian, Gay, Bisexual, and Transgender People*; Lambda Legal, New York City Bar, Human Rights Campaign Foundation. (2013). *Creating Equal Access to Quality Health Care for Transgender Patients: Transgender Affirming Hospital Policies*. New York: Lambda Legal, Accessed at www.lambdalegal.org/publications/fs_transgender-affirming-hospital-policies.

transgender patients who experience significant body dysphoria. In creating a plan for examination, it is of the upmost importance to approach each individual with clear, respectful communication and boundaries. Explain why you may want to do more sensitive genital or breast/chest exams, obtaining explicit consent for the exam procedure and explaining what specifically you are looking for. For all patients, a sensitive and gentle genital examination is essential to patient-centered care. For persons with severe dysphoria or histories of abuse, use of a relaxant or conscious sedation may provide some relief if they are experiencing severe distress.

Establishing a hospital nondiscrimination policy, which prohibits discrimination based on gender identity and expression, may help ensure delivery of trans-friendly care. All providers and staff must be educated about how they are expected to treat trans patients. Training staff on non-discrimination and trans-sensitive policies and patient care creates expectations for all providers and staff to provide gender diverse individuals with professionalism, courtesy, and respect. As with all personal health information, hospital workers should also keep a patient's gender identity private unless relevant or necessary for that person's care. It is acceptable and desirable for medical students to be involved in caring for transgender patients but with the same expectations for training and education as they would receive for cisgender patients. Individuals not involved in the direct care of the patient should not be included in the patient's care for voyeuristic or nonmedical purposes.

To ensure equal access to bathrooms, hospitals should allow individuals to use bathrooms and rooms based on their asserted gender. Hospitals can also provide unisex bathrooms. All patients placed in gender-specific rooms in the ED or on hospital admission should be roomed according to their identified gender unless they request otherwise.[16]

Case, Part 2

The patient reports that her symptoms began about six hours prior to coming to the ED. She has never had symptoms like this before. Review of systems is negative for fever, cough, leg swelling, travel or long trips. She has no prior history of asthma, COPD, cancer, heart disease, or pulmonary embolus. She has no family history of early stroke, cardiovascular disease, or clotting disorder. She says she is not prescribed any medications and does not have a medical provider. She is a one-pack-per-day smoker.

On exam, she is afebrile, tachycardic, with oxygen saturation is 91% on room air. She is in moderate respiratory distress with use of respiratory accessory muscles. Her heart rate is 120, with a regular rate rhythm, normal S1 and S2, no murmurs, rubs, or gallops. Lung fields are clear to auscultation bilaterally. Her abdomen is soft and nontender, but as you lift up the gown she becomes visibly distressed and you note voluntary guarding. She has no lower extremity swelling, erythema, or edema. She has male pattern face and body hair, no acanthosis, striae, or rashes.

Medical Therapies for Gender Actualization and Transition

Patients prescribed hormones have persistent, well-documented gender dysphoria and/or a strong desire to be another gender. Patients may receive hormonal therapies from a variety of primary care and specialty providers, often depending on available local resources. Some patients will begin therapies independent of providers because of limited access to care, fear of discrimination, lack of insurance, failure of insurance to cover gender-affirming medical therapies, or prohibitive cost.[17] Barriers are often circumvented by taking pro-hormone supplements or foods, sharing a friend's prescription, or purchasing hormones from an unlicensed provider in person or over the Internet. Convenience samples in the United States have shown that 20% to 60% of transgender women and 3% to 58% of transgender men report using non-prescribed hormones,

---

[16] Lambda Legal, *Creating Equal Access to Quality Health Care for Transgender Patients.*

[17] Rotondo, N.K., Bauer, G.R., Scanlon, K., et al. (2013). Nonprescribed hormone use and self-performed surgeries: "Do-it-yourself" transitions in transgender communities in Ontario, Canada. *American Journal of Public Health,* **103**, 1830–18.

depending on geographic location.[18] Taking hormones without the help of a provider, as well as substances not subject to quality control, places patients at risk for suboptimal outcomes and potentially dangerous side effects resulting from improper dosing, lack of monitoring, adverse side effects, or drug contaminants.[19]

Adolescents. Most transgender adolescents who have begun puberty continue to identify as transgender into adulthood (80%–90%).[20] To avoid the worsening gender dysphoria and distress that accompany the development of pubertal physical changes,[21] trans adolescents may halt or delay puberty with gonadotropic (GnRH) analogues or puberty "blockers" early in adolescence (Tanner stage 2). Hormone blockers prevent development of secondary gender characteristics (breasts, menses, face/body hair, voice, and musculoskeletal changes) that would require mediations with future hormones or surgical interventions. GnRH analogues are superior to progestin-only hormone-blocking treatments, but both are completely reversible and may be stopped at any time.[22] Initiating hormone blockers early in puberty allows individuals more time to explore and understand their gender, allows parents to come to terms with their child's evolving gender identity and outward expression, and allows families to create a safe and healthy approach to disclosure and support. Risks or adverse outcomes from puberty blockers are uncommon, but some patients later in puberty may experience menopausal-type symptoms (hot flashes, irritability, depression, fatigue) as their hormones return to prepubertal levels.

Feminizing Hormone Therapy (Table 13C.2). Feminizing hormone therapy typically includes a combination of estradiol and an antiandrogen. Sublingual, transdermal, or intramuscular (IM) b-17 estradiol is recommended over other estrogen formulations and routes of administration to decrease risk of venous thromboembolism (VTE).

Estradiol is the main feminizing hormone. Unlike with contraception, typical estrogen contraindications such as prior thromboemoblic event or thrombophilia, migraine with aura, or other estrogen sensitive diseases (previous neoplasm or end-stage liver disease) may not be an absolute contraindication to estradiol use. Most providers now use sublingual, intramuscular, or dermal routes to minimize VTE risk as the oral route, and ethinyl estradiol formulations in particular, increase the risk of thromboembolism. Unlike contraceptive technologies that offer non-estrogen alternatives, at present, feminization may only occur with estrogen compounds. Prolonged estrogen use has been

[18] Xavier, J. (2000). *Final Report of the Washington Transgender Needs Assessment Survey.* Washington, DC: Administration for HIV and AIDS, Government of the District of Columbia; Xavier, J., Honnold, J.A., and Bradford, J. (2007). *The Health, Health-Related Needs, and Lifecourse experiences of Transgender Virginians: Virginia Transgender Health Initiative Study Statewide Survey Report.* Richmond, VA: Virginia Department of Health, Division of Disease Prevention through the Centers for Disease Control and Prevention; Garofalo, R., Deleon, J., Osmer, E. et al. (2006). Overlooked, misunderstood and at-risk: Exploring the lives and HIV risk of ethnic minority male-to-female transgender youth. *Journal of Adolescent Health,* **38**(3), 230–6; Clements-Nolle et al., HIV prevalence, risk behaviors, health care use, and mental health status of transgender persons;Sanchez, N.F., Sanchez, J.P., and Danoff, A. (2009). Health care utilization, barriers to care, and hormone usage among male-to-female transgender persons in New York City. *American Journal of Public Health,* **99**(4), 713–9.

[19] Mueller, A., and Gooren, L. (2008). Hormone-related tumors in transsexuals receiving treatment with cross-sex hormones. *European Journal of Endocrinology,* **159**(3), 197–202; Moore, E., Wisniewski, A., and Dobs, A. (2003). Endocrine treatment of transsexual people: A review of treatment regimens, outcomes, and adverse effects. *Journal of Endocrinology and Metabolism,* **88**(8), 3467–73.

[20] Hembree, W.C. (2011). Guidelines for pubertal suspension and gender reassignment for transgender adolescents. *Child and Adolescent Clinics of North America,* **20**, 725–32; Drummond, K.D., Bradley, S.J., Peterson-Bidali, M. et al. (2008). A follow-up study of girls with gender identity disorder. *Developmental Psychology,* **44**, 34–45; Zucker, K.J. (2005). Gender identity disorder in children and adolescents. *Annual Review of Clinical Psychology,* **1**, 467–92.

[21] Delemarre-Van de Waal, H.A. and Cohen-Kettenis, P.T. (2006). Clinical management of gender identity disorder in adolescents: A protocol on psychological and paediatric endocrinology aspects. *European Journal of Endocrinology,* **155** (Suppl 1): S131–7.

[22] Hembree, W.C., Cohen-Kettenis, P., Delemare-van de Waal, H.A. et al. (2009). Endocrine treatment of transsexual persons: an Endocrine Society clinical practice guideline. *Journal of Clinical Endocrinology and Metabolism,* **94**(9), 3132–54.

Table 13C.2 Feminizing Medical Therapies

	Type	Effects	Possible Increased Risk
Estrogen 17 Beta-estradiol	Oral tablets Sublingual tablets Topical gel Transdermal patch Implants (less common)	Body fat redistribution (to hips, buttocks) Breast development Decreased muscle mass Testosterone suppression Emotional and sexuality changes	Thromboemoblic disease (Oral) Cardiovascular disease Hypertension Hypertriglyceridemia Gallstones Weight gain Mood changes Hyperprolactinemia Prolactinomas
Antiandrogen	Spironolactone Finasteride Dutasteride	Reduces endogenous testosterone levels and activity	Hyperkalemia Hypotension

associated with testicular atrophy, but the effect of estrogens and antiandrogens on sperm production is inconsistent.[23] In some, use may cause permanent sterility, but others may still have erectile function and produce semen; therefore, estradiol should not be considered effective birth control.

The primary risks and side effects associated with feminizing hormones are usually tolerable or desired and may include: erectile dysfunction, skin, muscle and body fat changes, and mood liability. Serious adverse outcomes are more rarely seen but include: weight gain, hypertriglyceridemia, gallstones, elevated liver enzymes, and increased risk of venous thromboembolic events.[24] For the transgender woman, the benefits of achieving feminization typically outweigh these potential risks. Individuals using estrogen may also be at greater risk of hyperprolactinemia or prolactinomas and, in the presence of other risk factors, non-insulin-dependent diabetes mellitus. While there are cases of breast cancer in both cismales and transgender

females, evidence is lacking as to whether individuals taking feminizing hormones are at increased risk for breast cancer.

Antiandrogens block testosterone effects on male pattern hair growth and have some minor effect in reducing endogenous testosterone levels. Common medications include spironolactone, which blocks testosterone synthesis and action, and finasteride (5-alpha reductase inhibitors), which blocks peripheral conversion of DHT to testosterone. Cyproterone acetate is a progestin commonly used as an antiandrogen outside of the United States but is not approved for use in the United States because of concerns for hepatotoxicity.[25] When using spironolactone, patients are typically monitored closely as the dose is increased over time to avoid side effects such as hyperkalemia or hypotension.

Masculinizing Hormone Therapy (Table 13C.3). Testosterone is the primary masculinization therapy for asserted male patients. It is typically given as an injection or topical application.[26] It is important to discuss correct injection technique and sterile needle use with patients using injectable

[23] Lübbert, H., Leo-Rossberg, I., and Hammerstein, J. (1992). Effects of ethinyl estradiol on semen quality and various hormonal parameters in a eugonadal male. *Fertility and Sterility*, **58**, 603–8; Schulze, C. (1988). Response of the human testis to long-term estrogen treatment: Morphology of Sertoli cells, Leydig cells and spermatogonial stem cells. *Cell Tissue Research*, **251**, 31–43.

[24] Asscheman, H.G.E., Megens, J.A.J., de Ronde, W. et al. (2011). A long-term follow-up study of mortality in transsexuals receiving treatment with cross-sex hormones. *European Journal of Endocrinology*, **164**, 635–42.

[25] World Professional Association for Transgender Health (WPATH). (2012). *Standards of Care for the Health of Transsexual, Transgender, and Gender-Nonconforming People*, version 7, 48.

[26] Gorton, R., Buth, J., and Spade, D. (2005). *Medical Therapy and Health Maintenance for Transgender Men: A Guide For Health Care Providers*. San Francisco: Lyon-Martin Women's Health Services.

Table 13C.3 Masculinizing Medical Therapies

	Type	Effects	Possible Increased Risk
Testosterone	Topical Intramuscular or subcutaneous Subcutaneous implants	Deepening of voice Hair growth Increased muscle mass Body fat redistribution (hips and buttocks to abdomen)	Polycythemia Alopecia Sleep apnea Elevated liver enzymes Hyperlipidemia Diabetes Mellitus Hypertension Cardiovascular disease Mood changes
Progestin	Medroxyprogesterone Depo-Provera®	Cessation of menses Weight gain	Hypertriglyceridemia

Table 13C.4 Masculinizing Surgeries and Procedures

Procedure	Description
Mastectomy	Breast removal
Hysterectomy	Removal of uterus
Salpingo-oophrectomy	Removal of fallopian tubes and ovaries
Vaginectomy	Vaginal removal.
Phalloplasty	Penile construction or reconstruction; may include erectile prosthesis
Scrotoplasty	Scrotal construction or reconstruction; may include testicular prosthesis
Facial masculinization	Procedures include chin implants and lip reduction
Pectoral implants	Implants to create a male-appearing chest contour
Liposuction +/– Lipofilling	Removal and redistribution of fat, especially from hips, to diminish feminine features, enhance masculine appearance

preparations. Caution against needle sharing to prevent transmission of blood-borne diseases such as HIV and hepatitis C. Early in hormone therapy, some individuals may also take progestins, specifically medroxyprogesterone, to aid in menstrual cessation. Testosterone is likewise not an effective method of contraception for transmen exposed to semen, sperm, and unprotected vaginal intercourse. Testosterone is contraindicated in transmen who are pregnant due to risk of masculinizing a fetus.

Masculinizing hormones increase the risk of polycythemia, alopecia, sleep apnea, and weight gain. Other possible side effects include elevated liver enzymes and hyperlipidemia. In the absence of testosterone use, there has been a noted increased prevalence of polycystic ovarian syndrome (PCOS) or endogenous hyperandrogenism among transmen,[27] and the effect of prolonged testosterone use on ovarian function is unknown.[28] Additional use of testosterone may place individuals with PCOS at additional risk for developing diabetes mellitus, hypertension, and cardiovascular disease. Evidence is inconclusive whether taking masculinizing hormones results in loss of bone density or increased risk for breast, cervical, ovarian, or uterine cancer.[29]

[27] Balen, A., Schacter, M.E., Montgomery, D. et al. (1993). Polycystic ovaries are a common finding in untreated female to male transsexuals. *Clinical Endocrinology*, **38**(3), 325–9.
[28] Hembree et al. Endocrine treatment of transsexual persons.
[29] World Professional Association for Transgender Health (WPATH), *Standards of Care for the Health of Transsexual, Transgender, and Gender-Nonconforming People*, version 7, 45.

Table 13C.5 Feminizing Surgeries and Procedures

Procedure	Description
Breast augmentation	Breast implants or lipofilling
Penectomy	Removal of penis
Orchiectomy	Removal of testes
Vaginoplasty	Creation of a neo-vagina
Clitoroplasty	Creation of a clitoris
Vulvoplasty	Creation of a neo-vulva
Facial feminization	Bony and soft tissue procedures of the face include brow lift, rhinoplasty, cheek implants, lip augmentation
Laryngeal modification	Thyroid chondroplasty, to reduce laryngeal prominence; laryngeal shortening or shaving to create higher-pitched voice
Lipofilling	For creation of feminine features, may get filling in face, breasts, hips, gluteal area
Electrolysis	Removal of undesired hair, especially on face, back, chest, arms
Gluteal augmentation	Filling, implants, or liposculpting to create feminine appearance

Additional Hormone Therapy Considerations. The changes of transitioning, including the shifting to endogenous hormone suppression and institution of cross-gender hormones may create some changes in mood and affect, especially early in the course of transition. Most trans patients report feeling more emotionally stable and happy after hormonal treatment takes effect. Psychological and physiologic goals of cross-gender hormone therapy include gaining desired physical characteristics of their gender identity, improved confidence and comfort in their own physical habitus and presentation, and minimizing side effects or adverse events. Dosing of hormones is based on these clinical features as well as maintaining hormone levels in the average range for asserted gender. Labs are followed regularly until a patient is established on a regular dose of hormones, with good levels and affect, as well as fewest side effects.

Surgical methods for gender actualization

Surgeries of the chest are commonly referred to as "top" surgeries and surgeries involving genitalia are commonly referred to as "bottom" surgeries. Not all transgender individuals seek surgery in their gender transition, either due to not wanting to have surgery, unavailability of a surgeon, lack of insurance coverage and prohibitive cost. It is important to not assume what procedures trans patients have or have not had in their gender transition.

Feminizing Surgeries and Procedures. Breast augmentation is also utilized to increase breast cup size for those transwomen who do not get the desired breast contour or size with hormones. Transwomen uncomfortable with their genitals may desire an orchiectomy and construction of a neovulva and vagina. Prior to or instead of surgery, transwomen may tuck their genitals to create a female type vulva profile or opt for a less expensive orchiectomy. Many women prioritize facial feminization therapy, including tracheal shave, as this may help with "passing" in the gender they assert. For a list of feminizing procedures, see Table 13C.5.

Complications of these procedures are often related to the surgeon's experience and more often associated with bottom surgery as opposed to the more commonly done top surgery. Top surgeries are high value, low risk, with relief from dysphoria and affirming cosmetic outcomes usually outweighing risk can be postsurgical infection and dissatisfaction with cosmetic outcomes. Post operative courses for trans male hysterectomy or vaginoplasty, include vaginal prolapse (7.5%), and some may also have fecal urgency (9.4%) or incomplete bowel emptying (7.6%). Nearly a quarter of individuals included in this study were dissatisfied with their sexual function.[30] Bottom surgeries that construct neo-vaginas and neophaloplasty, are more complicated and require more surgical expertise to avoid distressing complications and need for additional surgeries. One small cross-sectional study showed that almost half of individuals undergoing both male and female genitourethral reconstruction had bladder symptoms, including difficulty voiding (47%), urgency (24.6%), urge incontinence (17%), and stress incontinence (23%).[31]

Masculinizing Surgeries and Procedures. The removal of breasts and construction of a male chest eliminates significant body and breast dysphoria for many transmen. Chest binders and wraps are nonsurgical methods employed to promote the appearance of a male chest. Similarly, instead of or prior to having a phalloplasty, transmen may use packers (prosthetic testicles and penis) and or "stand-to-pee" devices. For a list of masculinizing procedures, see Table 13C.4.

At times, individuals will seek procedures from unlicensed practitioners because of lack of access to care, lack of insurance, failure of insurance to cover gender-affirming surgeries, or prohibitive cost. Rarely, individuals will perform surgeries on themselves, such as self-removal of testes, penis, or breasts.[32] Case reports also

underrepresent incidence of and poor outcomes related to self-injection of silicone,[33] corn, or castor oil[34] for breast, gluteal, or facial augmentation. Procedures performed by unlicensed providers can result in poor cosmetic outcomes as well as complications that range from routine postsurgical infections to disfigurement, migration of injected substances, infection, multisystem organ failure, fat embolization, pain syndromes, and transmission of HIV and hepatitis C from contaminated needles.[35]

Case, Part 3 – Conclusion

As the physician continues the interview, the patient is asked to identify gender, name, and pronoun preferences. The patient reports that she is a transgender woman, early in her transition from male to female. She has not been able to change her driver's license so it has her birth name on it. She tells you she has been taking estrogen pills orally for four months. She does not have a primary care provider and gets these from a friend. Lab work and chest X-ray are unrevealing. You have high suspicion for pulmonary embolus given concurrent oral estrogen use and cigarette smoking. CT pulmonary embolus study reveals bilateral submassive, segmental pulmonary emboli. You discuss your findings, initiate heparin treatment, and admit her to the hospital. The patient requests a private room, which the hospital is able to accommodate.

---

[30] Kuhn et al. Vaginal prolapse, pelvic floor function, and related symptoms 16 years after sex reassignment surgery in transsexuals.

[31] Kuhn, A., Santi, A., and Birkhäuser, M. (2011). Vaginal prolapse, pelvic floor function, and related symptoms 16 years after sex reassignment surgery in transsexuals. *Fertility and Sterility*, **95**, 2379–82.

[32] Conacher, G.N. and Westwood, G.H. (1987). Autocastration in Ontario federal penitentiary. *British Journal of Psychiatry*, **150**, 565–6; McGovern, S.J. (1995). Self-castration in a transsexual. *Journal of Accident & Emergency Medicine*, **12**(1), 57–8; Brown, G.R. (2010). Autocastration and autopenectomy as surgical self-treatment in incarcerated persons with gender identity disorder. *International Journal of Transgenderism*, **12**(1), 31–3.;Stunnell, H., Power, R.E., Floyd, M., and Quinlan, D.M. (2006). Genital self-mutilation. *International Journal of Urology*, **13**(10), 1358–1360; Baltieri, D.A. and Guerra de Andrade, A. (2005). Transsexual genital self-mutilation. *American Journal of Forensic Medicine and Pathology*, **26**(3), 268–270; Murphy, D., Murphy, M., and Grainger, R. (2001). Self-castration. *Irish Journal of Medical Sciences*, **170**(3), 195; Rana, A. and Johnson, A.D. (1993).

Sequential self-castration and amputation of penis. *British Journal of Urology*, **71**(6), 750.

[33] Reback, C., Simon, P., Bemis, C., and Gatson, B. (2001). *The Los Angeles Transgender Health Study: Community Report*. Los Angeles: University of California at Los Angeles.

[34] Smith, S.W., Graber, N.M., Johnson, R.C. et al. (2009). Multisystem organ failure after large volume injection of castor oil. *Annals of Plastic Surgery*, **62**, 12–14; Hain, J.R. (2009). Subcutaneous corn oil injections, fat embolization, and death. *American Journal of Forensic Medicine and Pathology*, **30**(4), 398–402.

[35] Smith et al., Multisystem organ failure after large volume injection of castor oil; Hain, Subcutaneous corn oil injections, fat embolization, and death; Tom Waddell Health Center. (2006). Protocols for Hormonal Reassignment of Gender. Accessed January, 2013 at http://sfdph.org/dph/comupg/oservices/medSvs/hlthCtrs/TransGendprotocols122006.pdf.

Table 13C.6 Trans Health Resources

- Callen-Lorde Health Center (NYC):
  http://callen-lorde.org
- Center for Disease Control:
  http://www.cdc.gov/lgbthealth/transgender.htm
- Fenway Health:
  ww.fenwayhealth.org
- Fenway LGBT help line: 888.340.4528
- Gay and Lesbian Medical Association:
  www.glma.org
- Lyon-Martin Health Center:
  http://lyon-martin.org/
- National Center for Transgender Equality:
  http://transequality.org/Issues/health.html
- Trans-Health:
  http://www.trans-health.com
- UCSF Center of Excellence for Trans Health:
  http://transhealth.ucsf.edu/
- World Professional Association for Transgender
  Health:
  http://www.wpath.org/

Conclusion

Transgender patients have unique medical and mental health needs and trans health disparities are intimately linked to societal stigma, discrimination, socioeconomic status, and denial of rights. Emergency medical providers can help address these disparities not only by treating trans patients with respect and dignity but also by understanding medical and surgical methods of transitioning that may be key to establishing the correct diagnosis and plan of care.

Take Home Points

A. Birth or biologic sex and gender identity are separate concepts that may or may not be congruent and may change with time, experience, and development.

B. Gender dysphoria is the distress transgender and gender nonconforming individuals may experience as a result of incongruence between their birth sex, body characteristics, and gender identity. Transgender identity is not considered a psychiatric pathological condition.

C. Ask your gender-nonconforming patients their preferred name and pronoun–and then use them consistently.

D. EMRs should use a two-step process to collect sex and gender information and have fields to note preferred name and pronouns.

E. Hospitals and EDs should adopt a nondiscrimination policy to prevent discrimination based on gender identity and expression.

F. All hospital floors should have unisex bathrooms to ensure universal bathroom access.

G. Transgender related past medical and sexual histories are important when diagnostically relevant to presenting concern but should not be elicited out of curiosity.

H. Screen transgender individuals for mental health and social risks when appropriate as transgender individuals are at higher risk for substance use, anxiety, depression and suicidality, interpersonal violence and assault, HIV.

I. Discuss need for sensitive physical exams with patient and obtain consent.

J. Multiple therapeutic and medical and surgical interventions are available to help individuals with gender dysphoria. Long-term outcomes of these therapies are still being studied but seem to offer benefit in helping transgender patients pass and live in their asserted gender.

Gaps in Knowledge, Future Research Questions

- Long-term effects of hormone-blocking and adjunctive hormone therapies.
- Effect of masculinizing hormones on bone density in FtM individuals.
- Effect of masculinizing hormones on incidence of breast, cervical, ovarian, or uterine cancer among FtM individuals.
- Effect of feminizing hormones on breast cancer risk among MtF individuals.
- Relative risk of pulmonary embolus in MtF individuals taking estrogen.
- Incidence of cardiovascular disease after initiation of testosterone therapy.

- Incidence of diabetes mellitus and PCOS after initiation of testosterone therapy.
- Potential surgical issues for genital reconstruction following the use of puberty blockers.
- Frequency of postsurgical complications.

- Barriers to ED care and access patterns; opportunities to improve care for gender-nonconforming persons in ED settings.
- Clinical and cultural competency of emergency physicians and physicians in training.

Chapter 14

Sex and Gender in Medical Education: The Next Chapter

Marjorie R. Jenkins

Sex and Gender in Medical Education Begins with Research

Sex- and gender-specific medicine is based on the science of how normal human function and the experience of the same disease vary as a function of biological sex and gender. It is not women's health under a different label. Indeed, sex- and gender-specific medicine is now a burgeoning field of scientific inquiry and is a cornerstone of "individualized medicine."

The question for many is, "Why consider sex and gender differences?" Because sex and gender are two universal variables that every patient will have without fail, a more appropriate question is how can we not consider sex and gender when an abundance of science has revealed that differences matter. According to the American Medical Association,[1] "a patient's gender plays an appropriate role in medical decision making when biological differences between the sexes are considered."

More than 50,000 PubMed articles from basic science to clinical trials currently include sex and/or gender considerations. The bridge from this massive repository of evidence to the patient – "the bench" to "the bedside" – is the education of health professionals (Figure 14.1). Research will fall far short of its promise to usher in an era of personalized medicine unless the contribution of biological sex to the diversity of in which health outcomes are better understood and this knowledge applied to the next generation of interventions and medical technologies.[2] A research discovery cannot save lives without making the journey through the health professionals' classroom.

Points of Engagement: Creating Culture Change

Altering the culture of a one-sex model within medicine will require engagement on many

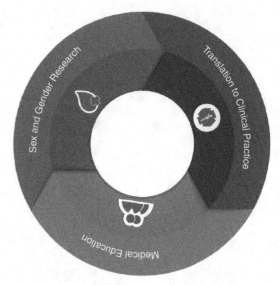

Figure 14.1 From the bench to the bedside: translational education

fronts. Figure 14.2 represents proposed points of engagement required to create real and lasting change. As stated in the Introduction, there is a growing momentum to ensure sex balance in research. This momentum has been increasing over the past two decades, as evidenced by the development of sex- and gender-based medicine (SGBM) professional organizations, textbooks, and online resources (Table 14.1). For example, in the United States, a group of academic and nonprofit organizations, researchers, clinicians, and educators have come together to create the Sex and Gender Women's Health Collaborative (www.sgwhc.org). This group's mission is to ensure integration of sex and gender knowledge into medical education to improve health care for all. Such programs will gradually increase the visibility of sex and gender topics in medicine and facilitate the integration of these topics into

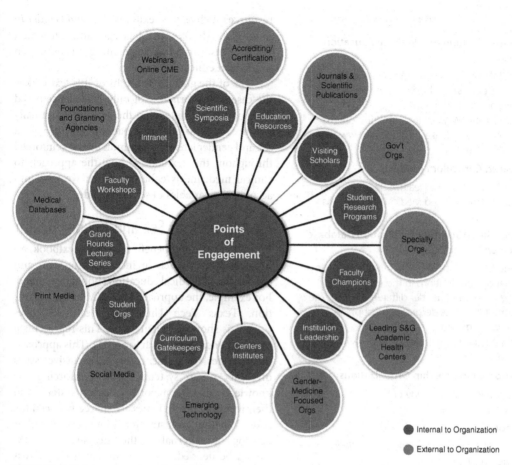

Figure 14.2 Defining sex and gender health

○ Internal to Organization
○ External to Organization

medical school and continuing medical education curricula.

Translational Health Education

What is translational education? Before answering this question, let us review the definition of translational research from Merriam-Webster: "medical research that is concerned with facilitating the practical application of scientific discoveries to the development and implementation of new ways to prevent, diagnose, and treat disease, also called translational medicine."[3] We propose the following definition for translational health education: health care education that integrates the practical application of scientific discoveries to improve the health and well-being of patients through prevention, diagnosis, and treatment of disease. Coupling SGBM with translational health

education ensures that practitioners first consider, and then apply, sex and gender evidence to health and disease.

A Paradigm Shift in Medical Education: The Lifelong Learner

If we accept the presented premise, then the need for clinically relevant, evidence-based educational resources becomes imperative. Physicians have long practiced within the "see one, do one, teach one" framework, and much of our health professions' education is learning through hands-on application of principles. Educational works that provide an abundance of text without application have significant limitations within an evolving paradigm of medical education that focuses on developing lifelong independent learners. To continue along this evolution of medical education,

Table 14.1 Sex- and Gender-Based Medicine Resources

Web Based Continuing Medicine Education Courses

- NIH ORWH The Science of Sex and Gender in Health. Courses 1–3. http://sexandgender course.od.nih.gov/
- TTUHSC Laura W. Bush Institute for Women's Health. Y Does X Make A Difference? www.laur abushinstitute.org

Web Based Curriculum Products

- Texas Tech University Health Sciences Center Sex and Gender-Based Medicine. www.texas techsgbm.org

Evidence Based Scientific Publication Database and Search Engine Tools

- GenderMed Database is a systematic collection of scientific publications in the medical field analyzing sex and gender differences. http://ge ndermeddb.charite.de/protected.php?site =home&;lang=eng
- SGBM PubMed Search Engine Tool www.texas techsgbm.org

Professional Membership Organizations

- Organization for the Study of Sex Differences. www.ossdweb.org

Textbooks

- Legato M. *Principles of Gender-Specific Medicine.* Elsevier. 2011. 2nd ed.
- Oertelt-Prigione, Regitz-Zagrosek. *Clinical Aspects of Gender Specific Medicine.* Springer. 2012.
- Schenk-Gustafsson K, DeCola PR, Pfaff SW, Plsetsky DS. *Handbook of Clinical Gender Medicine.* Karger. 2012.
- Regitz-Zagrosek V. *Sex and Gender Differences in Pharmacology.* Springer. 2012.

Web Based Research and Educational Resources

- Sex and Gender Women's Health Collaborative. www.sgwhc.org
- Stanford University's Gendered Innovations. http://genderedinnovations.stanford.edu/
- Canadian Institute of Gender Health. What a Difference Sex and Gender Make. www.cihr-irsc .gc.ca/e/44082.html

Gender and Medication Effects

- Karolinska Instituet. www.genderedreactions .com

resources such as this textbook, *Sex and Gender in Acute Care Medicine* by McGregor and colleagues, are vital resources in transforming our approach to medical education.

One of the greatest strengths of this textbook is the case-based format. Not only is evidence-based information presented, but the authors continually reinforce how to approach patient care through a sex and gender lens. The common thread reinforced throughout this textbook is how the approach to clinical medicine is enhanced when we take into account the variables of sex and gender.

An Approach to Sex and Gender Health

To obtain maximal benefit from this textbook, an institution's approach to incorporating sex- and gender-based medical education should be defined. For example, the approach to SGBM at my institution, Texas Tech University Health Sciences Center, is shown in Figure 14.3. This represents a more expansive approach to SGBM. This approach incorporates the influence of sex-exclusive issues on other organ systems, while reinforcing the knowledge that the majority of organ systems and their resulting health issues are shared between the sexes. Whether an institution adopts this model or develops an alternative, the message of SGBM should be defined, and remain consistent, across research and educational programs; otherwise, both researchers and learners can be confused by ambiguous terminology.

Once the institution has committed to incorporating SGBM into medical education, resources such as this text become a mainstay to achieving defined educational program goals and objectives. Although this text focuses on acute care settings, the topics presented here are also addressed throughout a variety of primary and specialty care, making this text a versatile resource for student, resident, and fellowship training programs.

SGBM Federal Initiatives

One of the most interesting aspects in the growth of SGBM is that it is not being driven by a large influx of monetary resources such as expansive grant programs and private foundation funding. Rather, it is a discipline that first emerged within the work of the Women's Health Movement, a movement that brought forth irrefutable evidence

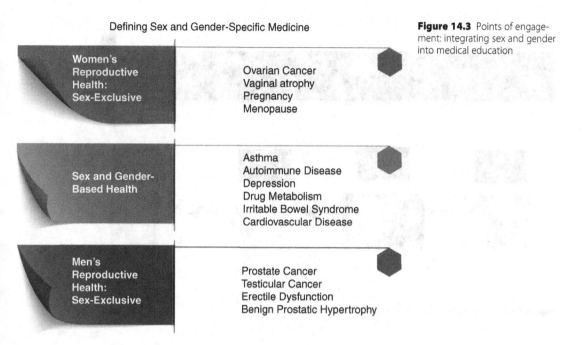

Defining Sex and Gender-Specific Medicine

Figure 14.3 Points of engagement: integrating sex and gender into medical education

that differences exist between males and females across the biological and societal spectra. It has gained traction through continued grassroots efforts in academia, federal agencies, and increasing consumer awareness.

In 2014, publicized action was taken within the National Institutes of Health (NIH) to ensure sex and gender inclusion in research and from the Food and Drug Administration (FDA) to ensure sex and gender inclusion and data analysis in drug and device applications.[4,5] These efforts are vital to ensure that the pipeline of knowledge from the lab to the patient is balanced to include all. Figure 14.4 shows that preclinical and clinical trials lack sex and gender balance. Yet research outcomes are utilized to drive clinical care. When the research pipeline is biased toward one sex or gender, the results cannot be applied with certainty to a global population.

The NIH began its process of creating new mandates involving sex and gender balance in preclinical research subjects and, as applicable, scientifically sound evaluation of data by sex and/or gender. The commentary regarding the need and outline of the initiative was coauthored by the NIH Director Dr. Francis Collins and Director of the Office of Research in Women's Health Dr. Janine Clayton and published in

Nature.[4] The FDA published an action plan to improve the inclusion of women and minorities in drug and device development and subsequent analysis of efficacy and outcomes in diverse populations by including sex and gender.[5] These federal initiatives impact medical education through improving the body of knowledge required to teach evidence-based medicine. Expanding reporting outcomes among diverse populations provides findings that are more applicable to real-world populations. Within sex- and gender-based medicine, initiatives such as these move medicine toward inclusion and away from the current "one-sex" model.

The Future of Sex- and Gender-Based Medicine

Efforts must continue on all fronts represented in Figure 14.1. Scientific journal editors and editorial boards must provide authors with instructions that ignoring sex or gender is unacceptable. The current practice of omitting the reporting of the sex of cells, tissue, and animals should not be the status quo. Along these lines, the ubiquitous reporting of "subjects" omits sex and gender completely. Ultimately, sex and gender transparency in published works should be set as a measure of

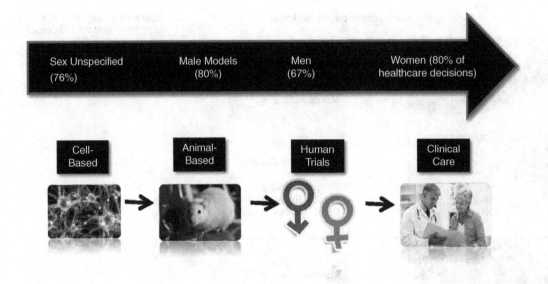

Figure 14.4 Sex and gender bias in the research pipeline

the quality of the journal. Accrediting bodies such as the Liaison Committee on Medical Education (LCME) and the Accreditation Council for Graduate Medical Education (ACGME) have the potential to impact the integration of SGBM significantly by creating requirements for its inclusion into medical education. We may one day see the establishment of postgraduate SGBM certificate or fellowship programs. Any and all of this is possible.

Rarely are health care professionals given the opportunity to be instrumental in transformational change. That is exactly what SGBM promises to be in breaking down the myths, assumptions, and misrepresentations that have evolved over thousands of years. In doing so, the medical researcher, educator, learner, and practitioner can all play a part in the process.

Utilizing This Resource: Where When and How

Mainstays of medical education delivery exist throughout US medical schools, such as lectures, case-based or problem-based learning, simulation, and the Objective Structured Clinical Exam (OSCE). This textbook can be utilized to create educational activities in each of these environments. In the case of the 54-year-old female patient presenting with acute coronary syndrome in Chapter 2, not only are the pertinent epidemiology, clinical presentation, and underlying pathophysiology presented in a direct and straightforward manner, the prompt of "*What are the gender-specific elements in diagnosis and management that you should consider?*" lends itself to several educational opportunities.

Although medical education is moving away from passive learning, as represented by didactics, to more active learning such as the flipped classroom, PowerPoint lectures remain a foundation of current educational programs. Utilizing the educational pearls listed throughout this book, educators can readily create one to two clinically relevant slides for a multitude of disease states. The case presentations lend themselves to the development of small-group exercises and clinical-case simulations. Threading sex and gender differences into established OSCE exams is achievable given the available evidence-based information contained here. Across the spectrum of medical education delivery methods, this textbook represents an extremely adaptable resource.

The millennials and the generations after them will continue to live within a digitally native environment. Their learning environment is one that expands at the touch of a button. Textbooks are important adjuncts to learning but even more important is helping the learner develop an approach to the application of bodies of evidence. In this respect, *Sex and Gender in Acute Care Medicine* is transformational.

References

1. The American Medical Association (AMA) Opinion 9.122 – Gender Disparities in Health Care: (I, IV). Available at www.ama-assn.org/ama/pub/ physician-resources/medical-ethics/code-medical -ethics/opinion9122.page.

2. NIH ORWH, U.S. Department of Health and Human Services. Publication No. 10–7606.

3. "Translational Research." Merriam-Webster.com. Merriam-Webster, n.d. Web. 2014. www.merriam -webster.com/dictionary/translational research.

4. Clayton J. Collins F. NIH to balance sex in cell and animal studies. *Nature* 2014; **509**:282–283.

5. FDA. Action Plan to Enhance the Collection and Availability of Demographic Subgroup Data. Available at www.fda.gov/downloads/RegulatoryIn formation/Legislation/FederalFoodDrugandCosme ticActFDCAct/SignificantAmendmentstotheFDCA ct/FDASIA/UCM410474.pdf.

Moving into the Future with New Dimensions and Strategies: A Vision for 2020 for Women's Health Research. Available at http://orwh.od.nih.gov/res earch/strategicplan/ORWH_StrategicPlan2020 _Vol1.pdf.

Index

AAU (Amateur Athletic Union),
101
Abdominal aortic aneurysm (AAA),
diagnostic imaging and, 170
Abdominal disorders. *See*
Gastroenterological disorders
Abdominal pain
adnexal torsion (AT), 204–205
(*See also* Adnexal torsion (AT))
appendicitis (*See* Appendicitis)
in children, 199–206
computed tomography (CT) and,
169–170
constipation (*See* Constipation)
diagnostic imaging and, 169–170
ecoptic pregnancy, 205 (*See also*
Ecoptic pregnancy)
functional abdominal pain
syndrome (FAPS), 143
future research topics, 206
nephrolithiasis, 201 (*See also*
Nephrolithiasis)
ovarian cysts, 204 (*See also*
Ovarian cysts)
overview, 200, 206
patient case study, 199, 206
pelvic inflammatory disease
(PID), 202–204 (*See also* Pelvic
inflammatory disease (PID))
testicular torsion, 206 (*See also*
Testicular torsion)
ultrasound and, 170
Absorption of drugs, 65
Accreditation Council for
Graduate Medical Education
(ACGME), 234
ACE-inhibitors/ARB, 11
ACEP. *See* American College of
Emergency Physicians (ACEP)
Acetaminophen
migraines and, 93
overdoses of, 69
ACL injuries. *See* Anterior cruciate
ligament (ACL) injuries
ACTH (Adrenocorticotropic
hormone), 196
Acute coronary syndrome (ACS)
anticoagulants and, 10–11
aspirin and, 11
beta-blockers and, 11

biomarkers, 7–8
clinical conclusions, 12
clinical presentation, 7
depression as risk factor, 7
diabetes as risk factor, 7
diagnostic imaging and, 168
gender-specific diagnostic
approach, 7–9
investigative studies, 7–8
ischemic chest pain, 9–10 (*See
also* Ischemic chest pain)
overview, 9, 11
patient case study, 6
prevalence in women, 6
prognosis in women, 11
risk factors, 7–8
risk stratification scores, 8
spontaneous coronary artery
dissection (SCAD), 13–14
stress tests, 8, 168–169
Takotsubo's cardiomyopathy,
12–13 (*See also* Takotsubo's
cardiomyopathy)
tobacco use as risk factor, 7
treatment in women, 10–11
warning signs, 7
Acute liver failure, 139
Acute pain, 127
Adhesive capsulitis, 108
Adnexal torsion (AT), 204–205
acute management, 205
in children, 204–205
clinical presentation, 204
diagnosis, 205
ultrasound and, 205
Adolescents, medical therapies for
gender actualization and
transition, 223
Adrenergic agents, 33, 40
Adrenocorticotropic hormone
(ACTH), 196
Adverse drug reactions in elderly
persons, 180–181
AEI. *See* Athletic energy imbalance
(AEI)
AF. *See* Atrial fibrillation (AF)
Affordable Care Act of 2010,
164
African Americans
asthma and, 35

slipped capital femoral epiphysis
(SCFE) in, 207
substance abuse and, 53
Aged persons. *See* Elderly persons
AIDS. *See* Human
immunodeficiency virus (HIV)
Alcoholic acute pancreatitis, 140
Alcohol use
breast cancer and, 51–52
clinical consequences, 51–52
factors related to use, 50–51
fetal alcohol spectrum disorders
(FASD), 51–52
metabolism and, 51–52
motor vehicle collisions and, 53
prevalence in women, 50–51
sexual assault and, 54
"telescoping," 51
violence and, 53–54
Aldosterone, 196, 197, 198
Alvarado Score, 200
Alzheimer's disease in elderly
persons, 181–182
Amateur Athletic Union (AAU),
101
American Academy of Pediatrics
transgender persons and, 220
urinary tract infections (UTIs)
and, 193, 194, 195
American Association of Physicists
in Medicine, 165
American College of Cardiology, 17
American College of Emergency
Physicians (ACEP), 171–172
American College of Radiology,
164, 166
American College of Sports
Medicine, 108
American Congress of Obstetricians
and Gynecologists, 150
American Heart Association, 89
American Medical Association,
220, 230
American Psychiatric Association,
220
American Psychological
Association, 220
American Society of
Echocardiography, 164
American Stroke Association, 89

American Urological Association, 150

Amitriptyline, 64

Amphetamines, 68

Ampicillin, 64, 204

Aneurysms. *See* Subarachnoid hemorrhages (SAH)

Ankle injuries, 105

Annals of Emergency Medicine, 31

Anorectal disorders, 143

Anterior cruciate ligament (ACL) injuries
acute management, 209
in children, 208–209
clinical presentation, 103
diagnosis, 209
estrogen and, 103
hormones and, 103
magnetic resonance imaging (MRI) and, 209
osteoarthritis and, 104, 209
post-emergency department care, 209
prevalence, 102, 208
risk factors, 208
sex and gender differences in, 102–103, 208
sports medicine and, 102–104
x-rays and, 209

Antibiotics
chronic obstructive pulmonary disease (COPD) and, 40
urinary tract infections (UTIs) and, 187

Anti cholinergics, 33, 40

Anticoagulants
acute coronary syndrome (ACS) and, 10–11
atrial fibrillation (AF) and, 16
ischemic stroke and, 88
trauma and, 80

Anti convulsants, 64

Antidotes, 69–70

Antifungals, 64

Antiretroviral therapy (ART), 156–157

Anti tuberculars, 64

Apical ballooning syndrome. *See* Takotsubo's cardiomyopathy

Appendicitis
acute management, 201
in children, 200–201
clinical presentation, 200
complications, 201
computed tomography (CT) and, 170, 200
diagnosis, 200
diagnostic imaging and, 170
laparoscopic appendectomy, 201

magnetic resonance imaging (MRI) and, 200
obesity and, 201
open appendectomy, 201
during pregnancy, 173
ultrasound and, 170, 200

Arrythmia, 18

ART (Antiretroviral therapy), 156–157

Aspirin
acute coronary syndrome (ACS) and, 11
cardiovascular disease and, 1–2, 18
ischemic stroke and, 87
Takotsubo's cardiomyopathy and, 13

Assisted ventilation, 33, 40

Association of Medical Microbiology and Infectious Diseases – Canada, 150

Astemizole, 2

Asthma, 29–35
acute management, 33–35
African Americans and, 35
assisted ventilation and, 33
clinical manifestations, 31–32
clinical outcomes, 35
costs of, 29
diagnosis, 32–33
future research topics, 43
gender risk, 29–30
hormones and, 30
menstruation and, 43
morbidity and mortality, 30–31
natural history, 30–31
obesity and, 35
oral contraceptive pills (OCPs) and, 30
overview, 29, 35
pregnancy and, 30
prevalence, 29
prevention, 35
smoking cessation programs and, 35
spirometric testing, 33
testosterone and, 30
treatment options, 34
triggers, 33

AT. *See* Adnexal torsion (AT)

Athletic energy imbalance (AEI), 108–111
bone mineral density (BMD) and, 109–110
caloric intake and, 108–109
diagnosis, 110–111
hormones and, 109
low bone mass, 109–110
low energy availability, 108–109
menstrual irregularity, 109

patient case study, 108
prevalence, 110
"thin build" sports and, 110
treatment, 110–111

Atlantic Monthly, 24

Atrial fibrillation (AF), 15–17
anticoagulants and, 16
clinical conclusions, 17
complications, 16–17
heart failure as risk factor for, 15
hypertension and, 16
ischemic stroke and, 87, 88
overview, 17
patient case study, 15–16
prevalence, 16
prognosis in women, 16
treatment in women, 16
triggers, 16

Autoimmune hepatitis, 139

Avascular necrosis, 207

Back pain, 107

Bacteremia, 195

Bacteriuria, 150, 186

Barrett's esophagus, 138

Beasley, G.M., 52

Benzodiazepines, 64

Bernstein, S.L., 27

Beta-blockers
acute coronary syndrome (ACS) and, 11
Takotsubo's cardiomyopathy and, 13

Beta carotene, 1

Bias
in cardiovascular disease, 18
in substance abuse treatment, 52–53

Bilateral orchipexy, 206

Biliary tract, disorders of
biliary pancreatitis, 140
diagnostic imaging and, 170
overview, 139–140, 144

Bipolar disorder in elderly persons, 183

Bisphosphonates, 114

Blood pressure. *See* Hypertension

Bone mineral density (BMD), 109–110, 112–113

Bradykinins, 125

Brain
concussions, 115–117 (*See also* Concussions)
traumatic brain injury (TBI), 82–83 (*See also* Traumatic brain injury (TBI))

Brain organization theory, 199

Breast cancer, alcohol use and, 51–52

Broken heart syndrome. *See*
    Takotsubo's cardiomyopathy
Burkhart, S.S., 106

CAH. *See* Congenital adrenal
    hyperplasia (CAH)
Calcium, 114
Calcium channel blockers, 11
Camplyobacter, 151
Cancer
    alcohol use and, 51–52
    breast cancer, alcohol use and,
        51–52
    chemotherapeutics and, 87
    colorectal cancer, 141
    gastric cancer, 138
    lung cancer, tobacco use
        and, 25
    ovarian cancer, pelvic
        inflammatory disease (PID)
        and, 204
    pancreatic cancer, 140
    sex and gender differences
        in, 180
    transgender persons and, 221,
        224, 228
Carboplatin, 71
Cardiac catheterization, 17
Cardiovascular disease
    acute coronary syndrome (ACS)
        (*See* Acute coronary syndrome
        (ACS))
    arrythmia, 18
    aspirin and, 1–2, 18
    atrial fibrillation (AF), 15–17 (*See
        also* Atrial fibrillation (AF))
    feminizing hormone therapy and,
        224
    future research topics, 18
    gender bias in, 18
    heart failure, 14–15 (*See also*
        Heart failure)
    importance of sex and gender,
        1–2
    ischemic chest pain, 9–10 (*See
        also* Ischemic chest pain)
    masculinizing hormone therapy
        and, 225–226
    non-ST-elevation myocardial
        infarction (non-STEMI), 7,
        10–11
    overview, 6
    peripartum/postpartum
        cardiomyopathy (PPCM), 18
    pregnancy and, 17–18
    spontaneous coronary artery
        dissection (SCAD), 13–14
    ST-elevation myocardial
        infarction (STEMI), 7, 10–11,
        13–14, 17

structural heart disease (*See* Heart
    failure)
Takotsubo's cardiomyopathy,
    12–13 (*See also* Takotsubo's
    cardiomyopathy)
Carpal instability, 107
Carpal tunnel syndrome, 107
Catecholamines, 125, 198
CCTA (Coronary CT angiogram),
    8, 169
Cellulitis, 152
Census Bureau, 179
Center for Medicare and Medicaid
    Innovation, 164
Centers for Disease Control and
    Prevention (CDC)
    chlamydia and, 154
    pelvic inflammatory disease
        (PID) and, 203
    syphilis and, 155
    traumatic brain injury (TBI)
        and, 115
Cephalosporins, 64
Cerebrovascular emergencies
    epilepsy, 94
    future research topics, 95–96
    intra cerebral hemorrhages
        (ICH), 90–91 (*See also* Intra-
        cerebral hemorrhages (ICH))
    ischemic stroke, 87–90 (*See also*
        Ischemic stroke)
    migraines, 92–94 (*See also*
        Migraines)
    overview, 87, 94–95
    patient case study, 87, 95
    prevalence, 87
    seizures, 94
    status epilepticus, 94
    subarachnoid hemorrhages
        (SAH), 91–92 (*See also*
        Subarachnoid hemorrhages
        (SAH))
Chemotherapeutics, 87
Chenodeoxycholic acid, 65
Children. *See also specific disorder*
    abdominal pain in, 199–206
    adnexal torsion (AT) in, 204–205
        (*See also* Adnexal torsion (AT))
    anterior cruciate ligament (ACL)
        injuries, 208–209 (*See also*
        Anterior cruciate ligament
        (ACL) injuries)
    appendicitis in, 200–201 (*See also*
        Appendicitis)
    congenital adrenal hyperplasia
        (CAH) in, 196–199 (*See also*
        Congenital adrenal hyperplasia
        (CAH))
    constipation in, 202 (*See also*
        Constipation)

ecoptic pregnancy in, 205 (*See
    also* Ecoptic pregnancy)
fever without a source (FWS)
    in, 193
gender actualization and
    transition, medical therapies
    for, 223
knee injuries in, 206–210
nephrolithiasis in, 201 (*See also*
    Nephrolithiasis)
Osgood-Schlatter disease in, 208
    (*See also* Osgood-Schlatter
    disease)
ovarian cysts in, 204 (*See also*
    Ovarian cysts)
overview, 193
pelvic inflammatory disease
    (PID) in, 202–204 (*See also*
    Pelvic inflammatory disease
    (PID))
slipped capital femoral epiphysis
    (SCFE) in, 207–208 (*See also*
    Slipped capital femoral
    epiphysis (SCFE))
testicular torsion in, 206 (*See also*
    Testicular torsion)
urinary tract infections in,
    193–196 (*See also* Urinary tract
    infections (UTIs))
Chlamydia, 154–155, 202
Chlamydia trachomatis, 202
Choi, J., 8
Cholecystitis, 139–140
Cholelithiasis, 139–140
Chondrolysis, 207
Chronic bronchitis, 37
Chronic obstructive pulmonary
    disease (COPD), 36–42
    acute management, 39–41
    antibiotics and, 40
    assisted ventilation and, 40
    chronic bronchitis, 37
    classification by severity, 38
    clinical manifestations, 38–39
    clinical outcomes, 42
    costs of, 36
    definition, 37
    diagnosis, 39
    dyspnea, 38
    emphysema, 37
    future research topics, 43
    gender risk, 36–37
    morbidity and mortality, 42
    natural history, 37–38
    overview, 36, 42
    prevalence, 36
    prevention, 41–42
    risk factors, 36–37, 41–42
    sex and gender differences in,
        36–37

COPD (cont.)
  smoking cessation programs, 40–41
  tobacco use and, 36–37, 40–41
  treatment options, 40
Chronic pain, 127
Chronic regional pain syndrome (CRPS), 107–108
Cigarettes. See Tobacco use
Circumcision
  human immunodeficiency virus (HIV) and, 157
  sexually transmitted infections (STI) and, 154
  urinary tract infections (UTIs) and, 193–194
Cirrhosis, 139
Cisplatin, 70–71
Clark, N.M., 33–35
Clayton, Janine, 4, 233
Clindamycin, 204
Clinical trials, inclusion of women in, 2–4, 233
Clinton, Bill, 4
Clofibric acid, 64
Clostridium difficile, 151
Cocaine, 68
Collins, Francis, 4, 233
Colon, disorders of, 140–141
Colorectal cancer, 141
Computed tomography (CT)
  abdominal aortic aneurysm (AAA) and, 170
  abdominal pain and, 169–170
  appendicitis and, 170, 200
  coronary CT angiogram (CCTA), 8, 169
  CT pulmonary angiogram (CTPA), 169
  dose variability, 166–168
  measuring radiation from, 165–167
  migraines and, 172
  musculoskeletal pain syndromes and, 107
  overview, 163
  pregnancy and, 172, 173
  prevalence, 163–164
  pulmonary embolism (PE) and, 168, 169
  renal colic and, 170–171
  reporting radiation from, 165–167
  risk of radiation from, 166
  size specific dose estimate (SSDE), 165
  subarachnoid hemorrhages (SAH) and, 92
  thoracic aortic dissection (TAD) and, 168
  trauma and, 171–172

traumatic brain injury (TBI) and, 172
Computerized neuropsychological testing (NPT), 116–117
Comstock, R.D., 116
Concussions, 115–117
  computerized neuropsychological testing (NPT) for, 116–117
  definition, 115
  metabolic mismatch, 116
  patient case study, 115
  post-concussion syndrome (PCS), 116
  prevalence, 115
  sex and gender differences in, 115–116
  symptoms, 116
  testing for, 116–117
  treatment, 117
Condoms, human immunodeficiency virus (HIV) and, 157
Confronting COPD International Survey, 41
Congenital adrenal hyperplasia (CAH), 196–199
  acute management, 198
  in children, 196–199
  clinical manifestations, 196–197
  diagnosis, 197–198
  enzyme deficiency and, 196
  fertility and, 199
  future research topics, 199
  gender and, 198–199
  non-salt-wasting CAH, 197
  overview, 196, 199
  pathophysiology, 196
  patient case study, 196, 199
  post-emergency department care, 198–199
  prevalence, 196
  salt-wasting CAH, 197
  sexual orientation and, 199
Congenital anorectal malformations, 202
Congressional Women's Caucus, 3
Constipation
  in children, 202
  clinical presentation, 202
  diagnosis, 202
  sex and gender differences in, 140
Contraceptives. See Oral contraceptive pills (OCPs)
Contractures, 108
COPD. See Chronic obstructive pulmonary disease (COPD)
Copenhagen City Heart Study, 7
Coronary artery disease, diagnostic imaging and, 168–169
Coronary CT angiogram (CCTA), 8, 169

Corticosteroids, 33, 40, 64
Cortisol, 196
Crohn's disease, 141
CRPS (Chronic regional pain syndrome), 107–108
Cryptococcal meningitis, 153
CT. See Computed tomography (CT)
CT pulmonary angiogram (CTPA), 169
Cultural change, creating, 230–231
Cutaneous infections, 152
Cyclic adenosine, 125
Cyclophosphamide, 70–71
Cyclosporine, 64
CYP1A2 enzyme, 67
CYP2C9 enzyme, 67
CYP2C19 enzyme, 67
CYP2D6 enzyme, 67
CYP3A4 enzyme, 67, 139
CYP450 system, 66–67, 139
Cyproterone, 224
Cystectomy, 204, 205
Cystic fibrosis, 202
Cystitis, 150

Decompensated cirrhosis, 139
Defining sex and gender, 1
Dehydroepiandrosterone (DHEA), 30
Delirium in elderly persons, 182
Dementia in elderly persons, 181–182
Depression
  acute coronary syndrome (ACS), as risk factor for, 7
  in elderly persons, 183, 185
  hip fractures and, 185
  tobacco use and, 26–27
DHEA (Dehydroepiandrosterone), 30
Diabetes
  acute coronary syndrome (ACS), as risk factor for, 7
  diabetic foot infections, 152
  feminizing hormone therapy and, 224
  hypertension and, 92–93
  intra cerebral hemorrhages (ICH), as risk factor for, 90
  ischemic stroke, as risk factor for, 87, 88
  masculinizing hormone therapy and, 225–226
  migraines and, 92–93
  urinary tract infections (UTI) and, 186
Diagnostic and Statistical Manual of Mental Disorders (DSM-V), 220

Diagnostic imaging
    abdominal aortic aneurysm
        (AAA) and, 170
    abdominal pain and, 169–170
    acute coronary syndrome (ACS)
        and, 168
    appendicitis and, 170
    appropriateness of, 164–165
    biliary tract and, 170
    comparative effectiveness of, 165
    computed tomography (CT) (See
        Computed tomography (CT))
    coronary artery disease and,
        168–169
    coronary CT angiogram (CCTA),
        8, 169
    CT pulmonary angiogram
        (CTPA), 169
    dyspnea and, 168
    echocardiography (See
        Echocardiography)
    future research topics, 174
    of head, 172
    magnetic resonance imaging
        (MRI) (See Magnetic
        resonance imaging (MRI))
    migraines and, 172
    overview, 163–164, 173–174
    "pan-scanning," 171
    patient case study, 163, 174
    PET scans, 10
    pregnancy and, 172–173
    prevalence, 164
    pulmonary embolism (PE) and,
        168, 169
    renal colic and, 170–171
    sex and gender differences in, 164
    stress tests, 8, 168–169
    thoracic aortic dissection (TAD)
        and, 168
    trauma and, 171–172
    traumatic brain injury (TBI) and,
        172
    ultrasound (See Ultrasound)
    value of, 165
    ventilation perfusion (VQ) scan,
        173
    x-rays (See X-rays)
Diarrheal illnesses, 151
Diethylstilbestrol, 2
DIR (Dose Imaging Registry),
    166–168
Dischinger, P.C., 49
Distribution of drugs, 65–66
DLP (Dose length product),
    165–167
Docetaxel, 71
Dopamine neurotransmission, 52
Dorsal wrist capsulitis, 107
Dorsal wrist ganglion, 107

Dose Imaging Registry (DIR),
    166–168
Dose length product (DLP),
    165–167
Doxorubicin, 70–71
Drinkwater, B., 108
Drug use
    clinical consequences, 52
    factors related to use, 51
    intra cerebral hemorrhages (ICH)
        and, 90
    metabolism and, 52
    motor vehicle collisions and, 53
    opioids, 51
    prevalence in women, 51
    by prisoners, 51
    violence and, 54
DSM-V (Diagnostic and Statistical
    Manual of Mental Disorders),
    220
Duodenum, disorders of, 139
Dupuytren's contracture, 108
Dyspnea
    COPD and, 38
    diagnostic imaging and, 168
    echocardiography and, 168
Dysrhythmia, 68–69
Dysuria, 187

E. coli, 187, 188, 194–195
Echocardiography
    chest pain and, 168
    dyspnea and, 168
    heart failure and, 14
    ischemic stroke and, 89
Eclampsia
    ischemic stroke, as risk factor for,
        88
    seizures and, 94
Ecoptic pregnancy
    acute management, 205
    in children, 205
    clinical presentation, 205
    diagnosis, 205
    prevalence, 173
    ultrasound and, 205
EDCAS (Emergency Department
    Assessment of Chest Pain
    Score), 8
Education. See Medical education
Education Amendments of 1972,
    101
EGFR (Epithelial growth factor
    receptor), 71
Elbow injuries, 107
Elderly persons
    adverse drug reactions in, 180–181
    Alzheimer's disease in, 181–182
    bipolar disorder in, 183
    delirium in, 182

dementia in, 181–182
demographics, 179
depression in, 183, 185
emergency department care,
    180–181
falls by, 184–185
future research topics, 188
hip fractures by, 185
life expectancy, sex and gender
    differences in, 179–180
mental illness in, 182–183
osteoporosis in, 112
overview, 179–180, 188
patient case studies, 179,
    183–184, 185–186, 188
schizophrenia in, 183
substance abuse and falls in,
    54–55
suicide in, 183
trauma in, 79–80, 184–185
urinary tract infections in,
    186–188 (See also Urinary tract
    infections (UTIs))
Elimination of drugs, 67
Emergency care, focus on, 4
Emergency Department
    Assessment of Chest Pain
    Score (EDCAS), 8
Emphysema, 37
Endocarditis, 151
Endorphin system, 125, 126
Enterococcus faecalis, 187, 194
Enzyme deficiency, congenital
    adrenal hyperplasia (CAH)
    and, 196
Ephedrine as risk factor for intra-
    cerebral hemorrhages
    (ICH), 90
Epilepsy, 94
Epithelial growth factor receptor
    (EGFR), 71
Esophagus, disorders of, 138
    esophageal adenocarcinoma, 138
    esophageal squamous cell
        carcinoma, 138
Estriadol, 223–224
Estrogen
    anterior cruciate ligament (ACL)
        injuries and, 103
    in feminizing hormone therapy,
        223–224
    ischemic stroke and, 87
Ethanol, pharmacological effects of,
    65
Etoposide, 70–71
European Society for Microbiology
    and Infectious Diseases, 150
European Society of Cardiology, 17
Evirapine, 70
Expedited partner therapy, 154

Expert Panel Report on Guidelines for the Diagnosis and Management of Asthma (2007), 32

Falls by elderly persons, 184–185
FAPS (Functional abdominal pain syndrome), 143
FASD (Fetal alcohol spectrum disorders), 51–52
FAST (Focused assessment with sonograph in trauma), 172, 173
FDA. See Food and Drug Administration (FDA)
FDA Modernization Act of 1997, 4
Female athlete triad. See Athletic energy imbalance (AEI)
Feminizing hormone therapy, 223–224
Feminizing surgeries, 226
Fertility, congenital adrenal hyperplasia (CAH) and, 199
Fetal alcohol spectrum disorders (FASD), 51–52
Fever without a source (FWS), 193
Finasteride, 224
Fluoroquinolone, 187
Fluorouracil, 87
Focused assessment with sonograph in trauma (FAST), 172, 173
Follicular cysts, 204
Food and Drug Administration (FDA)
    absorption of drugs and, 65
    clinical trials, inclusion of women in, 2, 3–4, 233
    Guidance of General Considerations for the Clinical Evaluation of Drugs, 2
    importance of sex and gender, 2
    Office of Women's Health (OHW), 2
    pharmacology and, 63–64
    zolpidem and, 63
Foot injuries, 105
Fosfomycin, 150–151, 187
Framingham Risk Score, 8
Functional abdominal pain syndrome (FAPS), 143
FWS (Fever without a source), 193

Gallbladder disorders, 139–140, 144
Gallstones, 139–140, 143, 144, 224
Gan, W.Q., 36–37
GAO. See General Accounting Office (GAO)
Gastric cancer, 138
Gastroenterological disorders
    anorectal disorders, 143
    Barrett's esophagus, 138
    of biliary tract (See Biliary tract, disorders of)
    cirrhosis, 139
    of colon, 140–141
    colorectal cancer, 141
    constipation (See Constipation)
    Crohn's disease, 141
    of duodenum, 139
    esophageal adenocarcinoma, 138
    esophageal squamous cell carcinoma, 138
    of esophagus, 138 (See also Esophagus, disorders of)
    functional abdominal pain syndrome (FAPS), 143
    of gallbladder, 139–140, 144
    gallstones, 139–140, 143, 144
    gastric cancer, 138
    gastroesophageal reflux disease (GERD), 138
    HELLP (hemolysis, elevated liver enzymes, low platelets) syndrome, 143
    hepatitis, 139
    hypertensive upper esophageal sphincter (UES), 138
    irritable bowel syndrome (IBS), 139, 140–143
    of liver, 139
    nonalcoholic steatohepatitis (NASH), 144
    non-ulcer dyspepsia (NUD), 141
    overview, 136–137, 144
    of pancreas, 140 (See also Pancreas, disorders of)
    pancreatic cancer, 140
    pancreatitis, 140
    patient case studies, 136, 144
    peptic ulcer disease (PUD), 138
    pregnancy-related disorders, 143
    prevalence, 137
    of rectum, 140–141
    sex and gender differences, 137
    of small bowel, 139
    of stomach, 138
    of tongue, 138
    ulcerative colitis, 141
Gastroesophageal reflux disease (GERD), 138
Gay and Lesbian Medical Association, 220–221
GCS (Glasgow Coma Scale), 91–92
Gender
    congenital adrenal hyperplasia (CAH) and, 198–199
    definition, 1
    sex distinguished, 1, 219, 221, 229
    significance of, 1–2
    transgender persons (See Transgender persons)

General Accounting Office (GAO), 2, 3–4
Gentamicin, 204
GERD (Gastroesophageal reflux disease), 138
Geriatric care. See Elderly persons
Glasgow Coma Scale (GCS), 91–92
Global Initiative for Chronic Lung Disease (GOLD), 37, 38
Global Registry of Acute Coronary Events (GRACE) Risk Score, 8
Globus sensation, 138
Gluten enteropathy, 202
Gold, D.R., 37
Gonorrhea, 203
Grisso, J.A., 54
Guy, G., 139

H. pylori, 138
Hallux valgus, 105
Hamate fractures, 107
Hand injuries, 107
Head
    concussions, 115–117 (See also Concussions)
    diagnostic imaging of, 172
    traumatic brain injury (TBI), 82–83 (See also Traumatic brain injury (TBI))
Heart disease. See Cardiovascular disease
Heart failure, 14–15
    atrial fibrillation (AF), as risk factor for, 15
    clinical presentation, 15
    definition, 14
    echocardiography and, 14
    gender differences in, 15
    importance of, 14
    lack of evidence in women, 14
    overview, 14, 15
    physiology and, 14–15
    with preserved systolic function (HFPEF), 14
    with reduced systolic function (HFREF), 14
    sex differences in, 14–15
    types of, 14
HEART (History, ECG, Age, Risk factors, Troponin) Score, 8
HELLP (hemolysis, elevated liver enzymes, low platelets) syndrome, 143
Hemorrhages
    intra cerebral hemorrhages (ICH), 90–91 (See also Intra cerebral hemorrhages (ICH))

subarachnoid hemorrhages (SAH), 91–92 (*See also* Subarachnoid hemorrhages (SAH))
Hemorrhagic cysts, 204
Hemorrhagic strokes. *See* Intracerebral hemorrhages (ICH)
Heparin, 13, 18
Hepatic clearance of drugs, 67
Hepatitis C, 139, 152, 224–225
Hepatocellular carcinoma, 139
Hepatoxicity, 139
Hip fractures
    depression and, 185
    by elderly persons, 185
    trauma and, 80
Hirschsprung's disease, 202
Hispanics, slipped capital femoral epiphysis (SCFE) in, 207
Historical background, 2–3
HIV. *See* Human immunodeficiency virus (HIV)
H1N1 influenza, 150
Hormones
    ankle and foot injuries and, 105
    anterior cruciate ligament (ACL) injuries and, 103
    asthma and, 30
    athletic energy imbalance (AEI) and, 109
    estradiol, 223–224
    estrogen (*See* Estrogen)
    feminizing hormone therapy, 223–224
    ischemic stroke and, 88
    life expectancy and, 180
    longevity and, 180
    masculinizing hormone therapy, 224–226
    migraines and, 93
    pain and, 123, 129
    pharmacology and, 64
    QTc effects and, 68–69
    seizures and, 94
    testosterone (*See* Testosterone)
    transgender persons and, 221, 222–226
    trauma and, 81
Houry, D., 53
HPV (Human papilloma virus), 154
Human immunodeficiency virus (HIV), 155–157
    antiretroviral therapy (ART), 156–157
    circumcision and, 157
    condoms and, 157
    cryptococcal meningitis and, 153
    cultural factors, 156
    masculinizing hormone therapy and, 224–225

pharmacology and, 70
pregnancy and, 70
sex and gender differences in, 155–157
sexual violence and, 157–158
socioeconomic factors, 156
treatment, 156–157
Human papilloma virus (HPV), 154
Hydrocortisone, 198
Hyperkalemia, 197–198, 224
Hyperlipidemia, 225–226
Hyperprolactinemia, 224
Hypertension
    atrial fibrillation (AF) and, 16
    diabetes and, 92–93
    hypertensive upper esophageal sphincter (UES), 138
    intra cerebral hemorrhages (ICH) and, 90, 91
    ischemic stroke, as risk factor for, 87, 88
    masculinizing hormone therapy and, 225–226
    migraines and, 92–93
    subarachnoid hemorrhages (SAH), as risk factor for, 91
    tobacco use and, 7
Hypertriglyceridemia, 224
Hypoglycemia, 198
Hypothyroidism, 202
Hypovolemia, 197–198

IBS. *See* Irritable bowel syndrome (IBS)
ICD (International Coding and Diagnostic) Manual, 220
ICH. *See* Intra cerebral hemorrhages (ICH)
Imipramine, 11, 64
Immunology, trauma and, 81
Immunosuppression, trauma and, 78
Importance of sex and gender, 1–2
Incontinence, 186
Indanavir, 70
Infants. *See* Children
Infectious disease
    "behavioral hypothesis," 148
    camplyobacter, 151
    cellulitis, 152
    chlamydia, 154–155
    clostridium difficile, 151
    cryptococcal meningitis, 153
    cutaneous infections, 152
    diabetic foot infections, 152
    diarrheal illnesses, 151
    endocarditis, 151
    future research topics, 159
    hepatitis C, 152
    H1N1 influenza, 150

human immunodeficiency virus (HIV), 155–157 (*See also* Human immunodeficiency virus (HIV))
influenza, 150
leptospirosis, 152
Lyme disease, 152–153
malaria, 152
onchocerciasis, 153
overview, 147–148, 158
patient case studies, 147, 158–159
"physiologic hypothesis," 148
pneumonia, 149
respiratory infections, 148–150
river blindness, 153
salmonella, 151
sex and gender differences in, 148
sexually transmitted infections (STI) (*See* Sexually transmitted infections (STI))
shigella, 151
Staph aureus, 151
syphilis, 155
traveler's infections, 151
trichomonas, 155
tuberculosis, 149–150
urinary tract infections, 150–151 (*See also* Urinary tract infections (UTIs))
Infectious Diseases Society of America, 150
Influenza, 150
Injury Severity Score, 83
Institute of Medicine (IOM)
    clinical trials, inclusion of women in, 4
    Committee on the Ethical and Legal Issues Relating to the Inclusion of Women in Clinical Studies, 4
    Committee on Understanding the Biology of Gender Differences, 4
    defining sex and gender, 1
    importance of sex and gender, 1–2
    transgender persons and, 220–221
International Coding and Diagnostic (ICD) Manual, 220
International Conference on Concussion in Sport (2001), 115
Intimate partner violence during pregnancy, 80
Intra cerebral hemorrhages (ICH), 90–91
    acute management, 90–91
    clinical outcomes, 91
    diabetes as risk factor, 90
    drug use and, 90

(ICH) (cont.)
ephedrine as risk factor, 90
hypertension and, 90, 91
morbidity and mortality, 91
mutations and, 90
prevention, 90
risk factors, 90
tobacco use as risk factor, 90
treatment response, 90–91
Intravenous lipid emulsion, 69–70
IOM. *See* Institute of Medicine
(IOM)
Ireland, Mary Lloyd, 102
Irritable bowel syndrome (IBS), 139,
140–143
Ischemic chest pain, 9–10
magnetic resonance imaging
(MRI) and, 10
microvascular angina, testing
for, 10
non-obstructive coronary artery
disease, 10
overview, 10
PET scans and, 10
WISE study, 10
Ischemic stroke, 87–90
acute management, 89
anticoagulants and, 88
aspirin and, 87
atrial fibrillation (AF) and, 87, 88
clinical manifestations, 88–89
clinical outcomes, 90
clinical presentation, 88–89
diabetes as risk factor, 87, 88
diagnosis, 89
echocardiography and, 89
eclampsia as risk factor, 88
estrogen and, 87
hormones and, 88
hypertension as risk factor, 87, 88
migraines as risk factor, 88
physiology, 88
pregnancy and, 88
prevention, 87–88
risk factors, 87–88
sex and gender differences in, 88
treatment response, 89–90
ultrasound and, 89

Jacoby, S.F., 79

Katz, D.A., 27
Kidney stones. *See* Nephrolithiasis;
Renal colic
Klebsiella pneumoniae, 187, 194
Knee injuries
anterior cruciate ligament (ACL)
injuries (*See* Anterior cruciate
ligament (ACL) injuries)
in children, 206–210

future research topics, 209
Osgood-Schlatter disease, 208
(*See also* Osgood-Schlatter
disease)
overview, 104–111, 207, 209
patient case study, 206, 209
Q angle and, 104–111
slipped capital femoral epiphysis
(SCFE), 207–208 (*See also*
Slipped capital femoral
epiphysis (SCFE))
Kuhn, J.E., 106

Labral tears, 106
Laparoscopic appendectomy, 201
LCME (Liaison Committee on
Medical Education), 234
Ledderhose's contracture, 108
Leptospirosis, 152
Leukocyte esterase, 186
Leukocytopenia, 71
Leukotrienes, 125
Liaison Committee on Medical
Education (LCME), 234
Life expectancy, sex and gender
differences in, 179–180
Liver, disorders of, 139
Longevity, sex and gender
differences in, 179–180
Low impact fractures. *See*
Osteoporosis
Lucky Strikes (cigarette brand), 25
Lung cancer, tobacco use and, 25
Lung disease. *See* Pulmonary
disease
Lung Health Study (LHS), 26,
27, 41
Lyme disease, 152–153

Magnesium, 33
Magnetic resonance imaging (MRI)
anterior cruciate ligament (ACL)
injuries and, 209
appendicitis and, 200
ischemic chest pain and, 10
musculoskeletal pain syndromes
and, 107
ovarian cysts and, 204
overview, 163
pregnancy and, 173
Malaria, 152
Malignant liver masses, 139
Masculinizing hormone therapy,
224–226
Masculinizing surgeries, 225
Mayo Clinic, 13–14
McCune-Albright syndrome,
204
McGregor, Alyson J., 231–232
Mechanoreceptors, 124–125

Medical education, 230–235
accreditation organizations, 234
cultural change, creating,
230–231
federal initiatives, 232–233
future trends, 233–234
life-long learning, importance of,
231–232
recommended approach, 232
research, importance of, 230
resources, 232
translational health education,
231
utilizing book, 234–235
Medicare, transgender persons and,
220
Meningitis, 152, 193
"Menstrual migraines," 93
Menstruation, asthma and, 43
Mental health, substance abuse
and, 55
Mental illness in elderly persons,
182–183
Metabolism
alcohol use and, 51–52
of drugs, 66
drug use and, 52
Methyphenidate, 68
Metoclopramide, 68
Microvascular angina, testing for, 10
Migraines, 92–94
acetaminophen and, 93
acute management, 93–94
clinical manifestations, 93
clinical outcomes, 94
clinical presentation, 93
computed tomography (CT) and,
172
diabetes and, 92–93
diagnosis, 93
diagnostic imaging and, 172
hormones and, 93
hypertension and, 92–93
ischemic stroke, as risk factor
for, 88
"menstrual migraines," 93
natural history, 93
prevention, 92–93
risk factors, 92–93
treatment response, 93–94
Minority stress models, 218
Minors. *See* Children
Molecular drug transporters, 68
Monophosphate, 125
Morgan, C.D., 106
Morphine for treatment of pain,
122, 128, 130–131
Motor vehicle collisions
alcohol use and, 53
drug use and, 53

substance abuse and, 53
trauma and, 77
MRI. *See* Magnetic resonance
imaging (MRI)
Muhammad ibn Zakariya Razi, 115
Multicenter AIDS Cohort Study,
157
Multi-system organ dysfunction
syndrome (MSODS), 78
Musculoskeletal pain syndromes,
107–108
adhesive capsulitis, 108
back pain, 107
chronic regional pain syndrome
(CRPS), 107–108
computed tomography (CT) and,
107
contractures, 108
Dupuytren's contracture, 108
Ledderhose's contracture, 108
magnetic resonance imaging
(MRI) and, 107
Mutations, intra cerebral
hemorrhages (ICH) and, 90

NAAT (Nucleic Acid Amplification
Test), 203
NASH (Nonalcoholic
steatohepatitis), 139, 144
National Cancer Institute, 27
National Health Interview Study
(2011), 29
National Institute on Drug Abuse
(NIDA), 55
National Institute on Alcohol Abuse
and Alcoholism (NIAAA), 54
National Institutes of Health (NIH)
generally, 2
clinical trials, inclusion of women
in, 3–4, 233
Office of Research on Women's
Health (ORWH), 3, 4, 233
Public Health Service Task Force
on Women's Health, 3
National Osteoporosis Foundation,
112
National Quality Forum (NQF), 166
National Study on Drug Use and
Health (2011–2012), 50
National Trauma Data Bank, 79
Neisseria gonorrhea, 202
Nelfinavir, 70
Nephrolithiasis, 201
acute management, 201
in children, 201
clinical presentation, 201
complications, 202
diagnosis, 201
Neutropenia, 71
Nevirapine, 70

NIAAA (National Institute on
Alcohol Abuse and
Alcoholism), 54
Nicorette (gum), 26
NIDA (National Institute on Drug
Abuse), 55
NIH. *See* National Institutes of
Health (NIH)
NIH Revitalization Act of
1993, 4
Nitrates, 13
Nitrites, 186
Nitrofurantoin, 150–151, 187
Nitroglycerin, 18
Nociceptors, 124–125
Nonalcoholic steatohepatitis
(NASH), 139, 144
Non-nucleoside reverse
transcriptase inhibitors
(NNRTIs), 70
Non-obstructive coronary artery
disease, 10
Non-ulcer dyspepsia (NUD), 141
NPT (Computerized
neuropsychological testing),
116–117
NQF (National Quality Forum), 166
NTCP (Sodium taurocholate
contransporting polypeptide),
71
Nucleic Acid Amplification Test
(NAAT), 203
Nucleoside reverse transcriptase
inhibitors (NRTIs), 70
NUD (Non-ulcer dyspepsia), 141

"Obamacare," 164
Obesity
appendicitis and, 201
asthma and, 35
slipped capital femoral epiphysis
(SCFE) and, 207
tobacco use and, 27
Objective Structured Clinical Exam
(OSCE), 234
OCPs (Oral contraceptive pills)
asthma and, 30
pharmacology and, 64
OCT2 (Organic cation
transporter 2), 71
Oligoanalgesia, 123
Olympics, women in, 101
Onchocerciasis, 153
Oophorectomy, 204
Open appendectomy, 201
Opioids
overdoses, 69
substance abuse, 51
for treatment of pain, 127–128,
130–131

Oral contraceptive pills (OCPs)
asthma and, 30
pharmacology and, 64
Orchiectomy, 206
Organic cation transporter 2
(OCT2), 71
Orthopedics. *See also specific injury*
athletic energy imbalance (AEI),
108–111 (*See also* Athletic
energy imbalance (AEI))
concussions, 115–117 (*See also*
Concussions)
future research topics, 117
musculoskeletal pain syndromes,
107–108 (*See also*
Musculoskeletal pain
syndromes)
osteoporosis, 111–114 (*See also*
Osteoporosis)
overview, 101–102
patient case study, 102
sex and gender differences in,
101–102
OSCE (Objective Structured
Clinical Exam), 234
Osgood-Schlatter disease, 208
acute management, 208
in children, 208
diagnosis, 208
prevalence, 208
risk factors, 208
sex and gender differences in, 208
x-rays and, 208
Osteoarthritis, anterior cruciate
ligament (ACT) injuries and,
104, 209
Osteoporosis, 111–114
bone mineral density (BMD) and,
112–113
causes, 112
costs of, 112
definition, 112
diagnosis, 112–114
in elderly persons, 112
morbidity and mortality, 113
prevalence, 111–112
patient case study, 111
risk factors, 112–113
sex and gender differences in, 112
trauma and, 80
treatment options, 114
Ovarian cancer, pelvic inflammatory
disease (PID) and, 204
Ovarian cysts, 204
acute management, 204
in children, 204
clinical presentation, 204
diagnosis, 204
magnetic resonance imaging
(MRI) and, 204

Ovarian torsion. *See* Adnexal torsion (AT)
Overdoses
  acetaminophen, 69
  opioids, 69
  overview, 69

Paclitaxel, 71
Pain
  abdominal pain (*See* Abdominal pain)
  acute pain versus chronic pain, 127
  assessment of, 122–123
  catecholamines and, 125
  clinical evaluation of, 126
  detection of, 124–125
  endorphin system and, 126
  expression of, 125–126
  future research topics, 131
  hormones and, 123, 129
  measurement of, 126–127
  mechanoreceptors, 124–125
  modulation of, 125
  morphine for treatment of, 122, 128, 130–131
  musculoskeletal pain syndromes, 107–108 (*See also* Musculoskeletal pain syndromes)
  nociceptors and, 124–125
  oligoanalgesia, 123
  opioids for treatment of, 127–128, 130–131
  overview, 122–124, 130
  patient case study, 122, 130–131
  perception of, 124–126
  peripheral nerve fibers and, 125
  polymodal nociceptors (PMNs), 124–125
  prognosis, 128–129
  sex and gender differences in, 122–124, 127, 129–130
  stabilization of secondary pain factors, 128
  stress induced analgesia, 125
  stress induced hyperalgesia, 125
  subjectivity of, 129–130
  thermoreceptors, 124–125
  transduction of, 124–125
  transmission of, 125
  treatment options, 127–128
  wide dynamic range neurons (WDRNs), 125
Pancreas, disorders of, 140
  pancreatic cancer, 140
  pancreatitis, 140
"Pan-scanning," 171
PCOS (Polycystic ovarian syndrome), 225–226

PCS (Post-concussion syndrome), 116
PE. *See* Pulmonary embolism (PE)
Pediatric Appendicitis Score (PAS), 200
Pediatric care. *See* Children
Pediatric Emergency Care Applied Research Network (PECARN), 172
Pelvic inflammatory disease (PID), 202–204
  acute management, 203–204
  in children, 202–204
  chlamydia and, 202
  clinical presentation, 202
  complications, 204
  diagnosis, 203
  gonorrhea and, 203
  ovarian cancer and, 204
Penicillin, 64
Peptic ulcer disease (PUD), 138
Percutaneous nephrolithotomy, 202
Perinephric abscess, 195
Peripartum/postpartum cardiomyopathy (PPCM), 18
Peripheral nerve fibers, 125
Peters, E.N., 53
Peters, M.G., 139
PET scans, 10
Pglycoprotein, 68, 70–71
Pharmacodynamics, 68
Pharmacology
  absorption of drugs, 64–65
  adverse effects, 69
  antidotes, 69–70
  chemotherapeutics, 87
  CYP1A2 enzyme, 67
  CYP2C9 enzyme, 67
  CYP2C19 enzyme, 67
  CYP2D6 enzyme, 67
  CYP3A4 enzyme, 67
  CYP450 system, 66–67
  differential drug dosing, 64
  distribution of drugs, 65–66
  drug–drug interactions, 64
  elimination of drugs, 67
  ethanol, pharmacological effects of, 65
  future research topics, 71
  hepatic clearance of drugs, 67
  hormones and, 64
  human immunodeficiency virus (HIV) and, 70
  intravenous lipid emulsion, 69–70
  metabolism of drugs, 66
  molecular drug transporters, 68
  oral contraceptive pills (OCPs) and, 64
  overdoses, 69 (*See also* Overdoses)

overview, 63–64, 71
  patient case study, 63, 71
  pharmacodynamics, 68
  placebo effect, 64
  QTc effects, 68–69
  renal clearance of drugs, 67
  sex and gender differences in, 64, 71
  site of action effects, 68
Phenytoin, 64
Physicians' Health Study, 1
PID. *See* Pelvic inflammatory disease (PID)
Piovesan, D.M., 32
PIs (Protease inhibitors), 70
Placebo effect, 64
Pneumonia, 149, 193
Polycystic ovarian syndrome (PCOS), 225–226
Polymodal nociceptors (PMNs), 124–125
Post-concussion syndrome (PCS), 116
Post-traumatic stress disorder (PTSD), 84
PPCM (Peripartum/postpartum cardiomyopathy), 18
Pregnancy
  anorectal disorders, 143
  appendicitis during, 173
  asthma and, 30
  cardiovascular disease and, 17–18
  computed tomography (CT) and, 172, 173
  diagnostic imaging and, 172–173
  eclampsia, 94
  ecoptic pregnancy (*See* Ecoptic pregnancy)
  gallstones and, 143
  HELLP (hemolysis, elevated liver enzymes, low platelets) syndrome, 143
  human immunodeficiency virus (HIV) and, 70
  intimate partner violence during, 80
  ischemic stroke and, 88
  magnetic resonance imaging (MRI) and, 173
  pregnancy-related gastroenterological disorders, 143
  pulmonary embolism (PE) during, 173
  trauma during, 80–81, 173
  ultrasound and, 172–173
  venous thromboembolism (VTE) during, 173
Preventative Services Task Force (USPSTF), 1–2, 203

Primary biliary cirrhosis, 139
Primary sclerosing cholangitis, 139
Prisoners, drug use by, 51
Progesterone, 82–83
Prostaglandin, 125
Protease inhibitors (PIs), 70
Proteus mirabilis, 187, 194
Pseudomonas, 194
PTSD (Post-traumatic stress disorder), 84
PUD (Peptic ulcer disease), 138
Pulmonary disease
    asthma, 29–35 (*See also* Asthma)
    chronic bronchitis, 37
    COPD, 36–42 (*See also* Chronic obstructive pulmonary disease (COPD))
    dyspnea, 38
    emphysema, 37
    overview, 24, 44
    patient case study, 24, 43–44
    tobacco use, 24–29 (*See also* Tobacco use)
Pulmonary embolism (PE)
    computed tomography (CT) and, 168, 169
    diagnostic imaging and, 168, 169
    during pregnancy, 173
Pyelonephritis, 195
Pyuria, 186

Q angle, 104–111
QTc effects, 68–69
Quantitative Pretest Probability (QPTP) ACS Instrument, 8
Quinolones, 150–151

Radiation from computed tomography (CT)
    dose length product (DLP), 165–167
    dose variability, 166–168
    measuring, 165–167
    reporting, 165–167
    risk of, 166
Ranolazine, 11
Rectum, disorders of, 140–141
Reflex sympathetic dystrophy, 107–108
Relaxin, 103
Renal clearance of drugs, 67
Renal colic
    computed tomography (CT) and, 170–171
    diagnostic imaging and, 170–171
    ultrasound and, 171
Renal sodium loss, 197
Respiratory infections, 148–150
Reynolds Risk Score, 8

Rhodes, K., 54
Rifampin, 64
The Right Time, the Right Reasons: Dads Talk About Reducing and Quitting Smoking (University of British Columbia), 27
Ritonavir, 70
River blindness, 153
Rockett, I.R.H., 49
Rotator cuff injuries, 106–107

SAH. *See* Subarachnoid hemorrhages (SAH)
Salmonella, 151
SAMHSA (Substance Abuse and Mental Health Services Administration), 54
Saquinavir, 70
SCFE. *See* Slipped capital femoral epiphysis (SCFE)
Schizophrenia in elderly persons, 183
Screening, brief intervention, and referral to treatment (SBIRT), 50, 52
Seizures, 94
Selective serotonin reuptake inhibitors (SSRIs), 68, 139
Selegiline, 64
Serotonin, 125
Sex
    definition, 1
    gender distinguished, 1, 219, 221, 229
    significance of, 1–2
Sexual assault
    alcohol use and, 54
    substance abuse and, 54
Sexually transmitted infections (STI)
    chlamydia, 154–155
    circumcision and, 154
    diagnosis, 154
    future research topics, 159
    human immunodeficiency virus (HIV), 155–157 (*See also* Human immunodeficiency virus (HIV))
    long-term effects, 154
    patient case study, 147, 158–159
    prevalence, 153
    prevention, 154
    screening, 154
    sex and gender differences in, 153–154
    sexual behavior and, 154
    sexual violence and, 157–158
    syphilis, 155
    transmission of, 153–154
    trichomonas, 155

Sexual orientation
    congenital adrenal hyperplasia (CAH) and, 199
    definition, 217
    transgender persons (*See* Transgender persons)
Sexual violence
    human immunodeficiency virus (HIV) and, 157–158
    sexually transmitted infections (STI) and, 157–158
Shigella, 151
Shock wave lithotripsy, 202
Shoulder injuries, 105–107
    labral tears, 106
    patient case study, 105
    prevalence, 106
    rotator cuff injuries, 106–107
    sex and gender differences in, 105–106
    SLAP lesions, 106
Site of action effects, 68
SLAP lesions, 106
Slipped capital femoral epiphysis (SCFE), 207–208
    acute management, 207
    in African Americans, 207
    in children, 207–208
    clinical presentation, 207
    complications, 207
    diagnosis, 207
    in Hispanics, 207
    obesity and, 207
    prevalence, 207
    risk factors, 207
    sex and gender differences, 207
    x-rays and, 207
Small bowel, disorders of, 139
Smokefree Women, 27
Smoking. *See* Tobacco use
Smoking cessation programs, 26–27, 35, 40–41
Society for Academic Emergency Medicine, 150
Sodium taurocholate contransporting polypeptide (NTCP), 71
Spinal cord abnormality, 202
Spironolactone, 224
Spontaneous coronary artery dissection (SCAD), 13–14
Sports medicine. *See also* specific injury
    athletic energy imbalance (AEI), 108–111 (*See also* Athletic energy imbalance (AEI))
    concussions, 115–117 (*See also* Concussions)
    future research topics, 117

Sports medicine (cont.)
  musculoskeletal pain syndromes,
    107–108 (*See also*
    Musculoskeletal pain
    syndromes)
  osteoporosis, 111–114 (*See also*
    Osteoporosis)
  overview, 101–102
  patient case study, 102
  sex and gender differences in,
    101–102
SSRIs (Selective serotonin reuptake
    inhibitors), 68, 139
Staph aureus, 151
Statins, 11, 18
Status epilepticus, 94
STI. *See* Sexually transmitted
    infections (STI)
Stomach, disorders of, 138
Stress induced analgesia, 125
Stress induced hyperalgesia, 125
Stress tests for acute coronary
    syndrome (ACS), 8, 168–169
Strokes
  hemorrhagic strokes (*See* Intra
    cerebral hemorrhages (ICH))
  ischemic stroke, 87–90 (*See also*
    Ischemic stroke)
Structural heart disease. *See* Heart
    failure
Subarachnoid hemorrhages (SAH),
    91–92
  acute management, 92
  clinical manifestations, 91–92
  clinical outcomes, 92
  clinical presentation, 91–92
  computed tomography (CT)
    and, 92
  diagnosis, 92
  hypertension as risk factor, 91
  natural history, 91
  prevention, 91
  risk factors, 91
  tobacco use and, 91
Substance abuse
  African Americans and, 53
  alcohol use (*See* Alcohol use)
  brief intervention protocols,
    52–53
  chronic intoxication, sex and
    gender differences and, 55
  costs of, 49
  drug use (*See* Drug use)
  elderly persons, and falls in,
    54–55
  fetal alcohol spectrum disorders
    (FASD), 51–52
  gender bias in treatment of,
    52–53
  gender-specific treatment, 55

interventions, 52–53
  mental health comorbidities, 55
  motor vehicle collisions and, 53
  opioids, 51
  overview, 49–50, 56
  patient case study, 49, 56–57
  prevalence, 49
  recommended approach, 55–56
  screening, brief intervention, and
    referral to treatment (SBIRT),
    50, 52
  sex and gender differences in,
    52–53, 56
  sexual assault and, 54
  violence and, 53–54
Substance Abuse and Mental Health
    Services Administration
    (SAMHSA), 54
Suicide in elderly persons, 183
Sulfamethoxozole, 150–151
Sumatripan, 93
Surgeon General
  Report on Smoking and Health
    (1964), 25, 29
  Report on the Health
    Consequences of Smoking for
    Women (1980), 25, 26
  European Network for
    Understanding Mechanisms of
    Severe Asthma, 30
Syphilis, 155

TAD (Thoracic aortic dissection)
  computed tomography (CT) and,
    168
  diagnostic imaging and, 168
Takotsubo's cardiomyopathy,
    12–13
  acute management, 13
  angiography, 12–13
  aspirin and, 13
  beta-blockers and, 13
  catheterization, 12–13
  clinical presentation, 12
  diagnostic criteria, 12–13
  mechanisms, 13
  overview, 13
  prognosis, 13
  recurrence, 13
TBI. *See* Traumatic brain injury
    (TBI)
Tendinitis, 107
Terfenadine, 2
Testicular torsion, 206
  acute management, 206
  in children, 206
  clinical presentation, 206
  diagnosis, 206
  ultrasound and, 206
Testosterone

asthma and, 30
  longevity and, 180
  in masculinizing hormone
    therapy, 224–226
Tetracyclines, 64
Texas Tech University Health
    Sciences Center, 232
Theophylline, 64
Thermoreceptors, 124–125
Thoracic aortic dissection (TAD)
  computed tomography (CT)
    and, 168
  diagnostic imaging and, 168
Thromboembolism, 223–224
Thrombosis in Myocardial
    Infarction (TIMI) Risk Score, 8
Thromboxanes, 125
Tissue plasminogen activator (tPA),
    89–90
Title IX, 101
Tobacco use, 24–29
  acute coronary syndrome (ACS),
    as risk factor for, 7
  acute management, 27–28
  cancer and, 25
  clinical manifestations, 25–26
  COPD and, 36–37, 40–41
  costs of, 24
  depression and, 26–27
  future research topics, 43
  historical background, 24–25
  hypertension and, 7
  intra cerebral hemorrhages
    (ICH), as risk factor for, 90
  life expectancy and, 180
  lung cancer and, 25
  morbidity and mortality, 180
  obesity and, 27
  overview, 24, 29
  prevention, 28–29
  smoking cessation programs,
    26–27
  socioeconomic factors, 28–29
  subarachnoid hemorrhages
    (SAH) and, 91
  treatment options, 28
Tongue, disorders of, 138
Torsades de Pointes, 2, 16
Toward a Revolution in COPD
    Health (TORCH) Study, 42
Toxicology. *See* Pharmacology
tPA (Tissue plasminogen activator),
    89–90
Triangular fibrocartilage tears, 107
Transgender persons
  adolescents, 223
  cancer and, 221, 224, 228
  challenges in treatment of,
    217–218
  data collection, 220–221

emergency care for, 220–222
feminizing hormone therapy, 223–224
feminizing surgeries, 226
future research topics, 228
glossary of terms, 216–217
hormones and, 221, 222–226
masculinizing hormone therapy, 224–226
masculinizing surgeries, 225
medical therapies for gender actualization and transition, 222–226
Medicare and, 220
minority stress models, 218
non-discrimination policies, 222
overview, 216, 228
patient case study, 216, 222, 227
physical examinations, 221–222
prevalence, 219–220
removal from disorder categorization, 220
resources, 228
sex and gender distinguished in context of, 219, 221
surgical methods for gender actualization, 226–227
trauma in, 81–82
Transient left ventricle apical ballooning. See Takotsubo's cardiomyopathy
Translational health education, 231
Trauma
anticoagulants and, 80
clinical presentation, 78–79
computed tomography (CT) and, 171–172
concussions, 115–117 (See also Concussions)
diagnostic imaging and, 171–172
in elderly persons, 79–80, 184–185
focused assessment with sonograph in trauma (FAST), 172, 173
hip fractures and, 80
hormones and, 81
immunology and, 81
immunosuppression and, 78
long-term effects, 83–84
mechanisms of, 77–78
morbidity and mortality, 80
motor vehicle collisions and, 77
multi-system organ dysfunction syndrome (MSODS), 78
National Trauma Data Bank, 79
osteoporosis and, 80
overview, 84
patient case study, 77, 84

post-traumatic stress disorder (PTSD), 84
during pregnancy, 80–81, 173
prevalence, 77
provider differences, 83
sex and gender differences in, 77–78
team differences, 83
in transgender persons, 81–82
traumatic brain injury (TBI), 82–83 (See also Traumatic brain injury (TBI))
Traumatic brain injury (TBI), 82–83
See also Concussions
computed tomography (CT) and, 172
diagnostic imaging and, 172
long-term effects of, 83–84
sex and gender differences in, 77
Traveler's infections, 151
Trichomonas, 155
Trimethoprim, 150–151
Troponin, 7–8
Tuberculosis, 149–150
21-hydroxylase, 196

UES (Upper esophageal sphincter), 138
Ulcerative colitis, 141
Ulnar collateral ligament (UCL) injuries, 107
Ulnar impaction syndrome, 107
Ulnar nerve compression, 107
Ultrasound
abdominal aortic aneurysm (AAA) and, 170
abdominal pain and, 170
adnexal torsion (AT) and, 205
appendicitis and, 170, 200
ecoptic pregnancy and, 205
ischemic stroke and, 89
overview, 163
pregnancy and, 172–173
renal colic and, 171
testicular torsion and, 206
Upper esophageal sphincter (UES), 138
Upper extremity injuries, 138
Ureteroscopy, 202
Urinary tract infections (UTIs)
acute management, 195
antibiotics and, 187
bacteriuria, 150, 186
in boys, 193–194
in children, 193–196
circumcision and, 193–194
complications, 195

cystitis, 150
diabetes and, 186
diagnosis, 194–195
dysuria, 187
E. coli and, 187, 194–195
in elderly persons, 186–188
fluoroquinolone and, 187
fosfomycin and, 187
future research topics, 196
in girls, 193
incontinence, 186
nitrofurantoin and, 187
overview, 150–151, 195
patient case studies, 188, 193, 195–196
post-emergency department care, 195
prevalence, 193–194
prevention, 187–188
pyuria, 186
retention, 186
risk factors, 193–194
sexual behavior and, 187
testing, 186, 187
treatment, 187
vesicoureteral reflux (VUR) as risk factor for, 194
Urosepsis, 195
USPSTF (Preventative Services Task Force), 1–2, 203
UTIs. See Urinary tract infections (UTIs)

Vancouver Chest Pain Rule, 8
Venous thromboembolism (VTE) during pregnancy, 173
Ventilation perfusion (VQ) scan, 173
Vesicoureteral reflux (VUR) as risk factor for urinary tract infections, 194
Vincristine, 70–71
Violence
alcohol use and, 53–54
drug use and, 54
pregnancy, intimate partner violence during, 80
sexually transmitted infections (STI), sexual violence and, 157–158
substance abuse and, 53–54
Viral hepatitis, 139
Vitamin D, 114
VQ (Ventilation perfusion) scan, 173
VTE (Venous thromboembolism) during pregnancy, 173
VUR (Vesicoureteral reflux) as risk factor for urinary tract infections, 194

Warfarin, 16, 64
WHO. *See* World Health
    Organization (WHO)
Wide dynamic range neurons
    (WDRNs), 125
Wilcox, B., 116
Wilson's disease, 139
Women's Estrogen Stroke Test, 88
Women's Health Initiative Study, 88
Women's Health Movement,
    232–233

Women's Interagency HIV Study,
    157
World Health Organization (WHO)
    migraines and, 94
    osteoporosis and, 112
    tobacco use and, 24, 26, 28
    trauma and, 77
World Professional Association
    for Transgender Health,
    220–221
Wrist injuries, 107

X-rays
    anterior cruciate ligament
        (ACL) injuries and,
        209
    Osgood-Schlatter disease and,
        208
    overview, 163
    slipped capital femoral epiphysis
        (SCFE) and, 207

Zolpidem, 2, 63, 71

Printed in the United States
by Baker & Taylor Publisher Services

Printed in the United States
by Baker & Taylor Publisher Services